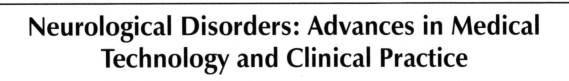

Neurological Disorders: Advances in Medical Technology and Clinical Practice

Neurological Disorders: Advances in Medical Technology and Clinical Practice

Editor: Particia Garcia

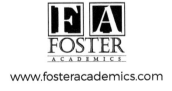

www.fosteracademics.com

www.fosteracademics.com

Cataloging-in-Publication Data

Neurological disorders : advances in medical technology and clinical practice / edited by Particia Garcia.
    p. cm.
Includes bibliographical references and index.
ISBN 978-1-64646-613-9
1. Nervous system--Diseases. 2. Medical technology. 3. Nervous system--Diseases--Diagnosis.
4. Nervous system--Diseases--Treatment. 5. Nervous system--Diseases--Diagnosis--Technological
innovations. 6. Nervous system--Diseases--Treatment--Technological in I. Garcia, Particia.
RC346 .N48 2023
616.8--dc23

Foster Academics,
118-35 Queens Blvd., Suite 400,
Forest Hills, NY 11375, USA

ISBN 978-1-64646-613-9 (Hardback)

Contents

Preface

The purpose of the book is to provide a glimpse into the dynamics and to present opinions and studies of some of the scientists engaged in the development of new ideas in the field from very different standpoints. This book will prove useful to students and researchers owing to its high content quality.

A neurological disorder refers to a type of disorder that affects the nervous system. These disorders include multiple sclerosis, Alzheimer's disease and other dementias, Parkinson's disease, brain tumors, epilepsy, neuroinfections, and cerebrovascular diseases. There are several signs and symptoms of these disorders, such as muscle weakness, seizures, loss of sensation, paralysis and poor coordination. Neurological disorders are diagnosed using a variety of medical techniques, including positron emission tomography (PET), electroencephalography (EEG), single-photon emission computed tomography (SPECT), computerized tomography (CT scan) and magnetic resonance imaging (MRI scan). These medical technologies generate massive amounts of complex and high-dimensional data, which is a crucial source for planning therapies and treatments. Various advances in clinical practice and medical technologies are being developed, such as therapies with the potential to detect and treat Alzheimer's disease before its symptoms manifest, usage of stem cells for replacement therapy, and development of implantable wireless brain devices. This book unravels the recent studies on neurological disorders. It elucidates the advances in medical technology and clinical practice with respect to these disorders. Those in search of information to further their knowledge will be greatly assisted by this book.

At the end, I would like to appreciate all the efforts made by the authors in completing their chapters professionally. I express my deepest gratitude to all of them for contributing to this book by sharing their valuable works. A special thanks to my family and friends for their constant support in this journey.

Editor

Immunoadsorption and Plasma Exchange in Seropositive and Seronegative Immune-Mediated Neuropathies

Alexander J. Davies [1], Janev Fehmi [1], Makbule Senel [2], Hayrettin Tumani [2], Johannes Dorst [2,†] and Simon Rinaldi [1,*,†]

[1]   Nuffield Department of Clinical Neurosciences, University of Oxford, Oxford OX3 9DU, UK; alexander.davies@ndcn.ox.ac.uk (A.J.D.); janev.fehmi@sjc.ox.ac.uk (J.F.)

[2]   Department of Neurology, University of Ulm, 89081 Ulm, Germany; makbule.senel@uni-ulm.de (M.S.); hayrettin.tumani@uni-ulm.de (H.T.); johannes.dorst@uni-ulm.de (J.D.)

*   Correspondence: simon.rinaldi@ndcn.ox.ac.uk

†   These authors contributed equally to this work.

Abstract: The inflammatory neuropathies are disabling conditions with diverse immunological mechanisms. In some, a pathogenic role for immunoglobulin G (IgG)-class autoantibodies is increasingly appreciated, and immunoadsorption (IA) may therefore be a useful therapeutic option. We reviewed the use of and response to IA or plasma exchange (PLEx) in a cohort of 41 patients with nodal/paranodal antibodies identified from a total of 573 individuals with suspected inflammatory neuropathies during the course of routine diagnostic testing (PNAb cohort). 20 patients had been treated with PLEx and 4 with IA. Following a global but subjective evaluation by their treating clinicians, none of these patients were judged to have had a good response to either of these treatment modalities. Sequential serology of one PNAb+ case suggests prolonged suppression of antibody levels with frequent apheresis cycles or adjuvant therapies, may be required for effective treatment. We further retrospectively evaluated the serological status of 40 patients with either Guillain-Barré syndrome (GBS) or chronic inflammatory demyelinating polyneuropathy (CIDP), and a control group of 20 patients with clinically-isolated syndrome/multiple sclerosis (CIS/MS), who had all been treated with IgG-depleting IA (IA cohort). 32 of these patients (8/20 with CIDP, 13/20 with GBS, 11/20 with MS) were judged responsive to apheresis despite none of the serum samples from this cohort testing positive for IgG antibodies against glycolipids or nodal/paranodal cell-adhesion molecules. Although negative on antigen specific assays, three patients' pre-treatment sera and eluates were reactive against different components of myelinating co-cultures. In summary, preliminary evidence suggests that GBS/CIDP patients without detectable IgG antibodies on routine diagnostic tests may nevertheless benefit from IA, and that an unbiased screening approach using myelinating co-cultures may assist in the detection of further autoantibodies which remain to be identified in such patients.

Keywords: Inflammatory neuropathy; chronic inflammatory demyelinating polyneuropathy; Guillain-Barré syndrome; multiple sclerosis; paranodal antibodies; plasmapheresis; plasma exchange; immunoadsorption

1. Introduction

The inflammatory neuropathies are a heterogeneous group of disorders in which peripheral nerve function and structure are disturbed by largely ill-defined immunological mechanisms [1]. They can broadly be divided into acute and chronic forms, typified by the umbrella terms Guillain-Barré syndrome (GBS) and chronic inflammatory demyelinating polyneuropathy (CIDP), respectively.

Humoral and cellular immunity are likely to play a role in the pathogenesis of both syndromes. For some clinically defined subtypes, a role for the humoral immune system and pathogenic autoantibodies appears to be more prominent [2,3], but particularly at the level of the individual patient, a direct and consistent link between the clinical syndrome, serological profile, and underlying immunopathological mechanism remains difficult to establish.

Randomised controlled trials have demonstrated that therapeutic plasma exchange (PLEx) speeds up recovery from GBS [4], and provides at least a short-term improvement in disability in CIDP [5]. In both conditions there is evidence that intravenous immunoglobulin (IVIg) has similar efficacy [6,7]. Two small, randomised studies have compared immunoadsorption (IA) with PLEx or IVIg in CIDP. Response rates to IA (6/9 using tryptophan-based columns [8] and 4/5 using protein A [9]) were not significantly different to their respective comparators. The trial comparing IA (using protein A) with IVIg had a high drop-out rate and was excluded from the relevant Cochrane review due to a high risk of bias [9]. Two further reports described the crossover from PLEx to IA in CIDP, in a single patient each, reaching opposite conclusions about which was more efficacious [10,11]. A number of retrospective case series and case reports have favourably evaluated immunoadsorption in both GBS and CIDP [12–21]. A retrospective Japanese report of IA in GBS found that patients who received IA within 6 days of onset of their neuropathy had a more rapid improvement in disability compared to those who received supportive care alone, whereas patients who received IA later than this in their disease course did not [22]. However, high-quality evidence demonstrating the efficacy of IA in the inflammatory neuropathies is lacking [23]. There is also some evidence that apheresis can improve recovery from multiple sclerosis relapses, and these approaches are often used after inadequate responses to corticosteroids [24,25].

Certain subtypes of GBS are associated with immunoglobulin (Ig) G ganglioside antibodies [26], with a handful of small studies showing an effective reduction of antibody titres using IA [19,27]. More recently a subset of CIDP-like neuropathies have been linked to predominantly IgG4-subclass antibodies directed against nodal or paranodal cell-adhesion molecules [28–32]. It has been speculated that patients with such antibodies may respond particularly well to selective IgG immunoadsorption [33]. A recent case series of four patients with CIDP and neurofascin-155 (NF155) antibodies reported that PLEx was effective in 3, and partially effective in 1, whilst tryptophan-based IA was ineffective in one such patient [34].

There are of course substantial differences between PLEx and IA. The former removes a broad range of circulating molecules and requires the use of replacement fluid, typically fresh frozen plasma, or albumin. Replacement fluid is not required in IA, and the range of circulating factors removed is more limited. This is advantageous in reducing complications, such as those due to the unwanted removal of coagulation factors [35], but may also lead to a loss of therapeutic effect if this depends on the removal of pro-inflammatory cytokines, or other pathogenically-relevant molecules, rather than immunoglobulins. It is also important to appreciate that there are variations in the biological effects between the different types of IA, which may also influence their clinical efficacy. For example, Yuki and colleagues have previously demonstrated that tryptophan-based columns are more effective than phenylalanine for adsorbing anti-ganglioside antibodies [36]. IA using protein A or synthetic ligands has been proposed as a method to remove a larger fraction of circulating IgG more selectively and quickly, whilst more modestly affecting IgM and IgA levels, and leaving complement, albumin and fibrinogen largely unaffected [37].

Intuitively, it may be assumed that patients who respond to "Ig-selective" IA do so because pathogenic Ig is being removed from the circulation. However, previous assessments of IA efficacy rarely report serological status. It is therefore currently unclear as to whether the presence of known serum autoantibodies in GBS and CIDP prospectively identifies a subpopulation of patients who are likely to respond more favourably to IA. It is also unclear as to whether any particular IA system or treatment programme is more likely to produce a positive outcome.

In this study we provide a retrospective evaluation of apheresis in two serologically-defined patient cohorts. We first reviewed the subjective clinician-reported overall impression of response to IA or PLEx in a cohort of neuropathy patients identified during routine diagnostic testing (PNAb cohort), and compared patients in which nodal/paranodal antibodies were or were not detected. We present the detailed case history and parallel serological analysis of a patient with NF155 antibodies who was treated with IA. Finally, we perform a retrospective analysis of the serological status of a sample of 60 patients who had been treated with IgG-depleting IA (IA cohort) and compare this with clinician-reported outcomes.

2. Experimental Section

2.1. Paranodal Antibody (PNAb) Patient Cohort

Since 2015, 88 patients with confirmed or suspected inflammatory neuropathies presenting to the neuropathy clinic in Oxford have been recruited to an observational study. This study was approved by the National Health Service (NHS) National Research Ethics Service Committee (South Central–Oxford A, 14/SC/0280). Patients recruited prior to 2017 were tested retrospectively, and those recruited from 2017 prospectively, for nodal/paranodal antibodies by the methods described in Appendix A. Since August 2017, serum samples from a further 537 external patients with confirmed or suspected inflammatory neuropathies have been received for diagnostic nodal/paranodal antibody testing by the Oxford laboratory. Clinical information was requested for all patients, including details of treatments used, and a clinician-led, subjective, overall impression of their efficacy.

2.2. IA Patient Cohort

The IA cohort consisted of 60 subjects (20 with CIDP, 20 with GBS, and a control group of 20 with multiple sclerosis/clinically-isolated syndrome, MS/CIS) who were selected from patients treated with IA between June 2013 and January 2018 in the University of Ulm, Department of Neurology based on the inclusion criteria outlined below. The study was reviewed by the appropriate ethics committee of the University of Ulm (approval number 20/10) and was performed in accordance with the ethical standards of the Declaration of Helsinki from 1964. Written informed consent for the sample collection was obtained from all patients participating in this study.

2.2.1. CIDP

All patients with CIDP fulfilled the EFNS criteria for possible, probable, or definite CIDP, had a continuously progressive course of disease, and had previously received several cycles of steroids ($n = 5$), IVIg ($n = 2$) or both ($n = 13$), with insufficient response. Fifteen patients who had previously received IVIg showed further disease progression under IVIg therapy, therefore we opted for a new therapeutic approach with IA. In 5 patients who had never received IVIg we chose IA instead of IVIg based on our favourable clinical experience with IA in CIDP. Two patients had never been treated with prednisolone because of severe diabetes mellitus. Further treatments included azathioprine ($n = 5$), cyclophosphamide ($n = 1$), mycophenolate mofetil ($n = 2$), and methotrexate ($n = 1$). Assessment of the clinical outcome directly and 2 weeks after IA was based on the Inflammatory Neuropathy Cause and Treatment (INCAT) score [38] and the Ulmer CIDP score, which includes the INCAT, the Oxford muscle strength grading scale (Medical Research Council, MRC), and vibration sensitivity testing [33].

2.2.2. GBS

All patients with GBS showed the typical clinical picture including rapidly progressive bilateral limb weakness and sensory deficits, hypo-/areflexia, electrophysiological signs of demyelination, and increased protein levels in cerebrospinal fluid. Anti-ganglioside antibodies were not tested prospectively. In contrast to CIDP and MS, IA was a first-line therapy in 4 GBS patients, and used as an escalation therapy in 9 more. In order to establish equally sized subgroups, the GBS group included

7 patients who received PLEx rather than IA. Classification of the clinical outcome (no improvement, equivocal improvement, partial improvement, large improvement) directly after the last treatment was retrospectively based on the neurological examination as documented in the medical records (discharge letter) of each patient.

2.2.3. MS/CIS

All patients fulfilled the 2017 MacDonald diagnostic criteria for MS [39] or CIS. All patients treated with IA suffered from a steroid-refractory relapse, i.e., an acute relapse without complete remission after one or more cycles of high dose intravenous methylprednisolone (IVMP) therapy (at least 3×1000 mg). Assessment of the clinical outcome directly after the last treatment was based on the Expanded Disability Status Scale (EDSS).

2.3. IA Treatment

One cycle of IA consisted of five treatments on 5 consecutive days. The total plasma volume of each patient was calculated using body weight, height, and haematocrit. Two plasma volumes were processed during the first treatment, and 2.5 plasma volumes were processed during all the subsequent treatments. The Adsorber system (ADAsorb, medicap clinic GmbH, Ulrichstein, Germany) contained two regenerating protein A columns (Immunosorba, Fresenius Medical Care, Bad Homburg, Germany).

2.4. Sample Collection and Storage

Eluate samples were obtained during each IA treatment and buffered with bicarbonate (pH 7.0). Serum samples were obtained before and after each IA treatment. A standardized protocol for serum and eluate collection was applied as previously recommended [40]. All biosamples were stored according to the predefined standard operating procedure (SOPs) at the local biobank in Ulm at minus 80 °C within two hours. Later they were transferred for measurement on dry ice to Oxford for further analysis.

2.5. Serological Analysis

Sera and eluates from the 3 patient cohorts and from control subjects were analysed using a nodal/paranodal antibody cell-based assay, paranodal, ganglioside and sulfatide ELISA, and against myelinating co-cultures. Methodological details for these experiments are given in Appendix A.

3. Results

3.1. Nodal/Paranodal Antibody (PNAb) Diagnostic Cohort

3.1.1. Demographics, Clinical and Serological Characteristics

Since August 2018, serum samples from 537 different patients with confirmed or suspected inflammatory neuropathies have been received for diagnostic nodal/paranodal antibody testing by the Oxford laboratory, and we have tested a further 88 patients from our own research cohort. Overall, 42/625 patients (6.7%) were positive for nodal/paranodal antibodies (PNAb+), comprising 16 (2.6%) with NF155 specific antibodies, 1 (0.2%) with NF186 specific antibodies, 6 (1%) with pan-neurofascin antibodies, 12 (1.9%) with contactin-1 (CNTN1) antibodies and 7 (1.1%) with contactin-associated protein (Caspr1) or CNTN1/Caspr1-complex antibodies. The median age of the PNAb+ patients was 58 (range 15 to 79) and 30/42 (71.4%) were male. The initial clinical diagnosis was CIDP in 28 (66.6%), GBS in 13 (31.0%) and atypical multifocal motor neuropathy in 1 (2.4%). In one patient, the diagnosis of CIDP was subsequently revised to motor neuron disease; the diagnosis of an inflammatory neuropathy was retained at follow up in all other antibody positive cases. The remaining 583 patients were paranodal antibody negative (PNAb-negative), with clinical data available for 185 patients. The median age of the PNAb-negative patients was 62 (range 4 to 90) and 120/185 (64.9%) were male. The initial clinical diagnosis was CIDP in 100 (53.8%), combined central and peripheral demyelination in 3 (1.6%), GBS in 38 (20.4%), and multifocal motor neuropathy in 16 (8.6%). In 9/131 (6.9%) patients for whom follow up data was available, the diagnosis was subsequently revised away from that of an inflammatory neuropathy. Summary demographic and clinical details of the subgroups of apheresis treated PNAb-positive and PNAb-negative patients are given in Table 1. There was no significant difference in the median age, sex distribution, clinical diagnosis, or other serological results between the 2 subgroups. There was a non-significant trend towards more severe disease and more frequent IgG and less frequent IgM paraprotein detection in PNAb-positive patients. The frequencies of prior IVIg, steroid, PLEx and immunosuppressant use was also similar between the groups, while rituximab and IA were significantly more likely to have been used in the PNAb-positive group. PLEX aside, there was, however, no statistically significant difference in the clinician reported responses to these therapies between the 2 groups, although there was a trend to rituximab being more often judged effective in the PNAb-positive compared to PNAb-negative group.

Table 1. Summary characteristics of apheresis treated patients from the PNAb cohort.

	PNAb Positive (n = 21)	PNAb Negative (n = 33)	Significance (PNAb+ v PNAb-neg)		
Age: median, (range)	58 (35–79)	62 (5–90)	ns	$p = 0.94$	Mann-Whitney
Male sex: n, (%)	16 (76.2%)	23 (69.7%)	ns	$p = 0.76$	Fisher's exact
Initial clinical diagnosis:					
• GBS: n (%)	6 (28.6%)	10 (30.3%)	ns	$p > 0.99$	Fisher's exact (GBS or not)
• CIDP: n (%)	14 (66.7%)	18 (54.5%)	ns	$p = 0.41$	Fisher's exact (CIDP or not)
• Other: n (%)	1 (4.7%)	5 (15.1%)	ns	$p = 0.39$	Fisher's exact (Other or not)
Peak severity/nadir mRs (median, range)	5 (2–6)	4 (2–5)	ns	$p = 0.10$	Mann-Whitney
Other serology: n/n (%)					
Any ganglioside Ab	1/16 (6.3%)	3/18 (16.7%)	ns	$p = 0.60$	Fisher's exact
• GM1	1/16 (6.3%)	2/18 (11.1%)	ns	$p > 0.99$	Fisher's exact
• GQ1b	0/16	1/18 (5.6%)	ns	$p > 0.99$	Fisher's exact
MAG	0/4	1/8 (12.5%)	ns	$p > 0.99$	Fisher's exact
Paraprotein	2/17 (11.8%)	6/26 (23.1%)	ns	$p = 0.45$	Fisher's exact
• IgM	0/17	5/26 (19.2%)	ns	$p = 0.14$	Fisher's exact
• IgG	2/17 (11.8%)	1/26 (3.8%)	ns	$p = 0.55$	Fisher's exact
Treatment % treated (% of those judged to have good response)			Difference in proportion treated/proportion with good response		
IVIg	90.5 (5.3%)	87.9% (3.4%)	ns/ns	$p > 0.99/p > 0.99$	Fisher's exact
Steroids	85.7% (0)	75.8% (8%)	ns/ns	$p = 0.50/p = 0.50$	Fisher's exact
PLEx	95.2% (0)	100% (24.2%)	ns/*	$p = 0.39/*p = 0.01$	Fisher's exact
IA	19% (0)	0 (0)	***/ns	$***p < 0.001/p > 0.99$	Fisher's exact
Rituximab	66.7% (64.3%)	18.2% (16.7%)	***/ns	$***p < 0.002/p = 0.14$	Fisher's exact
Other immuno-suppression	33.3% (28.6%)	24.2% (12.5%)	ns/ns	$p = 0.54/p = 0.47$	Fisher's exact

GBS, Guillain-Barré syndrome; CIDP, chronic inflammatory demyelinating polyneuropathy; GM1, monosialoganglioside GM1; GQ1b, tetrasialoganglioside GQ1b; MAG, myelin associated glycoprotein; IVIg, intravenous immunoglobulin; PLEx, plasma exchange; IA, immunoadsorption, * and ***, indicate statistical significance.

3.1.2. Physician-Reported Subjective Evaluation of Responses to Plasma Exchange or Immunoadsorption

Of the PNAb+ patients, 17 were treated with PLEx alone, 1 with IA alone, and 3 with both modalities. Protein A columns were used for three of the IA treated patients, the other (described in detail below) was treated with a GAM-peptide-ligand-based column (Globaffin, Fresenius Medical Care (UK) Ltd, Sutton-in-Ashfield, UK). Serial disability measures are available for only one other PNAb+ patient: a 68-year-old lady with a clinical diagnosis of GBS. Neither her overall neuropathy limitations score (ONLS, 12/12) nor inflammatory neuropathy Rasch-built overall disability score (iRODS, 0/48) improved following 2 cycles 5 treatments of PLEx starting on days 40 and 69 of her illness, prior to her death on day 110 from infectious complications. For all other PNAb+ patients, only clinician-reported, retrospective, and subjective evaluations of response were available. None of the treating clinicians judged that either PLEx or IA had produced a subjectively "good" response in any of the PNAb+ patients. With PLEx, 5 patients (25.0%) were reported as having had a partial response, 2 (10.0%) an equivocal response, 12 (60.0%) no response, and one to have deteriorated (5.0%). With IA, 1 (25%) partial response, and 1 (25%) equivocal response were reported, with 2 patients (50%) reported as showing no response (Figure 1A,B). The proportion of PNAb+ patients subjectively judged as showing a partial or better response to PLEx (25.0%) versus IA (25.0%) was identical.

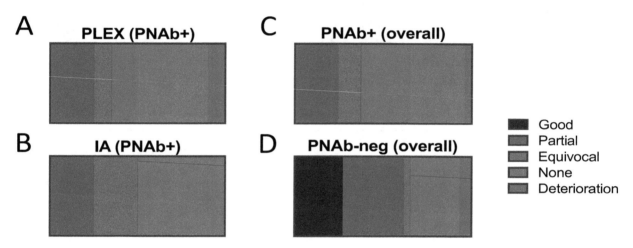

Figure 1. Physician-reported subjective evaluation of response to plasma exchange or immuno-adsorption in paranodal antibody positive and negative patients. Paranodal antibody positive patients treated with (**A**) plasma exchange ($n = 17$), (**B**) immunoadsorption ($n = 4$), or (**C**) either modality ($n = 21$), compared to (**D**) paranodal antibody negative patients ($n = 33$) (all treated with plasma exchange).

Of the PNAb-negative patients, 33 were treated with PLEx: 8 patients (24.2%) were subjectively reported as having a good response, 10 (30.3%) a partial response, 1 (3.0%) an equivocal response, 8 (24.2%) no response, and 2 (6.1%) as deteriorating. For 4 patients, the response to PLEx was not reported. Amongst the 3 ganglioside antibody positive patients, 2 were reported as having a partial response, and 1 no response, to PLEx. Apheresis, with or without IA, was significantly more likely to have been reported by treating clinicians to have produced partial or better response in the PNAb-negative patients (62.1%) compared to the PNAb+ patients (25.0%) ($p = 0.01$, Fisher's exact test, OR 4.9 (95% CI 1.52 to 14.88) (Figure 1C,D). It should be emphasised that this is a comparison of the physicians' subjective overall impression of response, rather than an evaluation of the true efficacy, or otherwise, of these treatments.

3.2. Detailed Profile of an NF155 Antibody Positive Patient Treated with Immunoadsorption

This 46-year-old male first presented to neurology in July 2019 with a 6-week history of ascending numbness and paraesthesia in his feet, then hands. He had lost the ability to run and found walking to be unsteady. On examination, power was full, but there was global areflexia with distal sensory loss to temperature, pin-prick, vibration and proprioception. His gait was broad-based and unsteady and Rhomberg's test was positive after 20 s of eye closure. There was a postural tremor of both hands without cerebellar or extrapyramidal signs. The presentation was felt to be consistent with sensory ataxic CIDP. Neurofascin-155 antibody mediated disease was high in the differential. A positive result on the NF155 CBA and ELISA was duly returned 2 days later, at an initial titre of 1:6400. IgG4 was the dominant subclass, with IgG1 and IgG2 also represented (Figure 2A,B). CSF was acellular with an elevated protein (1.8 g/L). Nerve conduction studies showed absent median but preserved sural sensory nerve action potentials. Distal motor latencies and F-wave latencies were significantly prolonged, with slowing of intermediate motor conduction velocities. There was conduction block without temporal dispersion in the sampled peroneal nerve between the ankle and fibular head. Pulsed dexamethasone was commenced 4 days later (40mg per day for 4 days every 4 weeks for 3 cycles). There was no change in the examination findings. A progressive deterioration in symptoms and disability measures prompted a trial of IVIg (2 g/kg over 5 days) which resulted in a pompholyx-type skin rash, and no neurological benefit over the next 6 weeks. Approval was then sought for rituximab, and IA was arranged as a potential temporising measure.

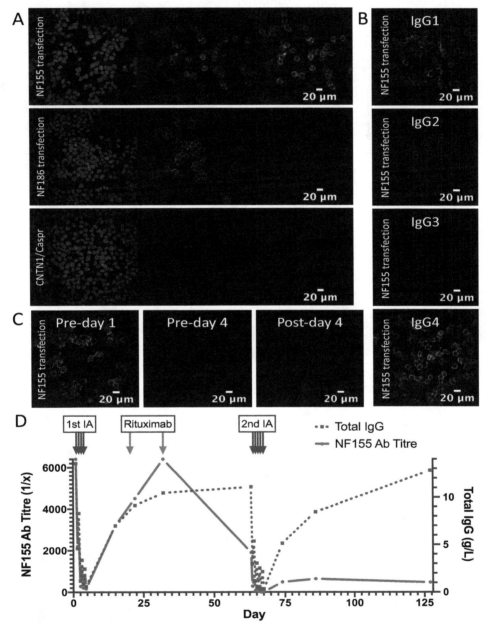

Figure 2. Serological results of NF155 antibody positive patient at baseline and during IA treatment. (**A**) Serum contains IgG (green) which binds to the cell membrane of NF155-transfected HEK293T cells, and co-localises with a commercial pan-neurofascin antibody (red). No signal is seen with NF186 or CNTN1/Caspr1-transfected cells. (**B**) The predominant IgG subclass of the NF155 antibodies is IgG4, with IgG1>IgG2 also represented. (**C**) The antibody signal intensity at 1:100 before, during and immediately after the first cycle of IA shows a progressive decline. (**D**) NF155 antibody titre (red) and total IgG levels (blue) over 2 cycles of IA, before and after rituximab.

Four treatment sessions of 2–2.5 plasma volumes were given on 4 consecutive days using a multiple pass, GAM-peptide-ligand-based column (Globaffin, Fresenius Medical Care Ltd, Sutton-in-Ashfield, UK). IA was effective in rapidly and substantially reducing the NF155 antibody titre (Figure 2C), but this had returned to baseline by 1 month (Figure 2D) and there was no observed clinical benefit. Rituximab was then given (1g on 2 occasions 2 weeks apart) followed by a second cycle of 5 treatments sessions of IA 1 month later. This was again associated with a rapid and substantial reduction in NF155 antibody titre, which on this occasion recovered more slowly and incompletely (Figure 2D). This more persistent suppression of antibody titres was associated with a progressive improvement in symptoms and disability, which is currently ongoing (Figure 3).

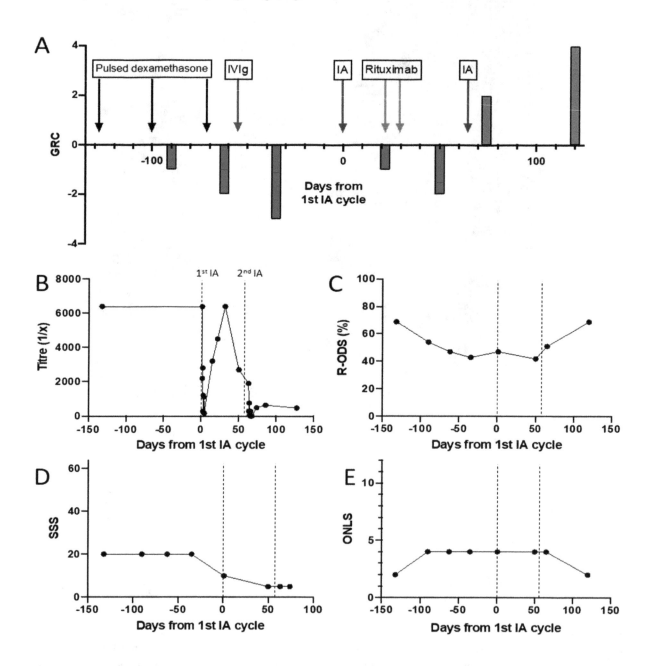

Figure 3. Antibody titres and outcome/disability measures during treatment of a patient with an NF155-antibody-mediated neuropathy. (**A**) Patient global rating of change after treatment with dexamethasone, IVIg, IA and rituximab. (**B**) NF155 antibody titre. (**C**) Inflammatory neuropathy Rasch-built Overall Disability Score. (**D**) Sensory sum score. (**E**) Overall neuropathy limitations score.

3.3. Demographics and Clinical Characteristics of the IA Treated Cohort

3.3.1. CIDP

Details of this cohort are given in Appendix B (Table A1). Sixteen of these 20 CIDP patients have been described in a previous publication [33]. 16/20 (80%) were male. At the start of IA treatment, the cohort had a median age of 66 (range 27 to 80), and a median disease duration of 95.5 months (range 63 to 139). All had progressive disease and met the European Federation of Neurological Societies (EFNS) criteria for definite, probable, or possible CIDP [41]. 18/20 had been previously treated with corticosteroids and 14/20 with IVIg, with sub-optimal responses. Six patients were treated with at least one of azathioprine, cyclophosphamide, mycophenolate mofetil or methotrexate. Nine patients received multiple (range 2–9) cycles of IA. Five patients showed improvements in their Inflammatory Neuropathy Cause and Treatment (INCAT) disability score when assessed 2 weeks after initial IA treatment, and 8 patients showed substantial improvements (at least 10 points) in the CIDP score.

3.3.2. GBS

Details of this cohort are given in Appendix B (Table A2). 10/20 patients (50%) were male. At the start of IA or PLEx treatment, the cohort had a median age of 66 (range 31 to 89). IA was applied to 13/20 patients. IA was used as a first-line therapy in 3, as a second-line therapy (after unsuccessful treatment with IVIg) in 9, and as a third-line therapy (after both IVIg and PLEx) in 1 patient. This subgroup was supplemented with 7 patients who received PLEx, instead of IA. In these patients, PLEx was used as a first-line therapy in 6, and as a second-line therapy (after IVIg) in 1 patient. 18/20 patients received 1 cycle of IA or PLEx, and only 2 patients received 2 cycles. 4/20 (3/13 IA, 1/7 PLEx) patients showed no clinical improvement after the last treatment, 3 patients (2/13 IA, 1/7 PLEx) showed equivocal improvement, 8 patients (4/13 IA, 4/7 PLEx) showed partial improvement, and 5 patients (4/13 IA, 1/ PLEx) showed large improvement.

3.3.3. MS/CIS

Details of this cohort are given in Appendix B (Table A3). 15/20 patients (75%) were female. At the start of IA treatment, the cohort had a median age of 29 (range 15 to 57). Patients were diagnosed with MS (16/20) or CIS (4/20), and had all been treated unsuccessfully with at least one cycle of high-dose intravenous methyl prednisolone (MP). 8 patients had received 2 or more cycles of high-dose IVMP. 11/20 patients showed an improvement of EDSS after the last IA treatment, while 9/20 patients did not improve.

3.4. Glycolipid and Nodal/Paranodal Antibodies in the IA Cohort

Pre-treatment serum samples from the IA cohort were tested for sulfatide and GM1- and GQ1b-ganglioside IgG antibodies by ELISA. None of these sera were positive on these assays. Serum samples taken pre and post-treatment, as well as first treatment session eluates from the IA cohort (20 CIDP, 20 GBS and 20 MS/CIS patients), were tested by both cell-based assay (CBA) and ELISA for antibodies to nodal (neurofascin-186) and paranodal (neurofascin-155, contactin-1 and Caspr) cell adhesion molecules. None of the sera were positive on either assay. One eluate from the MS/CIS cohort (patient 09) was positive on the neurofascin-155 CBA (blind scored as '2+' at 1:100, end-point titre 1:200, Figure 4A) (For scoring method see Appendix A.1). The sole detected subclass was IgG1. The corresponding pre-treatment serum was negative for NF155 antibodies at 1:100, the standard screening titre for this assay, but scored 3+ when repeated at 1:20. Two further eluates, one from the MS/CIS cohort and one from the CIP cohort, also produced faint membrane binding (1+) on the neurofascin-155 CBA that was not sufficient to be called positive at 1:100. Repeat testing of these eluates at 1:20 increased the signal to 2+ and 3+ respectively. However, this titre is below the usual positivity cut-off for this assay, and no signal was produced with any of the IgG subclass-specific secondary antibodies. All of these eluates were negative on the neurofascin-155 ELISA and negative for all other antigens by both CBA (including neurofascin-186, Figure 4B) and ELISA (results not shown).

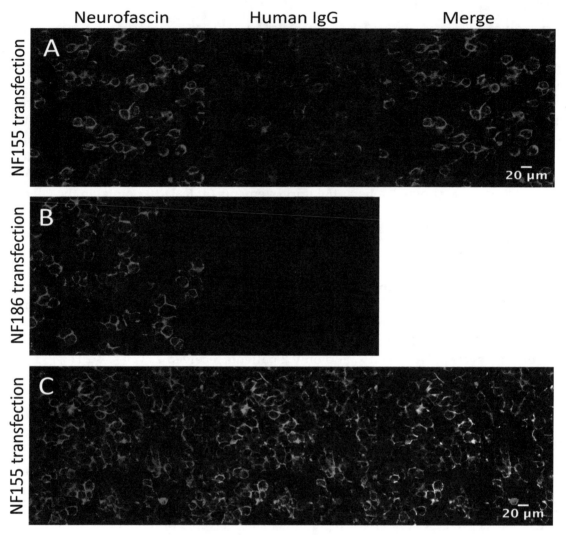

Figure 4. Nodal/paranodal cell-based assays. (**A**) MS/CIS eluate weakly positive on the neurofascin-155 CBA at 1:100 (Score 2+, end-point titre 1:200) and (**B**) negative on the neurofascin-186 CBA. (**C**) Strong positive at 1:100 (Score 4+, end-point titre 1:3200) from the antibody positive CIDP cohort shown for comparison.

3.5. Screening the IA Eluates for Novel Antibodies Using Myelinating Co-Cultures

In this experiment, eluates from the first treatment session of each IA cohort were compared with purified IgG from the serum of 22 healthy control volunteers (gratefully received from A/Prof Sarosh Irani, University of Oxford) isolated by Protein G purification. Serum was not available in sufficient quantities from PNAb cohort to purify IgG and these samples were therefore not tested in this experiment. IgG from IA eluates (1:50 dilution) and protein G purification (1:12.5 dilution) were applied to myelinated human sensory neuron cultures in a 96 well, flat-bottom imaging plate format enabling high-throughput staining and imaging. The mean IgG concentration after dilution was not significantly different between the groups (One-Way ANOVA: $F(3,78) = 1.500$, $p = 0.2211$) (Figure 5A). Out of 82 samples tested, 1 CIDP (patient 11), 1 GBS (patient 07, who was also concurrently identified as HIV positive, see Appendix B.2 for further detail) and 1 MS/CIS (patient 13) sample were scored as 'positive' for either axonal, glial or nodal IgG deposition by an observer blinded to the patient group; a further 1 MS/CIS patient sample with weak IgG labelling was marked 'equivocal'. All 4 of these sera and IA eluates were negative on the glycolipid and paranodal antibody assays, as above. Pre-treatment serum from MS patient 13 was also negative on our in-house live CBAs for aquapaorin-4 and MOG antibodies. Neither of the MS/CIS eluates which produced a weak signal on the neurofascin-155 CBA were positive on the co-culture assay.

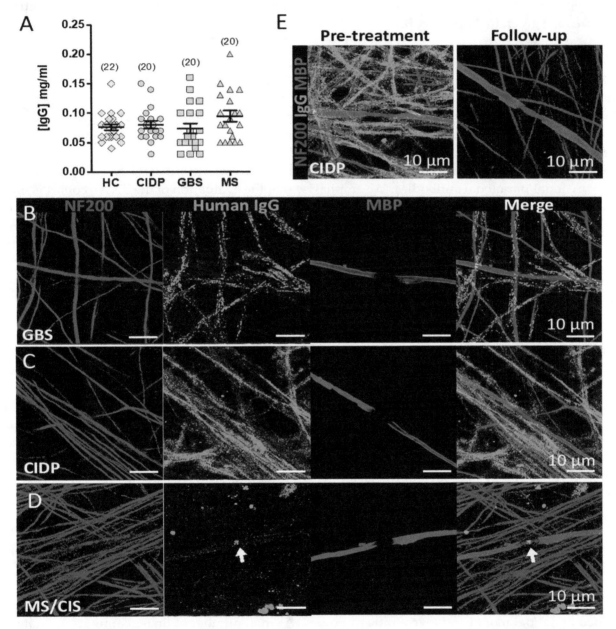

Figure 5. IgG deposition in myelinated co-cultures. (**A**) IgG concentration of dilution-adjusted eluates used for screening on myelinated cultures. (**B–D**) Immunofluorescence images of IgG binding patterns in myelinating co-cultures of IA eluates (1:50) from three patients with neurological disease identified in the screening assay: B) GBS (patient 07), C) CIDP (patient 11), and D) MS/CIS (patient 13) (arrow indicates IgG deposition at the node of Ranvier). (**E**) IgG labelling in myelinated co-cultures of serum (1:50) sampled from the CIDP (patient 11) before (Pre-treatment) and after IA (Follow-up). Note all IgG immunoreactivity is lost at follow-up. NF200, neurofilament 200; MBP, myelin basic protein.

Serum samples taken pre- and post-IA from the four candidate patients (1:50 dilution) were further validated on myelinated cultures plated on 13 mm coverslips with careful attention paid to media changes and washing steps. Strong IgG deposition aligned with neurofilament positive axons was observed in the serum and IA eluate of the GBS (patient 07) (Figure 5B) and CIDP (patient 11) (Figure 5C) patients. We confirmed nodal reactive IgG in the serum and IA eluate of one MS patient

(Figure 5D and Video S1), which was absent from post-IA serum. The post-treatment follow-up serum from the CIDP (patient 11) patient was negative for any IgG reactivity (Figure 5E). No IgG reactivity was observed in the serum or eluate of the MS/CIS patient 13 previously marked as equivocal, confirming this as a false positive. Clinical vignettes describing the patients with IgG deposition on co-cultures are given in Appendix B.

4. Discussion

In the PNAb cohort, we found that PLEx or IA were more often subjectively judged to have been effective in seronegative cases, and that in contrast, detection of at least one of the known nodal/paranodal antibodies in patients with inflammatory neuropathies was not associated with clinicians perceiving a positive response to either treatment. The proportion of PNAb-negative patients judged to have had a partial or better response (62.1%) was similar to the proportion of patients judged to have had a partial or better response in the IA cohort (52.5% overall), all of whom were also negative for known nodal/paranodal antibodies. We emphasise that the evaluation of the PNAb cohort is limited by the retrospective and subjective nature of the patient assessment. In addition, the small number of cases precludes us from reaching any conclusions regarding the objective benefits of one treatment modality compared to the other in this setting. In addition, improvement in neurological symptoms following IA/PLEX may occur after a delay, which may not be reflected in the immediate judgement of the treating physician. Blinding, randomisation, standardised follow up, as well as a control group to judge the natural history of these heterogeneous diseases, are required for a definitive evaluation of apheresis treatment efficacy in these patient groups. However, it is notable that treating physicians were less likely to think that apheresis had been effective in PNAb-positive patients.

Why seropositive patients were rarely assessed to have responded positively to either IA or PLEx is unclear. Our close monitoring of a prospectively-identified neurofascin-155 positive individual showed that while IA given as a mono-therapy was able to effectively reduce antibody titres, levels quickly rebounded and reached pre-treatment levels inside 4 weeks. This transient serological effect was not sufficient to reduce disability. More prolonged suppression of antibody titres, with frequent apheresis cycles or adjuvant therapies, may therefore be required for effective treatment in such cases.

Rituximab has previously been suggested as an effective treatment for paranodal antibody positive patients [42,43], but may take several weeks (or even months) to produce benefit. In this case, a second cycle of IA, 4 weeks after a course of rituximab, produced a more persistent suppression of antibody titres, which was associated with clinical improvement. The extent to which IA contributed to this effect is unclear. Theoretically, the more rapid action of IA might be complementary to the delayed but more sustained effects of rituximab. Whether this combination of treatment offers significant benefit over rituximab alone requires further investigation.

Retrospective analysis of serum samples from 60 IA-treated patients failed to identify any individuals who would have been classified as positive on routine diagnostic testing for previously described nodal/paranodal and glycolipid antibodies. A small number of first-treatment IA eluates did produce a low-level signal on the neurofascin-155 CBA. Whilst the diagnostic importance of low-titre, non-IgG4 results has been doubted [44], a pathogenic role for these antibodies cannot be ruled out.

The apparently better response of seronegative patients to apheresis, particularly IA, has several possible explanations. One is that these differences simply reflect variation in the disease characteristics and natural progression of seropositive versus seronegative inflammatory neuropathies: Overall, seropositive patients tend to have more severe, aggressive disease that is refractory to treatment [30–32]. Conversely, less severely affected, seronegative, patients may be more likely to have a monophasic disease course and stabilise or improve, independent of any particular therapy. Indeed, the median peak disability, measured by nadir modified Rankin score (mRs), of apheresis-treated PNAb+ patients in our series was higher, albeit non-significantly, than that of the apheresis-treated seronegative group (median nadir mRs 5 v 4, $p = 0.1$, Mann-Witney test, Table 1), although there was no significant difference in the use of, or clinician evaluated response to, other treatment modalities. There was also no significant difference in the proportion of patients initially diagnosed as GBS (28.6% and 30.3%, $p > 0.99$) compared to CIDP (66.7% and 54.5%, $p = 0.41$) in the PNAb+ and PNAb-negative groups, respectively (Fisher's exact test, Table 1). However, this does not exclude the possibility that patients in the seronegative group may often have a shorter disease course, with less irreversible axonal degeneration.

Another explanation for perceived apheresis efficacy in seronegative patients is the presence of antibodies below the threshold for positive detection on diagnostic testing, leading to a correspondingly slower rebound in titres following PLEx/IA and a more sustained suppression of antibody levels. A further possibility is that the response to IA in diagnostically seronegative patients is due to the therapeutic removal of as-yet uncharacterised, pathologically relevant antibodies in these patient groups. We therefore tested for further nerve-related antigens by screening eluates from the IA cohort against myelinating co-cultures. Three positive IA eluate samples were identified in the original 96-well co-culture screen and were further validated in a larger 24-well format, confirming similar binding patterns. IgG from one GBS patient co-localised with NF200 suggesting an axonal antigen. One CIDP patient serum and IA eluate showed IgG binding that aligned with NF200-positive axons but may also reflect deposition on non-myelinating Schwann cells.

One patient's serum and IA eluate from the MS/CIS group revealed nodal specific IgG binding. The presence of antibodies against nodal antigens such as neurofascin, has precedence in MS, and although uncommon, is more predominant in chronic progressive forms of the disease [45]. However, this sample was negative for antibodies against both the glial/paranodal and nodal/axonal isoforms of neurofascin (NF155 and NF186, respectively). The original focus on peripheral neuropathies led us to use a sensory neuron system for the myelinating cultures. Nevertheless, multiple peripheral nerve antigens are also found in the CNS (and vice versa), including NF155, CNTN1 and the ganglioside GM1. Therefore, it is quite feasible for the unknown antigen targeted by IgG in this CIS/MS patient to be mutually expressed in the peripheral and central nervous systems (CNS). Other autoantibodies against nerve and glial structures in the CNS including myelin basic protein, myelin-associated lipids, contactin-2, and KIR4.1 are among those proposed in MS patients [46]; however, their presence may not be specific to the disease [47]. For this reason, the inclusion of MS/CIS patients as a control group is potentially problematic. However, as patients with non-autoimmune neurological disease essentially never receive apheresis treatment, the inclusion of this group was a pragmatic way to obtain non-neuropathy IA eluates for use in our unbiased screening assays. With some similarity to the discovery of nodal/paranodal antibodies in chronic neuropathies, MS has recently been separated from other distinct, serologically-defined disorders, characterised by the presence of aquaporin-4 or myelin oligodendrocyte glycoprotein (MOG) directed autoantibodies. Whether the nodal antigen targeted by antibodies in this MS patient has a pathogenic role and might similarly define a non-MS disease entity is currently unknown. Further investigation using brain tissue may help elucidate the antigen target, pathological potential, and clinical relevance. Unfortunately, purified Ig/eluate was not available from the PNAb-negative apheresis cohort, and it is possible that novel autoantibodies are also present in some of these patients.

The two patients for whom follow-up samples were available (CIDP and MS/CIS) had no detectable IgG labelling in their serum after IA compared to pre-treatment. Thus, IA is effective at removing both established and potentially novel pathogenic autoreactive IgG from the circulation. Follow-up serum samples at later time points will help correlate any changes in disease progress with antibody titres.

Development of myelinated hiPSC-derived neuronal cultures in a 96-well format allowed for efficient simultaneous screening of >80 IgG eluates from patients and controls. The benefits of using live cultures for screening are the presence of complex structures including nodes of Ranvier, paranodal and juxtaparanodal regions, and compact myelin internodes, that provide an unbiased substrate for antibody screening against nerve-related antigens in their native conformation. IgG binding patterns ranged from broad axonal coverage to focal nodal localisation, reflecting morphologically distinct antigens. Images were acquired by an experienced observer who was blind to the sample identity.

Although time-consuming, acquisition in such a supervised manner aids the detection of localised signals, such as the node-specific labelling identified in one MS/CIS patient.

A single sample that was marked as 'equivocal' on the 96-well assay was subsequently confirmed as negative. The minimal occurrence of non-specific IgG labelling in the 96 well format may reflect a lower washing efficiency in the smaller volume of the 96-well plate. Nevertheless, no healthy control samples were identified as positive in the screen, suggesting the cultures are useful as a selective substrate for nerve-targeted autoantibodies.

IA is rarely performed on healthy subjects; therefore control IgG were prepared from the sera of healthy volunteers by protein G purification. IgG concentrations in the healthy samples were normalised to the patient IA eluates such that the mean IgG concentrations were not significantly different, however the variation within each group was maintained in order to reflect the original sample. The detection of specific signals in both the serum and IA eluate of each of the three positive patients suggests that a uniform dilution of 1:50 is sufficient for antibody screening within IA eluates. We cannot, however, exclude the possibility of further antibodies below the level of detection. In summary, our findings of nerve antigen reactive antibodies in three 'seronegative' neurological patients suggest the utility of an unbiased screening system such as we have described here for the myelinating co-cultures. The development of equivalent cultures containing CNS antigens and cell-types may be of further benefit to relevant MS cases.

5. Conclusions

Currently available serological tests do not unambiguously identify patients who are likely to respond to IA or PLEx. In patients with nodal/paranodal antibody associated neuropathies, frequent plasmapheresis and/or additional therapies may be required to produce an acceptable level and duration of clinical improvement. Prospective longitudinal studies involving standardized and validated outcome measures, with serial monitoring of auto-antibodies, are needed to optimise apheresis treatment regimens and accurately assess efficacy.

Author Contributions: Conceptualization, S.R. and J.D.; methodology, A.J.D., J.F., H.T., J.D., S.R., M.S.; validation, A.J.D., J.F., H.T., M.S., J.D., S.R.; formal analysis, A.J.D., J.D., S.R.; investigation, A.J.D., J.F., H.T., M.S., J.D., S.R.; resources, J.D., S.R.; data curation, A.J.D., J.F., J.D., S.R.; writing—original draft preparation, A.J.D., S.R.; writing—review and editing, A.J.D., J.F., H.T., J.D., S.R., M.S.; visualization, A.J.D., S.R.; supervision, S.R.; project administration, S.R.; funding acquisition, S.R. All authors have read and agreed to the published version of the manuscript.

Acknowledgments: The authors would like to thank Sarosh Irani, University of Oxford, for providing serum samples from control subjects used to prepare the control IgG, and all clinicians who sent samples and completed request forms for nodal/paranodal antibody testing.

Conflicts of Interest: S.R. runs a not-for-profit diagnostic testing service for nodal/paranodal antibodies. He has received a speaker's honorarium and travel expenses from Fresenius Medical Care. A.D. is named inventor on a patent for immune cell therapy in nerve injury and has received travel grants from IASP and Biolegend. M.S. has received consulting and/or speaker honoraria from Bayer, Biogen, Merck, Roche, and Sanofi Genzyme. She has received research funding from the Hertha-Nathorff-Program. J.D. reports research funds and speaker's honoraria from Fresenius Medical Care GmbH and Fresenius Medical Care Deutschland GmbH. The Globaffin IA column used to treat the NF155 PNAb+ patient was provided free of charge by Fresenius on a trial basis. The funders had no role in the design of the study; in the collection, analyses, or interpretation of data; in the writing of the manuscript, or in the decision to publish the results.

Appendix A. Detailed Experimental Methods

Appendix A.1. Nodal/Parnodal Cell-Based Assays

All sera and IA eluates were screened for IgG antibodies to neurofascin-155, neurofascin-186, contatctin-1 and Caspr1 using a live, cell-based assay (CBA), following previously described methods with slight modification [32]. In brief, HEK293T cells on poly-L-lysine coated 13mm coverslips at 80–90% confluence were transiently transfected with human neurofascin-155 (RC228652, Origene) or human neurofascin-186 (courtesy of Jerome Devaux, University of Marseille) mammalian-expression vectors, or co-transfected with both human contactin-1 (CNTN1, EXA1153-MO29 Genecopoeia, Maryland, US) and human Caspr1 (EXMO417-MO2 Genecopoeia, Maryland, US) at equimolar concentrations, using Jet-PEI transfection reagent (101-10; Polyplus). After 16 h, the cells were washed and replaced with Dulbecco's Modified Eagle Medium (DMEM) (Gibco) containing 10% fetal bovine serum (FBS). 24 hours later, sera and eluates diluted 1:100 in DMEM + BSA (1%) were incubated with the cells for 1 h at room temperature. Co-incubation with commercial chicken anti-neurofascin primary antibody, (1:1000) (Cat no. AF3235; R&D Systems, Bio-Techne) was used to confirm successful transfection and to assess for co-localisation with any bound human IgG. Following serum/eluate incubation, cells were washed 3 times with DMEM + HEPES (20 mM), and fixed for 5 minutes in 4% PFA. Secondary antibody incubation was with goat anti-human IgG-Fc specific-Alexa Fluor 488 (1:750) (Cat no. H10120; Life Tech) and goat anti-Chicken Alexa Fluor 546 1:1000 (Cat no. A11040; Life Tech). To determine antibody subclass unconjugated mouse anti-human IgG subclass 1-4 antibodies were used at 1:100 (Cat nos. I2513, I25635, I7260 I7385; Sigma-Aldrich, Merck) followed by a fluorescently tagged tertiary antibody goat anti-mouse Alexa Fluor 488 (1:750) (Cat no. A11029; Life Tech). Positivity was assessed by an observer blinded to the clinical data using fluorescence microscopy. Taking into account the intensity of the membrane signal and co-localisation of the human IgG signal with the commercial antibody, the assay was scored on a 5 point scale as follows: 4+ very strong positive, 3+ strong positive, 2+ positive, 1+ negative (non-specific background or faint/poorly co-localised human IgG signal only), 0 no human IgG binding seen.

Appendix A.2. Nodal/Paranodal ELISA

Individual wells of Nunc Maxisorp ELISA plates (Fisher Scientific) were coated overnight at 4 C with either human recombinant neurofascin-155 (NF155) (8208-NF; R&D systems), NF186 (TP329070; OriGene Technologies) or CNTN1 (10383-H08H; Sino Biological Inc) diluted to 1 g/ml in PBS. The coating solution was then removed and the plate blocked with 5% milk in PBS for 1 h at room temperature. Serum or eluates diluted 1:100 in 5% milk were then applied for 1h at room temperature then washed by 5 cycles of immersion in PBS. Anti-human IgG (Fc specific) peroxidase-conjugated anti-human IgG (A0170; Sigma) was used as the secondary antibody at 1:3000. The detection reaction was performed using 50 l o-Phenylenediamine dihydrochloride solution (OPD fast, Sigma), stopped after 20 minutes by the application of 25 l 4M sulphuric acid, and optical densities measured at 492 nm using a FLUOstar Omega plate reader (BMG Labtech). Wells with ODs greater than 0.1 above uncoated (PBS only) control wells were considered positive.

Appendix A.3. Ganglioside and Sulfatide ELISA

Ganglioside and sulfatide ELISAs were performed using Immunolon 2HB 96 well plates [48]. Wells were coated with 100 ul of GM1 or GQ1b bovine gangliosides diluted to 2 g/ml, or sulfatide to 5 g/ml, in methanol. Negative control wells contained methanol only. Plates were then air-dried overnight in the fume hood, placed at 4 C, and blocked with 2% BSA/PBS. Sera/eluates were diluted 1:100 in 1% BSA/PBS and incubated for 2 h at 4 C. Secondary antibodies and detection were the same as the nodal/paranodal ELISA, except that secondary antibody incubation was performed at 4 C.

Appendix A.4. Protein G IgG Purification

Healthy control sera (100 μl) were diluted 1:1 in sterile PBS, added to protein G columns (Cat. 28-4083-47, Ab SpinTrap, GE Healthcare) prepared according to the manufacturer's instructions. Briefly, samples were incubated 15 min at 4 °C on rollers to bind IgG. Serum was then removed by centrifugation (100 g, 30 s) and columns washed twice with binding buffer (20 mM Na_2PO_4, pH 7.0). IgG were eluted with 320 μl 0.1M glycine (pH 2.6) and neutralised with 80 μl Tris-HCl (pH 8.0). Elution was repeated once more and samples taken forward for IgG quantification.

Appendix A.5. IgG ELISA

IgG in serum and eluates was quantified by enzyme-linked immunosorbent assay (ELISA) using a human IgG ELISA quantification kit (Cat. E80-104, Bethyl Laboratories Inc. TX, US) according to the manufacturer's instructions. Briefly, 96 well plates (Maxisorp, Nunc) were coated with goat anti-human IgG-Fc capture antibody (10 μg/ml) in coating buffer (0.05M carbonate-bicarbonate, pH 9.6) (100 μl/well) for 1h at room temperature (RT). Plates were washed 5 times by immersion in wash buffer (50mM Tris, 0.14M NaCl, 0.05% Tween 20, pH 8.0), blocked for 1h at RT in blocking buffer (50mM Tris, 0.14M NaCl, 1% BSA, pH 8.0), followed again by immersion 5 times in washing buffer. Serum samples and IgG eluates were prepared at 1:10,000 dilution in sample diluent, as well as a dilution series of human reference serum standards (50mM Tris, 0.14M NaCl, 1% BSA, 0.05% Tween 20, pH 8.0). All samples and standards were prepared in duplicate (100 μL/well) and incubated 1h at RT. After 5x immersion washes 100 μL of HRP-conjugated goat anti-human IgG-Fc Detection Antibody (1:200,000) was incubated 1h at RT followed by 5 immersion washes. Plates were developed by the addition of 100 μL of TMB substrate solution (20 min, RT) and reaction stopped by adding equal volume of 0.18M H_2SO_4. Absorbance values were read immediately on a plate reader (FLUO Star Omega, BMG Labtech) at 450nm (signal) and 630nm (background). A standard curve was constructed from the background subtracted absorbance (OD) values obtained from the human serum standards using a 4-parameter function (https://mycurvefit.com/). IgG concentrations of each sample were calculated from averages of the duplicate, background-subtracted OD values, multiplied by the original dilution. All values for diluted samples fell within the standard curve (1–1000 ng/mL).

Appendix A.6. Myelinating Co-Cultures

Myelinating co-cultures were prepared using human induced pluripotent stem cells (hiPSC)-derived sensory neurons and primary rat Schwann cells with some modifications to previously described methods [49]. hiPSCs from control subjects were obtained via the StemBANCC consortium at the University of Oxford (https://www.ndcn.ox.ac.uk/research/stembancc). In brief, hiPSCs were differentiated to sensory neurons using a combination of small-molecule mediated dual-SMAD inhibition and wnt activation. On day 11 of differentiation, sensory neuron precursors were seeded onto 13 mm diameter glass coverslips (approximately 20,000 cells per coverslip) or 96-well flat, glass-bottom imaging plates (Sensoplate Microplate, Greiner-Bio) (approximately 5000 neurons per well) previously coated with poly-D-lysine (PDL) (10 μg/mL) overnight and reduced growth-factor matrigel (Corning). Neurons were maintained in neurobasal media supplemented with N2, B27, Glutamax and anti-anti (all Gibco, Life Technologies) ('complete' neurobasal) plus recombinant human β-NGF (rhNGF) (Cat. 450-01, Peprotech), NT3 (Cat. 450-03, Peprotech), GDNF (Cat. 450-10, Peprotech), and BDNF (Cat. PHC7074, Life Technologies) (all growth factors 25 ng/ml), supplemented with Rho-associated, coiled-coil containing protein kinase (ROCK) inhibitor (10 μM) (Tocris, Bio-Techne) on days 11–12, CHIR99021 (3 μM) (Sigma) on days 11–14 and cytosine arabinoside (Ara-C) (1 μM) (Sigma) on days 12–14. Neurons were incubated at 37 °C in 5% CO_2 for 4 weeks with twice-weekly medium changes prior to addition of Schwann cells for myelination.

Primary Schwann cells were isolated from the sciatic nerves of rat pups (P2-3). Mother and pups were killed by rising concentration of CO_2 in accordance with Schedule 1 of the UK Home Office

Animals (Scientific Procedures) Act 1986. Sciatic nerves were rapidly dissected and digested in a mixture of collagenase (3mg/ml) (Worthington, Lorne Labs) and dispase II (3.5mg/mL) (Roche) for 1 h at 37 °C with frequent gentle agitation. Nerves were washed in DMEM + FBS (10%) and gently triturated using a fire-polished glass Pasteur pipette. Dissociated cells were seeded into tissue culture flasks overnight and expanded in Schwann cell expansion medium containing charcoal-stripped FBS (10%) (Sigma), Forskolin (4 μM), recombinant human NRG1-β1 EGF domain (80 ng/mL) (Cat. 396-HB, R&D Systems) and recombinant murine NGF (10 ng/ml) (Cat. 450-34, Peprotech) in DMEM/F12 (Gibco). Cells were serially treated with 5–10 μM Ara-C to eliminate fibroblasts. Expanded Schwann cells were added to the neuronal cultures (25,000 cells per coverslip or 5000 cell per 96-well) and allowed to proliferate and align with the axons for 1 week in basal media containing: (CS-FBS) (10%), insulin (5 mg/ml) (Sigma), holo-transferrin (100 mg/mL) (Sigma), rhNGF (25 ng/mL) (Peprotech) (Sigma), Selenium (25 ng/mL) (Sigma), 25 ng/ml thyroxine (Sigma), progesterone (30 ng/ml) (Sigma), triiodothyronine (25 ng/mL) (Sigma) and putrescine 8 mg/mL (Sigma) in DMEM/F12 media (Gibco, Life Technologies). From this point on, cultures were maintained in 'myelination medium' containing: 5% CS-FBS, ascorbic acid (25 μg/mL), phenol-free matrigel (1:300) (Corning) and hrNGF (25 ng/mL) in 'complete' neurobasal medium. Myelinating cultures were matured for at least 4 weeks before use in subsequent experiments.

Appendix A.7. Myelinated Co-Culture Immunreactivity Screening

Sera or IgG eluates were diluted in neurobasal 'complete' media (including 1% BSA and human NGF, 50 ng/mL), added to myelinated co-cultures either in a 96 well plate (100 μL/well) or coverslips in a 24 well plate (300 μL/well) format and incubated for 1h at 37 °C. Serum containing antibodies to known antigens, as well as normal human serum, were run as positive and negative controls, respectively. For 96-well plate screening, serum samples were blinded by an independent investigator. Cultures were then washed 4x with pre-warmed PBS and fixed with 2% PFA in PBS for 30 min at RT. Wells were washed with PBS followed by DMEM plus HEPES (20 mM). Cultures were then labelled with Alex488-conjugated goat anti-human IgG (H+L) (A11013, Life Technologies) secondary antibody (1:750) in DMEM/HEPES plus 1% BSA, 1h at RT followed by washing 2x with DMEM/HEPES and 3x PBS. Cultures were then permeabilised with ice cold methanol (45 min on ice), blocked with 5% normal goat serum and incubated with chicken anti-neurofilament (NF)200 (1:10,000) (ab4680, Abcam) and rat anti-myelin basic protein (MBP) (1:500) (ab7349, Abcam) primary antibodies overnight at 4 °C. After washing in PBS antibodies were labelled with goat anti-chicken biotin (1:500) (BA-9010, Vector Laboratories) and goat anti-rat Alexa 546 (1:1000) (A11081, Life Technologies) secondary antibodies for 1h at RT, followed by streptavidin pacific blue (1:500) (S11222, Life Technologies) 45–60 min at RT. After washing in PBS coverslips were mounted onto glass slides (SuperFrost, ThermoScientific) with Vectorshield (H1000, Vector Laboratories) and stored at −20 °C prior to imaging. 96-well plates were flooded with PBS containing 0.02% NaN$_3$ and sealed with plate-sealing film. Plates were stored at 4 °C until imaging. Confocal images were acquired with a x63 oil-immersion lens (1024 × 1024 resolution) and exported as maximum intensity projection of 4–5 × 1 μm interval z-section images. Plates were allowed to reach room temperature before imaging.

Neurological Disorders: Advances in Medical Technology and Clinical Practice

Appendix B. Baseline Clinical Features of IA Cohorts and Clinical Vignettes of Patients with IgG Deposition in Co-Cultures

Table A1. Baseline characteristics and response to IA treatment of the CIDP cohort.

ID	Age	Sex	Disease Duration (mo)	Steroids Yes/No	IVIg Yes/No	Other Immunosuppression Used [1]	IA Cycles	CIDP-Score Baseline	CIDP Score at 2 Weeks	Progression before IA	Progression after IA
01*	59	M	83	Y	Y		1	296	298		
02*	61	M	114	Y	Y	AZA	3	376	416	2.9	0
03*	58	M	158	Y	N	AZA, CPM, MPM	9	102	118	4.1	0.1
04*	65	M	114	Y	N		1	434	438		
05*	67	F	112	Y	Y		1	435	435		
06*	60	M	104	Y	Y		1	268	313		
07*	80	M	66	Y	N	AZA	3	306	342	19.3	0.8
08*	62	M	73	N	Y		5	231	361	13.1	0.7
09*	68	M	67	Y	Y		4	373	364	6.7	0
10*	75	M	134	Y	Y		1	326	326		
11*	66	M	166	Y	Y	AZA, MTX	1	308	316		
12*	72	M	65	N	Y		3	314	330	8.7	2.0
13*	66	F	64	Y	N		1	314	282		
14*	60	M	102	Y	N		2	297	382	3.0	0
15*	66	F	86	Y	Y		1	393	405		
16*	68	M	62	Y	Y	MPM	1	264	264		
17	67	M	65	Y	N		3	N/A	N/A	N/A	N/A
18	53	M	97	Y	Y		1	N/A	N/A	N/A	N/A
19	67	F	94	Y	Y	AZA	2	N/A	N/A	N/A	N/A
20	67	M	201	Y	Y		1	N/A	N/A	N/A	N/A

* These patients were included in a previous publication [33]. [1] AZA=azathioprine, CPM=cyclophosphamide, MPM=mycophenolate-mofetil, MTX=methotrexate.

Table A2. Baseline characteristics and response to IA treatment of the GBS cohort.

ID	Age	Sex	1st/2nd/3rd-Line	PLEx Yes/No	IVIg Yes/No	PLEx / IA Cycles	Clinical Outcome
01	76	F	2	N	Y	1	0
02	73	M	3	Y	Y	2	(+)
03	36	F	2	N	Y	1	(+)
04	76	M	2	N	Y	2	++
05	64	M	2	N	Y	1	0
06	31	F	1	N	N	1	++
07	52	M	1	Y	N	1	+
08	33	F	1	N	N	1	0
09	53	F	2	N	Y	1	+
10	38	F	2	N	Y	1	++
11	89	M	2	N	Y	1	+
12	75	M	PLEx (1)	Y	N	1	+
13	66	F	PLEx (1)	Y	Y	1	0
14	66	F	PLEx (1)	Y	N	1	++
15	42	M	PLEx (1)	Y	N	1	+
16	77	F	PLEx (1)	Y	N	1	+
17	67	M	2	N	Y	1	++
18	77	M	PLEx (2)	Y	Y	1	(+)
19	62	M	PLEx (1)	Y	N	1	+
20	66	F	2	N	Y	1	+

Outcome: 0 no response; (+) equivocal response; + partial response; ++ good response.

Table A3. Baseline characteristics and response to IA treatment of the MS cohort.

ID	Age	Sex	Diagnosis	DMT	Symptoms	MP	IA Cycles	EDSS before IA	EDSS after IA
01	44	F	CIS	none	ON	5x1g iv 5x2g iv	1	2.0	0.0
02	21	M	MS	none	Sensory deficits UE+LE	5x1g iv	1	4.0	3.0
03	48	M	MS	none	Sensory deficits UE+LE	5x1g iv	1	4.0	3.0
04	18	F	CIS	none	ON	7x1g iv	1	1.0	1.0
05	30	F	MS	dimethyl fumarate	Sensory deficits UE	2x5x1g iv 2x5x1g it	1	1.0	1.0
06	46	F	MS	none	Sensory deficits UE+LE, gait ataxia	5x1g iv	1	6.5	6.5
07	28	F	MS	dimethyl fumarate	Sensomotoric deficits UE+LE	5x1g iv	1	6.5	6.5
08	26	F	MS	dimethyl fumarate	Sensory deficits UE	4x1g iv	1	3.0	3.0
09	19	M	MS	none	Organic psycho syndrome	5x1g iv	2	5.5	3.0
10	20	F	MS	none	ON	5x1g iv	1	2.0	1.0
11	47	F	MS	fingolimod	Motor deficits UE+LE	5x1g iv	1	7.0	6.0
12	19	F	MS	none	ON (bilateral), hemihypesthesia	5x1g iv	1	2.5	2.5
13	49	F	MS	fingolimod	ON, paraparesis	5x1g iv	1	4.5	4.5
14	23	F	CIS	none	ON	5x1g iv	1	2.0	1.0
15	50	F	MS	none	ON (bilateral), gait ataxia	5x1g iv 5x2g iv	1	5.0	4.0
16	15	M	MS	none	Dysarthria, dysphagia	12x1g iv	1	4.0	3.0
17	17	F	CIS	none	ON	5x1g iv	1	1.0	1.0
18	46	F	MS	interferon beta 1a	Sensory deficits UE+LE, gait ataxia	5x1g iv	1	3.5	3.0
19	57	F	MS	none	Paraparesis, hemihypesthesia	5x1g iv	1	4.0	4.0
20	37	M	MS	none	Paresis LE	5x1g iv 5x2g iv	1	6.0	5.5

MS—Multiple Sclerosis; CIS—Clinically Isolated Syndrome; ON—optic neuritis; UE—upper extremities; LE—lower extremities; MP—methyl prednisolone; DMT—actual disease-modifying treatment; EDSS—Expanded Disability Status Scale.

Appendix B.1. CIDP (Patient 11)

This 66-year-old male first developed sensory deficits, myalgia, and gait disturbance in 2007, followed in 2009 by asymmetric distal weakness in the legs then arms, and after 3 years, worsening neuropathic pain and trigeminal nerve dysfunction. Routine bloods, serum protein electrophoresis with immunofixation, and an extensive autoantibody screen revealed no abnormalities. Neve conduction studies showed a demyelinating, sensory-motor neuropathy (reduced nerve conduction velocities, prolonged motor distal latencies, prolonged F-wave latencies, and temporal dispersion in multiple nerves), meeting the EFNS criteria for definite CIDP. EMG showed no evidence of myopathy. First line treatment with high dose then tapering corticosteroids was initiated in 2007. This produced some improvement in myalgia but no other benefit and was stopped after a few weeks due to unacceptable side effects (multiple infections). Further progression in 2009 led to the use of IVIg and the introduction of azathioprine, which was again stopped after a few weeks due to adverse reactions. High-dose, pulsed, corticosteroids were again used in 2011, and methotrexate was also introduced. The clinical picture stabilised but these therapies could not be continued due to recurrent urosepsis. The patient then received 1 cycle (5 treatment sessions and 12 plasma volumes in total) of IA in 2015 without further improvement in his clinical picture after 2 weeks.

Appendix B.2. GBS (Patient 07)

This 52-year-old male presented in 2017 with neuropathic pain, limb-weakness, and facio-bulbar cranial nerve dysfunction. There was a rapid worsening over the next few days to complete tetraplegia, with autonomic involvement (bradycardia) and respiratory insufficiency, necessitating transfer to intensive care for ventilatory support. Nerve conduction studies showed a demyelinating, sensory-motor neuropathy. The CSF protein was elevated at 1.2 g/L, as was the CSF white cell count at 19 per mm^3. The white cells were classified as activated lymphocytes and monocytes. No infectious organisms were identified in the CSF despite extensive testing. A subsequent serological HIV test was positive, initially showing 376000 HIV RNA copies per ml. This confirmed a new diagnosis of HIV infection, and raises the possibility that this gentleman's GBS was associated with HIV seroconversion. However, in the absence of serial serological testing, we cannot confirm this unequivocally. The CD4/CD8 ratio was 0.34 (reduced). Standard IVIg treatment did not produce any immediate improvement. Antiretroviral therapy was commenced with an associated decline in viral load over the next few weeks, reducing HIV RNA copies to 100/ml. IA therapy had to be delayed multiple times due to recurrent infections and other complications. It was finally started about 6 weeks after onset of symptoms. Following 5 days of IA, there was a slow improvement in strength over the next 14 days, with a limited return of movement in the arms and legs. After a subsequent cycle of plasma exchange, this slow improvement continued. The patient was transferred to an early rehabilitation clinic about 3 months after onset of symptoms.

Appendix B.3. MS (Patient 13)

This 37-year-old male was diagnosed with highly active multiple sclerosis in 1998. This followed a relapsing-remitting course, with an accumulation of residual deficits producing a persistent spastic tetraparesis. Brain and spinal MRI were performed, showing multiple supra- and infratentorial, as well as spinal T2-hyperintense lesions with Gadolinum-enhancement in the cervical cord. Aquaporin-4- and MOG- antibodies were negative. The patient had previously received multiple disease modifying therapies, including beta-interferon, natalizumab, and currently fingolimod, but continued to experience relapses in the last year. A 2015 relapse with left sided optic neuritis was treated with high-dose prednisolone. This was associated with partial improvement and was followed with 5 days of IA. Further outcome data is not available.

References

1. Rinaldi, S.; Bennett, D.L. Pathogenic mechanisms in inflammatory and paraproteinaemic peripheral neuropathies. *Curr. Opin. Neurol.* **2014**, *27*, 541–551. [CrossRef] [PubMed]
2. Willison, H.J. The immunobiology of Guillain-Barre syndromes. *J. Peripher. Nerv. Syst.* **2005**, *10*, 94–112. [CrossRef] [PubMed]
3. Fehmi, J.; Scherer, S.S.; Willison, H.J.; Rinaldi, S. Nodes, paranodes and neuropathies. *J. Neurol. Neurosurg. Psychiatry* **2017**, *89*, 61–71. [CrossRef] [PubMed]
4. Chevret, S.; Hughes, R.A.; Annane, D. Plasma exchange for Guillain-Barré syndrome. *Cochrane Database Syst. Rev.* **2017**, *2017*, CD001798. [CrossRef]
5. Mehndiratta, M.M.; Hughes, R.A.C.; Pritchard, J. Plasma exchange for chronic inflammatory demyelinating polyradiculoneuropathy. *Cochrane Database Syst. Rev.* **2015**, *2015*, CD003906. [CrossRef]
6. Eftimov, F.; Winer, J.B.; Vermeulen, M.; De Haan, R.; Van Schaik, I.N. Intravenous immunoglobulin for chronic inflammatory demyelinating polyradiculoneuropathy. *Cochrane Database Syst. Rev.* **2013**, CD001797. [CrossRef]
7. Hughes, R.A.C.; Raphaël, J.C.; Swan, A.V.; A Doorn, P. Intravenous immunoglobulin for Guillain-Barré syndrome. *Cochrane Database Syst. Rev.* **2004**, CD002063. [CrossRef]
8. Lieker, I.; Slowinski, T.; Harms, L.; Hahn, K.; Klehmet, J. A prospective study comparing tryptophan immunoadsorption with therapeutic plasma exchange for the treatment of chronic inflammatory demyelinating polyneuropathy. *J. Clin. Apher.* **2017**, *32*, 486–493. [CrossRef]
9. Zinman, L.; Sutton, D.; Ng, E.; Nwe, P.; Ngo, M.; Bril, V. A pilot study to compare the use of the Excorim staphylococcal protein immunoadsorption system and IVIG in chronic inflammatory demyelinating polyneuropathy. *Transfus. Apher. Sci.* **2005**, *33*, 317–324. [CrossRef]
10. Hadden, R.D.M.; Bensa, S.; Lunn, M.; Hughes, R. Immunoadsorption inferior to plasma exchange in a patient with chronic inflammatory demyelinating polyradiculoneuropathy. *J. Neurol. Neurosurg. Psychiatry* **2002**, *72*, 644–646. [CrossRef]
11. Ullrich, H.; Mansouri-Taleghani, B.; Lackner, K.J.; Schalke, B.; Bogdahn, U.; Schmitz, G. Chronic inflammatory demyelinating polyradiculoneuropathy: Superiority of protein A immunoadsorption over plasma exchange treatment. *Transfus. Sci.* **1998**, *19*, 33–38. [CrossRef]
12. Galldiks, N.; Burghaus, L.; Dohmen, C.; Teschner, S.; Pollok, M.; Leebmann, J.; Frischmuth, N.; Höllinger, P.; Nazli, N.; Fassbender, C.; et al. Immunoadsorption in Patients with Chronic Inflammatory Demyelinating Polyradiculoneuropathy with Unsatisfactory Response to First-Line Treatment. *Eur. Neurol.* **2011**, *66*, 183–189. [CrossRef] [PubMed]
13. Yamawaki, T.; Suzuki, N. Can immunoadsorption plasmapheresis be used as the first choice therapy for neuroimmunological disorders? *Ther. Apher.* **1997**, *1*, 348–352. [CrossRef] [PubMed]
14. Pernat, A.M.; Svigelj, V.; Ponikvar, R.; Buturović-Ponikvar, J. Guillain-Barré Syndrome Treated by Membrane Plasma Exchange and/or Immunoadsorption. *Ther. Apher. Dial.* **2009**, *13*, 310–313. [CrossRef]
15. Arakawa, H.; Yuhara, Y.; Todokoro, M.; Kato, M.; Mochizuki, H.; Tokuyama, K.; Kunimoto, F.; Morikawa, A. Immunoadsorption therapy for a child with Guillain-Barre syndrome subsequent to Mycoplasma infection: A case study. *Brain Dev.* **2005**, *27*, 431–433. [CrossRef]
16. Okamiya, S.; Ogino, M.; Ogino, Y.; Irie, S.; Kanazawa, N.; Saito, T.; Sakai, F. Tryptophan-immobilized Column-based Immunoadsorption as the Choice Method for Plasmapheresis in Guillain-Barre Syndrome. *Ther. Apher. Dial.* **2004**, *8*, 248–253. [CrossRef]
17. Haupt, W.; Rosenow, F.; Van Der Ven, C.; Birkmann, C. Immunoadsorption in Guillain-Barré syndrome and myasthenia gravis. *Ther. Apher.* **2000**, *4*, 195–197. [CrossRef]
18. Uetakagaito, M.; Horikawa, H.; Yoshinaka, H.; Tagawa, Y.; Yuki, N. Two Patients with Acute Guillain-Barré Syndrome Treated with Different Apheresis Methods. *Ther. Apher.* **1997**, *1*, 340–342. [CrossRef]
19. Hirai, K.; Kihara, M.; Nakajima, F.; Miyanomae, Y.; Yoshioka, H. Immunoadsorption Therapy in Guillain-Barre Syndrome. *Pediatric Neurol.* **1998**, *19*, 55–57. [CrossRef]
20. Chida, K.; Takase, S.; Itoyama, Y. Development of facial palsy during immunoadsorption plasmapheresis in Miller Fisher syndrome: A clinical report of two cases. *J. Neurol. Neurosurg. Psychiatry* **1998**, *64*, 399–401. [CrossRef]

21. Ruiz, J.C.; Berciano, J.; Polo, J.M.; De Francisco, A.L.M.; Arias, M. Treatment of Guillain-Barré syndrome with protein-A immunoadsorption: Report of two cases. *Ann. Neurol.* **1992**, *31*, 574–575. [CrossRef] [PubMed]

22. Takei, H.; Komaba, Y.; Araki, T.; Iino, Y.; Katayama, Y. Plasma Immunoadsorption Therapy for Guillain-Barré Syndrome: Critical Day for Initiation. *J. Nippon. Med. Sch.* **2002**, *69*, 557–563. [CrossRef] [PubMed]

23. Mahdi-Rogers, M.; Brassington, R.; A Gunn, A.; A Van Doorn, P.; Hughes, R.A. Immunomodulatory treatment other than corticosteroids, immunoglobulin and plasma exchange for chronic inflammatory demyelinating polyradiculoneuropathy. *Cochrane Database Syst. Rev.* **2017**, *2017*, CD003280. [CrossRef] [PubMed]

24. Rolfes, L.; Pfeuffer, S.; Ruck, T.; Melzer, N.; Pawlitzki, M.; Heming, M.; Brand, M.; Wiendl, H.; Meuth, S. Ruck Therapeutic Apheresis in Acute Relapsing Multiple Sclerosis: Current Evidence and Unmet Needs—A Systematic Review. *J. Clin. Med.* **2019**, *8*, 1623. [CrossRef] [PubMed]

25. Lipphardt, M.; Wallbach, M.; Koziolek, M.J. Plasma Exchange or Immunoadsorption in Demyelinating Diseases: A Meta-Analysis. *J. Clin. Med.* **2020**, *9*, 1597. [CrossRef]

26. Willison, H.J.; Yuki, N. Peripheral neuropathies and anti-glycolipid antibodies. *Brain* **2002**, *125*, 2591–2625. [CrossRef]

27. Tagawa, Y.; Yuki, N.; Hirata, K. Ability to remove immunoglobulins and anti-ganglioside antibodies by plasma exchange, double-filtration plasmapheresis and immunoadsorption. *J. Neurol. Sci.* **1998**, *157*, 90–95. [CrossRef]

28. Ng, J.K.M.; Malotka, J.; Kawakami, N.; Derfuss, T.; Khademi, M.; Olsson, T.; Linington, C.; Odaka, M.; Tackenberg, B.; Prüss, H.; et al. Neurofascin as a target for autoantibodies in peripheral neuropathies. *Neurology* **2012**, *79*, 2241–2248. [CrossRef]

29. Querol, L.; Nogales-Gadea, G.; Rojas-García, R.; Martinez-Hernandez, E.; Diaz-Manera, J.; Suárez-Calvet, X.; Navas, M.; Araque, J.; Gallardo, E.; Illa, I. Antibodies to contactin-1 in chronic inflammatory demyelinating polyneuropathy. *Ann. Neurol.* **2012**, *73*, 370–380. [CrossRef]

30. Querol, L.; Nogales-Gadea, G.; Rojas-Garcia, R.; Diaz-Manera, J.; Pardo, J.; Ortega-Moreno, A.; Sedano, M.J.; Gallardo, E.; Berciano, J.; Blesa, R.; et al. Neurofascin IgG4 antibodies in CIDP associate with disabling tremor and poor response to IVIg. *Neurology* **2014**, *82*, 879–886. [CrossRef]

31. Doppler, K.; Appeltshauser, L.; Villmann, C.; Martin, C.; Peles, E.; Krämer, H.H.; Haarmann, A.; Buttmann, M.; Sommer, C. Auto-antibodies to contactin-associated protein 1 (Caspr) in two patients with painful inflammatory neuropathy. *Brain* **2016**, *139*, 2617–2630. [CrossRef]

32. Delmont, E.; Manso, C.; Querol, L.; Cortese, A.; Berardinelli, A.; Lozza, A.; Belghazi, M.; Malissart, P.; Labauge, P.; Taieb, G.; et al. Autoantibodies to nodal isoforms of neurofascin in chronic inflammatory demyelinating polyneuropathy. *Brain* **2017**, *140*, 1851–1858. [CrossRef] [PubMed]

33. Dorst, J.; Ludolph, A.C.; Senel, M.; Tumani, H. Short-term and long-term effects of immunoadsorption in refractory chronic inflammatory demyelinating polyneuropathy: A prospective study in 17 patients. *J. Neurol.* **2018**, *265*, 2906–2915. [CrossRef] [PubMed]

34. Kuwahara, M.; Suzuki, H.; Oka, N.; Ogata, H.; Yanagimoto, S.; Sadakane, S.; Fukumoto, Y.; Yamana, M.; Yuhara, Y.; Yoshikawa, K.; et al. ELectron microscopic abnormality and therapeutic efficacy in chronic inflammatory demyelinating polyneuropathy with anti-neurofascin155 immunoglobulin G4 antibody. *Muscle Nerve* **2017**, *57*, 498–502. [CrossRef] [PubMed]

35. Süfke, S.; Lehnert, H.; Gebauer, F.; Uhlenbusch-Körwer, I. Safety Aspects of Immunoadsorption in IgG Removal Using a Single-Use, Multiple-pass Protein A Immunoadsorber (LIGASORB): Clinical Investigation in Healthy Volunteers. *Ther. Apher. Dial.* **2017**, *21*, 405–413. [CrossRef] [PubMed]

36. Chida, K.; Watanabe, S.; Okita, N.; Takase, S.; Tagawa, Y.; Yuki, N. Immunoadsorption therapy for Fisher's syndrome: Analysis of the recovery process of external ophthalmoplegia and the removal ability of anti-GQ1b antibodies. *Rinsho Shinkeigaku* **1996**, *36*, 551–556.

37. Belak, M.; Borberg, H.; Jimenez, C.; Oette, K. Technical and clinical experience with Protein A Immunoadsorption columns. *Transfus. Sci.* **1994**, *15*, 419–422. [CrossRef]

38. Merkies, I.S.; Schmitz, P.I.M.; A Van Der Meché, F.G.; Samijn, J.; A Van Doorn, P. Clinimetric evaluation of a new overall disability scale in immune mediated polyneuropathies. *J. Neurol. Neurosurg. Psychiatry* **2002**, *72*, 596–601. [CrossRef]

39. Thompson, A.J.; Banwell, B.L.; Barkhof, F.; Carroll, W.M.; Coetzee, T.; Comi, G.; Correale, J.; Fazekas, F.; Filippi, M.; Freedman, M.S.; et al. Diagnosis of multiple sclerosis: 2017 revisions of the McDonald criteria. *Lancet Neurol.* **2017**, *17*, 162–173. [CrossRef]

40.   Teunissen, C.E.; Petzold, A.; Bennett, J.L.; Berven, F.S.; Brundin, L.; Comabella, M.; Franciotta, D.; Frederiksen, J.L.; Fleming, J.O.; Furlan, R.; et al. A consensus protocol for the standardization of cerebrospinal fluid collection and biobanking. *Neurology* **2009**, *73*, 1914–1922. [CrossRef]

41.   Pns, J.T.F.O.T.E.A.T.; Efns, J.T.F.O.T.; Pns, T. European Federation of Neurological Societies/Peripheral Nerve Society Guideline on management of chronic inflammatory demyelinating polyradiculoneuropathy: Report of a joint task force of the European Federation of Neurological Societies and the Peripheral Nerve Society-First Revision. *J. Peripher. Nerv. Syst.* **2010**, *15*, 1–9. [CrossRef]

42.   Querol, L.; Rojas-García, R.; Diaz-Manera, J.; Barcena, J.; Pardo, J.; Ortega-Moreno, A.; Sedano, M.J.; Seró-Ballesteros, L.; Carvajal, A.; Ortiz-Castellon, N.; et al. Rituximab in treatment-resistant CIDP with antibodies against paranodal proteins. *Neurol. Neuroimmunol. Neuroinflammation* **2015**, *2*, e149. [CrossRef] [PubMed]

43.   Demichelis, C.; Franciotta, D.; Cortese, A.; Callegari, I.; Serrati, C.; Mancardi, G.L.; Schenone, A.; Leonardi, A.; Benedetti, L. Remarkable Rituximab Response on Tremor Related to Acute-Onset Chronic Inflammatory Demyelinating Polyradiculoneuropathy in an Antineurofascin155 Immunoglobulin G4-Seropositive Patient. *Mov. Disord. Clin. Pr.* **2018**, *5*, 559–560. [CrossRef] [PubMed]

44.   Cortese, A.; Lombardi, R.; Briani, C.; Callegari, I.; Benedetti, L.; Manganelli, F.; Luigetti, M.; Ferrari, S.; Clerici, A.M.; Marfia, G.A.; et al. Antibodies to neurofascin, contactin-1, and contactin-associated protein 1 in CIDP: Clinical relevance of IgG isotype. *Neurol. Neuroimmunol. Neuroinflammation* **2019**, *7*, e639. [CrossRef]

45.   Stich, O.; Perera, S.; Berger, B.; Jarius, S.; Wildemann, B.; Baumgartner, A.; Rauer, S. Prevalence of neurofascin-155 antibodies in patients with multiple sclerosis. *J. Neurol. Sci.* **2016**, *364*, 29–32. [CrossRef] [PubMed]

46.   Häusser-Kinzel, S.; Weber, M.S. The Role of B Cells and Antibodies in Multiple Sclerosis, Neuromyelitis Optica, and Related Disorders. *Front. Immunol.* **2019**, *10*, 201. [CrossRef] [PubMed]

47.   Prineas, J.W.; Parratt, J.D. Multiple sclerosis: Serum anti-CNS autoantibodies. *Mult. Scler. J.* **2017**, *24*, 610–622. [CrossRef]

48.   Willison, H.J.; Veitch, J.; Swan, A.V.; Baumann, N.; Comi, G.; Gregson, N.A.; Iiia, I.; Jacobs, B.C.; Zielasek, J.; Hughes, R.A.C. Inter-laboratory validation of an ELISA for the determination of serum anti-ganglioside antibodies. *Eur. J. Neurol.* **1999**, *6*, 71–77. [CrossRef]

49.   Clark, A.; Kaller, M.; Galino, J.; Willison, H.J.; Rinaldi, S.; Bennett, D.L. Co-cultures with stem cell-derived human sensory neurons reveal regulators of peripheral myelination. *Brain* **2017**, *140*, 898–913. [CrossRef]

Functional Evaluation Using Inertial Measurement of Back School Therapy in Lower Back Pain

Claudia Celletti [1], **Roberta Mollica** [1], **Cristina Ferrario** [2,3], **Manuela Galli** [3] and **Filippo Camerota** [1,*]

[1]   Physical Medicine and Rehabilitation, Umberto I University Hospital, 00161 Rome, Italy; clacelletti@gmail.com (C.C.); roberta.mollica@uniroma1.it (R.M.)

[2]   Department of Mechanic, Politecnico di Milano, 20124 Milan, Italy; cristina.ferrario@polimi.it

[3]   Department of Electronics, Information and Bioengineering (DEIB) Politecnico di Milano, 20133 Milan, Italy; manuela.galli@polimi.it

*   Correspondence: filippo.camerota@uniroma1.it

Abstract: Lower back pain is an extremely common health problem and globally causes more disability than any other condition. Among other rehabilitation approaches, back schools are interventions comprising both an educational component and exercises. Normally, the main outcome evaluated is pain reduction. The aim of this study was to evaluate not only the efficacy of back school therapy in reducing pain, but also the functional improvement. Patients with lower back pain were clinically and functionally evaluated; in particular, the timed "up and go" test with inertial movement sensor was studied before and after back school therapy. Forty-four patients completed the program, and the results showed not only a reduction of pain, but also an improvement in several parameters of the timed up and go test, especially in temporal parameters (namely duration and velocity). The application of the inertial sensor measurement in evaluating functional aspects seems to be useful and promising in assessing the aspects that are not strictly correlated to the specific pathology, as well as in rehabilitation management.

Keywords: back school; inertial sensor; lower back pain; rehabilitation; stability; timed up and go test

1. Introduction

Lower back Pain (LBP) is a well described and extremely widespread health problem [1]. LBP is a pain that goes from the twelfth rib to the lower gluteal folds; pain can also spread to the lower limbs for one day or more [1]. This condition is the main cause of absence from work and activity limitations in much of the world. The consequence is a heavy economic burden for subjects, families, communities, industry, and governments [2]. Of the 291 conditions studied in the 2010 Global Burden of Disease (GBD) report, LBP had the highest load. LBP is the leading cause of disability globally [3].

The main components to treat this condition are education, reassurance, analgesic drugs, and non-pharmacological therapies. During the treatment, periodic check-ups are recommended based on individual patient needs, such as prognosis, treatment prescribed, and remaining concerns about serious pathological abnormality [4].

Chronic LBP is defined as lower back pain that lasts for over 12 weeks. Generally, one-third of the patients with LBP reported that in the year after an acute episode, lower back pain was of moderate intensity [2]. In patients with chronic back pain, a multidisciplinary approach leads to better results when combined with medical, rehabilitative, and psychological treatments [5].

Among other rehabilitation approaches, back schools (BS) are interventions that comprise an education component and exercises. BS are training programs with lessons given by a therapist to patients or workers, with the aim of treating or preventing lower back pain [6]. Several studies have demonstrated the efficacy of BS in reducing and managing lower back pain [7]. BS, due to the validity of their educational exercises, enhance the quality of life, reduce disability induced by LBP [8,9], and also improve mental well-being.

The aim of this study is to evaluate not only the efficacy of BS therapy in reducing pain but also in functional improvement, an aspect strictly related to pain but normally not evaluated in the studies that focus on assessing pain relief. A new and simple gait evaluation method is used to make the analysis. In particular, stability and ability to perform functional tests, such as the timed "up and go" test, are evaluated in order to verify if a rehabilitation program based on BS therapy is able to improve stability and walking.

2. Materials and Methods

Patients were recruited from the Rehabilitation Ambulatory Service of Umberto I University Hospital. All participants signed informed consent forms after receiving detailed information about the study's aims and procedures for the Declaration of Helsinki.

2.1. Eligibility Criteria

Patients were included in the study if they had lower back pain that had lasted for more than six weeks that was associated with limitations of motion. The presence of vertebral infections; tumoral metastasis; fractures and neoplasm; rheumatological, neurological, or oncological disease; previous back surgery; severe cognitive impairments; or pregnancy was considered an exclusion criterion.

2.2. Intervention

The BS program was supervised by a multidisciplinary professional team. A total of 10 one-hour sessions scheduled 3 times a week were carried out. The adopted rehabilitation program was chosen by considering the effectiveness of the BS on LBP reported in previous studies. The details of the program followed in this study are described below.

The first treatment session was used to provide subjects with basic anatomical knowledge of the spine and its functions; the correct ergonomic positions to be maintained in everyday life were also shown. During the following 9 sessions, the physiotherapists supervised the activities, which consisted of exercises based on diaphragmatic breathing (10 min), self-stretching of the trunk muscles (10 min), strengthening of erector muscles of the spine, abdominal strengthening, and postural exercises. The tasks were divided into 3 sets of 10 repetitions for each one; 3 min of rest was provided between each series. Explanations of the ergonomic position of the spine and how to introduce self-correction in daily life were provided for the whole duration of the treatment.

2.3. Health State: Clinical Evaluations

Patients were evaluated before and after physiotherapy treatment with the following clinical scales:

1. The *numeric rating scale* (NRS) is a rapidly administered 11-point numeric scale used to roughly measure any kind of pain, with a score ranging from 0 (no pain) to 10 (acute pain) [10];
2. The *Oswestry disability index* (ODI), also known as the Oswestry lower back pain disability questionnaire, is considered the "gold standard" of lower back functional outcome tools and consists of 10 sections, with a score varying from 0 to 5 for each one. A low score indicates minimal disability; the disability is more severe for higher scores [11];
3. The *performance-oriented mobility assessment* (POMA) scale was developed by Tinetti in 1986 to assess the mobility and risk of falling of the elderly [12]. This scale was chosen because it is very reliable and widely used. In this study, we used the balance scale of the POMA, which evaluates the positions and changes in position of the subject, assessing stability tasks. Each item is scored on a two- or three-point scale, where the maximum is 18 [13];

4.   The *timed up and go test* (TUG) is a clinical test that evaluates the balance and mobility of a subject [14,15]. In the traditional TUG test, a stopwatch is used to measure how long it takes a subject to lift off a chair, walk 3 m, turn 180°, return to the chair, and sit back down.

2.4. Biomechanical Evaluation

Instrumentation

In this study, we evaluated the TUG as both a time test and also using an inertial measurement unit (IMU). The commercial name of the device used is a G-Sensor instrument (BTS SpA, Milan, Italy). The communication with the receiving unit (personal computer) takes place via a Bluetooth connection. The associated software (BTS® G-Studio) is used to acquire, process, and archive data. In the IMU there is a triaxial accelerometer (16 bits/axes, up to 1000 Hz) with different sensitivities (±2, ±4, ±8, ±16 g), a triaxial 16-bit magnetometer (±1200 μT, up to 100 Hz), and a triaxial gyroscope (16 bits/axes, up to 8000 Hz) with multiple sensitivities (±250, ±500, ±1000, ±2000°/s). The G-Sensor is positioned at level L5 using an elastic belt. It is important to keep the power connector facing upwards and the logo outwards to correctly define the reference system (Figure 1a)

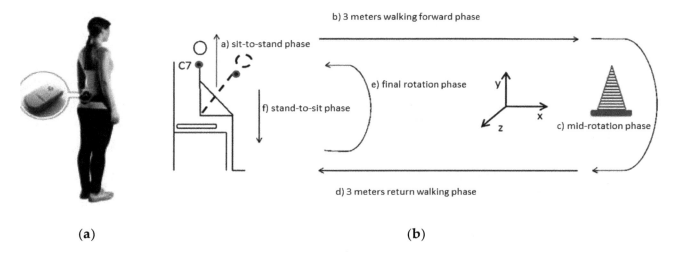

(a)   (b)

Figure 1. (a) Inertial measurement unit (IMU) position and (b) timed up and go test (TUG) phases.

The test begins with patients seated in a standard chair with their arms on either side of their body. After a signal from the clinician, the subject rises from the chair, walks three meters in a straight line at a speed that is normal for them, turns around an obstacle, and finally returns to the chair and sits down. The software used is BTS G-Studio, which has a specific protocol capable of analyzing the TUG test and automatically generates a TUG report with temporal parameters identifying the duration of the different sub-phases [16]. The mathematical method used to identify each sub-phase is the one described in the study by Salarian et al. [17]. Additionally, a detailed description of the practical operation of BTS G-Studio in iTUG analysis, as compared with an optoelectronic system, is provided in the study by Negrini [18].The test can, therefore, be divided into different phases: the first is that of rising from the chair (sit-to-stand sub-phase), walking for 3 m until reaching an obstacle (walking forward sub-phase), turning around the cone (mid-turning sub-phase), walking three m back towards the chair (return walking sub-phase), and then turning and sitting down on the chair (stand-to-sit sub-phase) without using the assistance of their arms, if possible. The test is concluded when the subject is seated again. The final report of the TUG test shows all the spatiotemporal parameters related to the walk for each sub-phase considered: the sit-to-stand, the steady-state gait, the turning, and the turn-to-sit phases [17]. The parameters supplied automatically by the IMU for each trial are: total time duration, sub-phase durations, mean velocity turning (mid-turning and final turning sub-phases), and the maximum trunk flexion angle and its range of motion during sit-to-stand and stand-to-sit sub-phases (Figure 1b).

Furthermore, an instrumental evaluation of stability was carried out using a baropodometric platform (P-Walk BTS Engineering). The stabilometry test measures the oscillations by evaluating the elliptical area containing 95% of sway points, velocities with closed eyes (CE) and opened eyes (OE), and the length of the excursion of the center of pressure. The test we performed had a duration of 30 s, within which the position of the CoP was recorded during quiet standing [19]. Patients were adequately informed about the procedure; the requirements were to maintain a natural standing position with the arms alongside the body, the feet open at an angle of about 30°, and the heels at a distance of about 3 cm. All tests were performed by the same examiner in order to reduce the inter-operator error and to increase the reproducibility of the test; thus, the subjects were given the same information before each test. For each trial condition (EO and EC), three tests were carried out, for which the median scores are reported. Considering the EO condition, subjects were required to stare at a mark fixed at eye level on a wall 1.5 m away.

2.5. Statistical Analysis

The statistical analysis was performed with SPSS software. To verify the normality of the parameters, the Kolmogorov–Smirnov test was used. When the normality assumption was not fulfilled, the median and range (minimum–maximum) were evaluated. The differences between variables were evaluated using the Friedman test for paired samples. The probability level for statistical significance in all tests was set at a $p < 0.05$.

3. Results

Forty-eight patients (mean age 71 ± 13.66) were recruited for this study; 4 patients did not complete the rehabilitation program and were excluded from the study; a total of 44 patients (34 female and 10 male, mean age 70 ± 14.02) were evaluated before and after back school treatment.

We observed a global pain reduction in patients with LBP that attended the back-school program. This reduction was also associated with clinical improvement of stability, as shown by the POMA balance score increase. When the postural analysis data were examined, a variation was not registered when considering the opened eyes test; instead, in the closed eyes test a significant reduction of the length of CoP was registered (Table 1).

Table 1. Clinical scale and instrumental evaluation before and after back school cycle.

		T0 (Median ± s.d.)	T1 (Median ± s.d.)	p	Chi Quadro	df
	POMA Balance	12.88 ± 2.00	13.86 ± 1.92	0.000	17.19	1
	NRS	6.11 ± 1.57	4.32 ± 1.99	0.000	33	1
	ODI	30.51 ± 13.29	28.72 ± 14.91	0.60	0.273	1
Stabilometria	Area OE (mm²)	210.27 ± 1012.07	231.84 ± 1007.86	0.75	0.1	1
	Lenght OE (mm)	115.24 ± 76.58	126.28 ± 99.40	0.15	2.07	1
	Area CE (mm²)	446.73 ± 2540.10	591.74 ± 3412.65	0.42	0.64	1
	Length OE (mm)	167 ± 308.20	162.33 ± 221.95	0.02	4.9	1
TUG	Total time (s)	13.37 ± 3.86	11.25 ± 2.16	0.00	19.70	1
	Stand up (s)	1.65 ± 0.37	1.47 ± 0.29	0.02	5.15	1
	Sitting (s)	2.20 ± 0.60	1.99 ± 0.42	0.50	0.44	1
	Rotation velocity (°/s)	77.71 ± 19.80	83.23 ± 22.45	0.04	8.52	1

Legend: POMA = performance-oriented mobility assessment; NRS = numeric rating scale; ODI = Oswestry disability index; OE = opened eyes; CE = closed eyes; TUG = timed up and go; s = second.

It is interesting to notice that there was a significant reduction of the total duration of the TUG test, and also of the stand-up and sitting phases (Table 1).

The BS groups showed significant improvement in several instrumental TUG (iTUG) parameters, especially in temporal (duration and velocity) parameters.

The BS treatment significantly reduced the total duration of the task and its sub-phases: the stand-to-sit sub-phase and the sit-to-stand phase, the mean velocity of TUG, and of mid-turning and final turning sub-phases increased at a significant level.

4. Discussion

As far as we know, this is the first paper to evaluate not only the pain aspect of lower back syndrome after treatment, but also the functional aspect that is not strictly related to this pathology (i.e., timed up and go evaluation). The TUG test provided in this study is an instrumented TUG. While the TUG test taken by an expert operator using a stopwatch has excellent reliability, accuracy, and precision, this measure is subjective and operator-dependent (i.e., a less experienced clinician could affect the quality of the measure). The use of the stopwatch in the clinical setting has several limitations: (a) the identification of the start time and the end time are not easily detectable by the operator; (b) the evaluation of the TUG time requires a high level of attention by the operator, which could decrease when many trials are required; (c) the quantification of sub-phases is not possible.

The instrumented TUG analysis is of considerable interest, as it evaluates the various sub-phases of the test (chair transition, straight-ahead gait, and 180° turn); this allows a better understanding of movement strategies. Considering, for example, the 180° turn, there is a variability between subjects with different gaits and with **or** without balance impairment. A further variation is introduced for patients using an assistive device, such as a walker.

Therefore, the IMU technology implementations for the iTUG quantification of pre- and post- specific therapies have several benefits, including additional performance parameters, generation of reports, fast assessment, and that the patient does not need to be undressed. In addition to this, it is important to consider the ability for self-administration at home and in a clinical environment. This could provide more details and insights about patient performance [16]. Although other variables could have been derived using the data provided by the wearable sensor, as the purpose of this work was to analyze the TUG, which is an automatic functional clinical test, the analysis focused mainly on the evaluation of the duration of the task included in the test. It is known that lower back pain is associated with functional impairment. In particular, the opportunity to analyze the different phases of this test using an inertial measurement instrument made it possible to assert that back school therapy may improve back function, increasing the promptness to position changes and speeding up movements. The changes observed with iTUG represent the effect of the reduction of LBP on functional ability. As the patients experience pain during the movement, the biomechanical result is a slow movement and a higher TUG time. After treatment, the patients feel better, experience less pain, and can get out of the chair faster. No changes are evidenced as far as postural acquisition is concerned. In maintaining postural control, pain in the lumbar area has a minor effect in terms of functional limitation, and therefore one can expect to have no obvious variations in postural control.

5. Conclusions

In conclusion, through the quantitative evaluation of the iTUG test, it is proven that the BS could be considered a promising new rehabilitative treatment for LBP in improving motor functional limitations. Moreover, as the IMU sensor can provide data that might provide many more temporal and kinematic measures after successive elaboration, future development of this study should provide additional data for a more detailed analysis, in order to show more important changes in patients' movement patterns after the treatment.

Author Contributions: Conceptualization, C.C. and F.C.; methodology, C.C., F.C., and R.M.; formal analysis, C.C., M.G., and C.F.; investigation, C.C. and F.C.; data curation, C.C. and F.C.; writing—original draft preparation, C.C.; writing—review and editing, F.C., M.G., and C.F.; supervision, R.M. and M.G. All authors have read and agreed to the published version of the manuscript.

Acknowledgments: We thanks Daniele Scilimati and Laura Venerucci for their contributions in evaluating and treating patients.

References

1. Hoy, D.; March, L.; Brooks, P.; Blyth, F.; Woolf, A.; Bain, C.; Williams, G.; Smith, E.; Vos, T.; Barendregt, J.; et al. The global burden of lower back pain: Estimates from the Global Burden of Disease 2010 study. *Ann. Rheum. Dis.* **2014**, *73*, 968–974. [CrossRef] [PubMed]

2. Rapoport, J.; Jacobs, P.; Bell, N.N.; Klarenbach, S. Refining the measurement of the economic burden of chronic diseases in Canada. *Chronic Dis. Can.* **2014**, *25*, 13–21.

3. Hoy, D.D.; March, L.; Brooks, P.; Woolf, A.; Blyth, F.; Vos, T.; Buchbinder, R. Measuring the global burden of lower back pain. *Best Pract. Res. Clin. Rheumatol.* **2010**, *24*, 155–165. [CrossRef] [PubMed]

4. Maher, C.; Underwood, M.; Buchbinder, R. Non-specific lower back pain. *Lancet* **2017**, *389*, 736–747. [CrossRef]

5. Urits, I.; Burshtein, A.; Sharma, M.; Testa, L.; Gold, P.A.; Orhurhu, V.; Viswanath, O.; Jones, M.R.; Sidransky, M.A.; Spektor, B.; et al. Lower back Pain, a Comprehensive Review: Pathophysiology, Diagnosis, and Treatment. *Curr. Pain Headache Rep.* **2019**, *23*, 23. [CrossRef] [PubMed]

6. Airaksinen, O.; Brox, J.J.; Cedraschi, C.; Hildebrandt, J.; Klaber-Moffett, J.; Kovacs, F.; Mannion, A.F.; Reis, S.; Staal, J.B.; Ursin, H.; et al. Chapter 4. European guidelines for the management of chronic nonspecific lower back pain. *Eur. Spine J.* **2006**, *15* (Suppl. 2), S192–S300. [CrossRef] [PubMed]

7. Heymans, M.M.; van Tulder, M.M.; Esmail, R.; Bombardier, C.; Koes, B.W. Back schools for non-specific low-back pain: A systematic view within the framework of the cochrane collaboration back review group. *Spine* **2005**, *30*, 2153–2163. [CrossRef] [PubMed]

8. Paolucci, T.; Morone, G.; Iosa, M.; Fusco, A.; Alcuri, R.; Matano, A.; Bureca, I.; Saraceni, V.M.; Paolucci, S. Psychological features and outcomes of the back-school treatment in patients with chronic non-specific lower back pain. A randomized controlled study. *Eur. J. Phys. Rehabil. Med.* **2012**, *48*, 245–253. [PubMed]

9. Morone, G.; Paolucci, T.; Alcuri, M.M.; Vulpiani, M.M.; Matano, A.; Bureca, I.; Paolucci, S.; Saraceni, V.M. Quality of life improved by multidisciplinary back school program in patients with chronic non-specific lower back pain: A single blind randomized controlled trial. *Eur. J. Phys. Rehabil. Med.* **2011**, *47*, 533–541. [PubMed]

10. Deschamps, M.; Band, P.P.; Coldman, A.J. Assessment of adult cancer pain: Shortcomings of current methods. *Pain* **1988**, *32*, 133–139. [CrossRef]

11. Fairbank, J.J.; Pynsent, P.B. The Oswestry Disability Index. *Spine* **2000**, *25*, 2940–2953. [CrossRef] [PubMed]

12. Tinetti, M.E. Performance oriented assessment of mobility problems in elderly patients. *J. Am. Geriatr. Soc.* **1986**, *34*, 119–126. [CrossRef] [PubMed]

13. Faber, M.M.; Bosscher, R.R.; van Wieringen, P.C. Clinimetric properties of the performance-oriented mobility assessment. *Phys. Ther.* **2006**, *86*, 944–954. [CrossRef] [PubMed]

14. Lin, M.; Hwang, H.; Hu, M.; Wu, H.; Wang, Y.; Huang, F. Psychometric comparisons of the timed up and go, one-leg stand, functional reach, and tinetti balance measures in community-dwelling older people. *J. Am. Geriatr. Soc.* **2004**, *52*, 1343–1348. [CrossRef] [PubMed]

15. Barry, E.; Galvin, R.; Keogh, C.; Horgan, F.; Fahey, T. Is the timed up and go test a useful predictor of risk of falls in community dwelling older adults: A systematic review and meta-analysis. *BMC Geriatr.* **2014**, *14*, 14. [CrossRef] [PubMed]

16. Kleiner, A.F.R.; Pacifici, I.; Vagnini, A.; Camerota, F.; Celletti, C.; Stocchi, F.; De Pandis, M.F.; Galli, M. Timed Up and Go evaluation with wearable devices: Validation in Parkinson's disease. *J. Body Mov. Ther.* **2018**, *22*, 390–395. [CrossRef] [PubMed]

17. Salarian, A.; Horak, F.F.; Zampieri, C.; Carlson-Kuhta, P.; Nutt, J.J.; Aminian, K. iTUG, a Sensitive and Reliable Measure of Mobility IEEE Trans. *Neural Syst. Rehabil. Eng.* **2010**, *18*, 303–310. [CrossRef] [PubMed]

18. Negrini, S.; Serpelloni, M.; Amici, C.; Gobbo, M.; Silvestro, C.; Buraschi, R.; Borboni, A.; Crovato, D.; Lopomo, N.F. Use of Wearable Inertial Sensor in the Assessment of Timed-Up-and-Go Test: Influence of Device Placement on Temporal Variable Estimation. In Proceedings of the 6th International Conference on Wireless Mobile Communication and Healthcare, MobiHealth 2016, Milan, Italy, 14–16 November 2016; Springer: Berlin/Heidelberg, Germany, 2017; Volume 192, pp. 310–317.

19. Scoppa, F.; Capra, R.; Gallamini, M.; Shiffer, R. Clinical stabilometry standardization: Basic definitions–acquisition interval–sampling frequency. *Gait Posture* **2013**, *37*, 290–292. [CrossRef] [PubMed]

Selective Apheresis of C-Reactive Protein for Treatment of Indications with Elevated CRP Concentrations

Stefan Kayser [1], Patrizia Brunner [2], Katharina Althaus [3], Johannes Dorst [3] and Ahmed Sheriff [1,4,*]

1   Pentracor GmbH, 16761 Hennigsdorf, Germany; kayser@pentracor.de
2   iAdsorb GmbH, 10787 Berlin, Germany; patrizia.brunner@gmx.de
3   Department of Neurology, University of Ulm, 89081 Ulm, Germany; katharina.althaus@uni-ulm.de (K.A.);
     johannes.dorst@uni-ulm.de (J.D.)
4   Medizinische Klinik m.S. Gastroenterologie/Infektiologie/Rheumatologie, Charité Universitätsmedizin,
     12203 Berlin, Germany
*   Correspondence: ahmed.sheriff@charite.de

Abstract: Almost every kind of inflammation in the human body is accompanied by rising C-reactive protein (CRP) concentrations. This can include bacterial and viral infection, chronic inflammation and so-called sterile inflammation triggered by (internal) acute tissue injury. CRP is part of the ancient humoral immune response and secreted into the circulation by the liver upon respective stimuli. Its main immunological functions are the opsonization of biological particles (bacteria and dead or dying cells) for their clearance by macrophages and the activation of the classical complement pathway. This not only helps to eliminate pathogens and dead cells, which is very useful in any case, but unfortunately also to remove only slightly damaged or inactive human cells that may potentially regenerate with more CRP-free time. CRP action severely aggravates the extent of tissue damage during the acute phase response after an acute injury and therefore negatively affects clinical outcome. CRP is therefore a promising therapeutic target to rescue energy-deprived tissue either caused by ischemic injury (e.g., myocardial infarction and stroke) or by an overcompensating immune reaction occurring in acute inflammation (e.g., pancreatitis) or systemic inflammatory response syndrome (SIRS; e.g., after transplantation or surgery). Selective CRP apheresis can remove circulating CRP safely and efficiently. We explain the pathophysiological reasoning behind therapeutic CRP apheresis and summarize the broad span of indications in which its application could be beneficial with a focus on ischemic stroke as well as the results of this therapeutic approach after myocardial infarction.

Keywords: CRP; apheresis; stroke; inflammation

1. General Introduction

Inflammatory processes involve a plethora of signaling pathways and affect the whole body, even if their origin is most often locally restricted in an acute setting. Mounting an inflammatory response is the body's strategy to primarily eliminate any cause of tissue damage and subsequently repair the injury [1]. This is rooted in the evolutionary background that damage is mainly caused by pathogens or at least exacerbated by them within an external wound. In this case the elicited inflammation is beneficial in fighting infiltrating bacteria or viruses as well as restoring tissue homeostasis. However, healing of injured tissue often happens at the cost of still healthy tissue/cells and involves additional cell death as collateral damage [2]. In specific situations, these negative effects outweigh the positive aspects of the inflammatory reaction. Whenever an injury is "sterile", meaning it occurred internally without pathogen involvement, inflammation aggravates deterioration by elimination of additional cells, which were either vital or only slightly and reversibly impaired. This happens for example after ischemic injury like stroke or myocardial infarction, leading to a larger extent of organ damage, increased scarring and thereby worsening clinical outcome [3,4]. Likewise, negative effects dominate in situations when the immune system produces an excessive general reaction that is not justified by the trigger [5]. For example, during acute pancreatitis, a systemic inflammatory response syndrome (SIRS), or an acute bacterial or viral infection (Sepsis) the inflammation might cause widespread tissue injury, which might result in multiple organ failure [6].

Although a plentitude of proteins is involved in inflammation, many of them are cytokines or modulators that do not actively participate in the elimination of pathogens or cells [1]. Several mediator proteins play a key role.

One of the acute-phase mediators directly involved in these pro-inflammatory processes is C-reactive protein (CRP) which was discovered by Tillett and Francis in 1930 [7]. CRP is well-established as one of the most reliable markers of inflammation, rising dramatically during any type of inflammation. It has been shown that CRP as an inflammatory mediator not only reflects tissue damage, but also aggravates the severity of damage and contributes causally to course and outcome of various diseases [8]. Therefore, CRP has to be regarded not only as a marker, but also as an active pro-inflammatory protein.

2. Role of CRP

CRP is a sensitive, reliable and early indicator of inflammation and infection. Evolutionarily highly conserved, this pentameric molecule is part of the ancient humoral immune response and involved in various immunological pathways as a key mediator [9,10]. It is predominantly synthesized and secreted into the blood circulation by hepatic cells as a response to trauma, inflammation, or infection. In these situations, the proinflammatory cytokines interleukin 6 (IL-6) and, to a lesser extent, interleukin 1β (IL-1β) as well as tumor necrosis factor @(TNF@) induce CRP expression on the transcriptional level [11–14]. Following an acute phase stimulus, serum CRP values increase up to levels a few thousand times higher than the normal (healthy) concentration of human CRP (0.05 to 3000 mg/L) [15,16]. The half-life in plasma is about 19 h [17,18].

After secretion, CRP efficiently detects and opsonizes bacteria upon their infiltration and initiates their phagocytosis by activation of complement [19,20]. This is probably its original purpose as one of the most ancient proteins within the humoral immune system.

However, CRP also detects and binds to endogenous cells [21,22]. Cells, which are either apoptotic, energy-depleted, or simply exposed to stressors like the acidic and often ischemic environment of inflammation display conformational and biochemical changes of their membrane [23]. One of these changes is the formation of lyso-phosphatidylcholine (LPC) by partial hydrolyzation of phosphatidylcholine (PC). To this end, one of its two fatty acid groups is removed by the secretory phospholipase A2 type IIa (sPLA2 IIa) [24,25]. This phospholipase is secreted and activated by inflammation (IL-6) and marks the beginning of detrimental destruction of still viable tissue after e.g., ischemia [26–29]. LPC is thereby accessible in the plasma membrane of dead, damaged, or inflamed cells. The CRP pentamer binds to LPC with high avidity in a so-called cooperative manner and subsequently mediates the elimination of these cells, similarly to infiltrating pathogens, by activating the classical complement pathway [30–35]. Complement C1q binds to CRP directly and mediates the binding of C2–C4 [36]. Thus, these cells are irreversibly marked for phagocytes which dispose the marked cells. Phagocytes in turn secrete IL-6 which induces the synthesis of additional CRP by the liver, subsequently amplifying the immune response. This way, more cells become marked by CRP (Figure 1).

Importantly, this mechanism facilitates binding of CRP to actually still vital cells, which may potentially regenerate with more CRP-free time. By interacting with complement, CRP triggers the destruction and therefore negatively affects the regeneration of tissue. By now, a large body of data obtained from animal experiments demonstrates that this CRP-mediated mechanism plays an active role in exacerbating ischemia and reperfusion-induced damage [37–43].

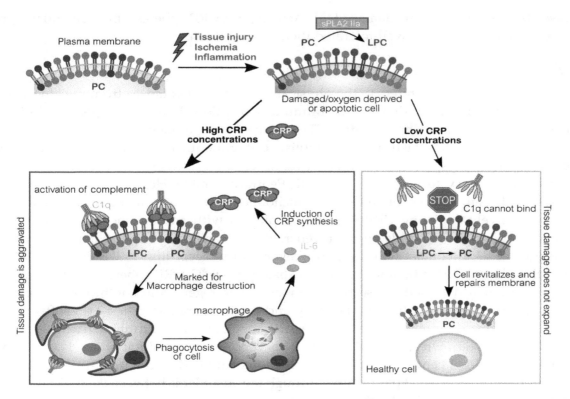

Figure 1. Molecular pathomechanism of CRP-mediated tissue damage. Upon inflammation or acute oxygen-deprivation, cells display a dramatic shortage of adenosine triphosphate (ATP). ATP is essential to prevent apoptosis which manifests in the outer cell membrane: Phosphatidylcholine (PC) is converted into lyso-phosphatidylcholine (LPC) by phospholipase (sPLA2 IIa). Due to the lack of ATP, this alteration cannot be reversed. CRP subsequently binds to LPC on anaerobic cells and recruits complement factors (C1q-C4). These opsonized cells will be disposed by phagocytes, which in turn induce CRP synthesis. Without CRP or in situations with low CRP concentrations (e.g., after CRP apheresis), energy deprived-cells are spared and may switch back to aerobic metabolism, repair molecular changes and revitalize again, leading to an overall reduced tissue damage [41,43–45]. CRP C-reactive protein; C1q Complement component 1q; IL-6 Interleukin 6; LPC Lysophosphatidylcholine; PC Phosphatidylcholine; sPLA2 IIa secretory phospholipase A2 type IIa.

On the molecular level it is not fully elucidated yet whether pro-inflammatory signaling is mediated by the pentameric, native form of CRP, or if CRP dissociates into its non-covalently bound monomers upon binding to LPC, which then exhibit novel binding capacities and other specific functions [46–48]. Publications which described anti-inflammatory actions of pentameric CRP hypothesized that CRP switches functions by undergoing structural changes. Although various quaternary structures of CRP are still not well proven in the physiological context, it might well be possible that CRP monomers exist in specific inflammatory microenvironments and represent different stages of inflammation [47,49]. It has been clearly shown that CRP is secreted in its native, pentameric form by the liver and-if at all-only dissociates locally within inflamed tissue. Hence, therapeutic interventions are more efficient targeting pentameric CRP as high circulating levels are the actual source for its detrimental action [50,51]. Its known physiological function is the disposal of cells (bacteria, necrotic and apoptotic cells).

To date, no pharmacologic inhibitor of inflammation has been proven to be successful in ischemia-related injuries, since they all featured unfavorable pharmacokinetic profiles or serious side effects. Therefore, a different strategy is needed to target the detrimental inflammatory response [43,52]. Specifically, targeting avoidable organ damage caused by the action of CRP represents a promising therapeutic option [43,53]. Decreasing CRP levels could potentially protect salvageable cells and give them more time to recover. Therefore, removing CRP from the blood circulation interrupts the innate cascade and reduces tissue damage [44]. Accordingly, CRP apheresis may potentially present a promising, highly efficient, and well-tolerated therapeutic option.

3. CRP Apheresis

Extracorporeal apheresis refers to the physical removal of substances from the blood by means of filtration, precipitation or adsorption. Immunoadsorption defines the specific binding of an immunologic protein by an adsorber matrix. The elimination of pathogenic substances from the blood in extracorporeal apheresis constitutes an established therapeutic measure in the clinical routine of numerous diseases.

The CRP adsorber system (PentraSorb® CRP, Pentracor GmbH, Hennigsdorf, Germany) features an agarose-based resin, which contains a phosphocholine-derivative as ligand for CRP and is thereby capable of selectively depleting CRP from blood plasma with an efficiency of up to 94% (under laboratory conditions) [54]. The adsorber is regenerable and can be used up to a maximum cumulative treatment time of 24 h (contact with human plasma ≤24 h, according to CE license). In between treatments the adsorber has to be stored in sodium azide at 2–8 °C. CRP apheresis is executed in cycles, alternating between loading of the adsorber with plasma and regeneration of the column, that follows a fixed sequence of washing solutions. Loading and washing are controlled by a software module for automatic plasma flow management (ADAsorb, medicap clinic GmbH, Ulrichstein, Germany; Figure 2). Blood can be drawn via central or peripheral venous access (cubital veins). Plasma separation is performed by a blood centrifuge and blood is anti-coagulated 1:15 with citrate buffer (ACD-A; 3% citrate) or heparin. The usual plasma flow through the adsorber is between 25 to 35 mL/min. Blood flow ranges between 40 and 65 mL/min.

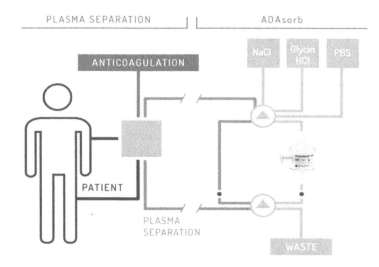

Figure 2. Schematic illustration of CRP apheresis. The procedure is described in detail by Ries et al. 2019 [45].

During one treatment, 6000 mL of plasma are usually processed in 12 cycles. A continuous monitoring of vital parameters, blood pressure and heart rate has to be carried out. Processing of 6000 mL blood plasma takes 4–5 h, depending on the blood flow. Patients can be treated an infinite amount of times with CRP apheresis, as the blood loss is only minimal. Depending on CRP level and indication, two to ten treatments on consecutive days are performed. So far, no side-effects have been reported [45,55–57].

The main advantages of CRP apheresis are the selective removal of the agent by the highly specific ligand and the good controllability of the process, since unlimited plasma volumes can be processed to achieve the desired CRP reduction. Drugs are not removed by CRP apheresis.

4. CRP Apheresis after Ischemic Tissue Damage

The extent of tissue damage during and after an acute traumatic incident defines outcome and follow-up health. Ischemic lesions, predominantly acute myocardial infarction (AMI) and ischemic stroke, generate initial organ damage in the acute zone by cell death due to oxygen deprivation and its magnitude is primarily determined by its duration [58]. Further, neighboring cells which are deprived of oxygen for a shorter duration or to a lesser extent are damaged but salvageable and constitute the area at risk (AMI) or penumbra (stroke) [58,59]. The first line of therapy constitutes the restoration of blood flow to limit the initial ischemic injury. This reperfusion, even though essential to decrease mortality and morbidity, is attended by an intense and maladaptive immune response, which augments and accelerates the organ damage and includes the still viable but damaged tissue [60,61]. The elimination of salvageable cells by CRP through this mechanism mediates reperfusion injury and critically contributes to the already existing deterioration [62,63]. CRP apheresis aims to remove circulating CRP after AMI and ischemic stroke in order to reduce acute tissue injury and ischemic reperfusion injury.

4.1. Myocardial Infarction

Patients who recover from AMI often suffer from reduced quality of life and very high risk of severe complications later on (e.g., second infarct), which implies a huge burden for the health system. This risk correlates significantly with the extent of myocardial injury and scarring [64,65].

It has long been established that inflammation especially mediated by the innate immune system extends myocardial injury, however, anti-inflammatory strategies to minimize myocardial necrosis have failed so far, maybe because these processes are also needed for healing and cardiac repair [3,4,52,66]. While baseline CRP levels in the healthy state are established as predictor of the incidence of cardiovascular disease [67–69], serum CRP concentration during and after AMI correlates with clinical outcome [16,17,70–74]. It is well known that high peak CRP levels during the acute phase response after AMI correlate with larger infarct size and higher mortality as well as incidence of major adverse events [17,74,75]. This has been described for more than two decades now and is in line with the described pathological function of CRP, eliminating cells in the area at risk [8,23,76]. This area contains cells, which could partially recover after revascularization and reperfusion, but are finally destroyed by immune-mediated mechanisms, as explained above and shown in detail in numerous experimental approaches focusing specifically on AMI [39,40,63,70,77,78]. Targeting CRP in AMI has therefore been proposed previously, but was never achieved due to non-functioning therapeutic approaches [43,79–81].

Preclinical studies on the efficacy of specific extracorporeal depletion of CRP have been successfully performed in a porcine animal model of AMI [41,42]. In this study, a mean reduction of CRP levels by about 50%, a significant reduction of the infarct size and a stabilization of the ejection fraction was observed. Interestingly, a completely different scar morphology was detected in animals after CRP apheresis compared to controls [41]. A smaller scar tissue and more vital heart muscle reflected the efficacy of this treatment strategy (Figure 3, previously published and taken from [41]). AMI was therefore selected as indication for the first clinical trial of CRP apheresis. CRP apheresis was applied in patients with ST-elevation myocardial infarction (STEMI) (CAMI-1 trial: "Selective depletion of C-reactive protein by therapeutic apheresis (CRP apheresis) in acute myocardial infarction", DRKS ID: DRKS00008988). Just recently, this multi-center clinical trial has been finished and first data were shown in Case reports and a publication describing 13 patients as a preliminary report [44,45,55,56].

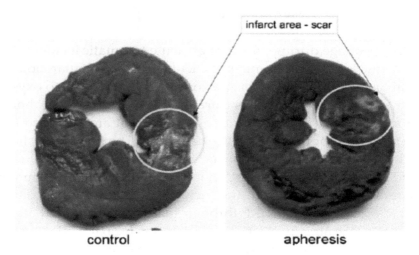

Figure 3. Porcine Heart Slices after AMI with and without CRP apheresis. Slices of the left ventricle 14 days after AMI. Slices were generated after an Evans Blue staining of the heart. Circles localize a characteristic transmural scar of a control animals (left) versus spotted scar morphology after CRP apheresis (right). Figure previously published and taken from [41].

The CAMI-1 trial tested the hypothesis whether specific depletion of CRP by CRP apheresis can reduce myocardial infarct size in humans. Endpoints were safety, myocardial infarct size and function as well as CRP concentration in patients with acute STEMI. A total of 83 patients were recruited at 8 study centers. Plasma CRP levels were reduced by approximately 60% over all performed apheresis procedures in the CAMI-1 trial. Treatments were safe and well tolerated. There were no serious adverse effects associated with the treatment [45]. The magnitude of increase of CRP concentration during the acute phase response after STEMI correlated significantly with the infarct size in control patients. Patients with similar initial CRP increase, who subsequently underwent CRP apheresis, showed smaller infarct sizes as well as improved left ventricular function and wall motion (strains) compared to control patients (*unpublished data-submitted*). Currently, a CAMI-1 registry is on-going, collecting more data (DRKS00017481) [44].

4.2. Ischemic Stroke

Stroke is the third most frequent cause of death and the leading cause of serious, long-term disability worldwide. This disease has a tremendous personal, familiar and socioeconomic impact. More than 80% of patients suffer from ischemic stroke [82]. To date, restoring rapid reperfusion of the brain constitutes the only established therapeutic strategy to reduce the size of the infarct and the consequences of the disease [83]. However, similar mechanisms to AMI take place and inflammation plays an important role in various stages of ischemic stroke, because several humoral and cellular mechanisms are set in motion by the occlusion and subsequent therapeutic reperfusion [84,85]. These mechanisms may explain why some patients with ischemic stroke suffer from severe neurological symptoms despite early and successful recanalization. Several findings substantiate the hypothesis that CRP plays a similar pathological role as shown in AMI, facilitating the elimination of energetically challenged and compromised cells in the penumbra.

First, various publications have shown an association between the early inflammatory response after ischemic stroke and the clinical outcome. The early inflammatory response after stroke has been identified as a key prognostic factor [86,87]. Patients with favorable clinical outcome feature significantly lower levels of inflammatory parameters, especially CRP, compared to patients with poor outcome. Previous studies have described an association between high CRP values after acute stroke and negative prognosis [88–91]. Muir et al. have shown that CRP levels measured within 72 h after stroke predict mortality over an observation period of up to 4 years [92]. According to Winbek et al., CRP levels 24 and 48 h after onset of symptoms affect prognosis, but not their concentration at admission [87]. In another stroke study, patients who died during the study period had significantly higher CRP levels at admission compared to survivors and CRP levels correlated with the clinical outcome after 3 months follow-up [86]. Further, studies in a rat animal model have shown that infusion of human CRP enlarges cerebral infarct areas after acute occlusion via a complement-dependent mechanism [37].

Based on this background, a clinical trial investigating selective CRP apheresis after ischemic stroke was initiated (CASTRO1 trial: "Selective Depletion of C-reactive Protein by Therapeutic Apheresis (CRP-apheresis) in Ischemic Stroke", ID: NCT0441723). The CASTRO trial is designed as a randomized, controlled, multicentric interventional pilot trial. The aim of the CASTRO trial is to evaluate if CRP apheresis can be applied safely in patients with ischemic stroke and efficiently lower the CRP level. Therefore, the primary endpoint is the type and frequency of adverse events and serious adverse events after apheresis. In addition, potential effects of CRP apheresis on clinical outcome parameters (cognitive measures, infarct volume, laboratory parameters) will be investigated.

Participants for this trial need to have an ischemic stroke with or without intravenous lysis and recanalization therapy. The National Institutes of Health Stroke Scale (NIHSS) has to be between 1–24 in order to exclude patients with severe, potentially complicated disease courses. CRP needs to increase ≥ 5 mg/L within 72 h after the incident and/or serum CRP concentration needs to be larger than 10 mg/L. We aim to include 20 patients which are 1:1 randomly assigned to either the control group (standard guideline therapy) or CRP apheresis in addition to the standard guideline therapy. The standard therapy of acute ischemic stroke is carried out according to the guidelines of the European Academy of Neurology [93].

Exclusion criteria are severe dysphagia (risk of aspiration pneumonia), clinical or laboratory evidence of systemic infection, contraindications against apheresis, Modified Rankin Scale (mRS) before index event ≥ 3, intracranial hemorrhage, epileptic seizure in the context of the acute event, pregnancy, and lactation. Treatment and study regime will be implemented into the clinical standard diagnostic and therapeutic regime after stroke. Since CRP levels begin to rise approximately 8 h after the ischemic incident and reach their peak after 24 h, the first CRP apheresis will be carried out within 72 h after onset of symptoms. Therefore, CRP apheresis will not delay acute guideline therapies of stroke, such as intravenous lysis and intraarterial thrombectomy. The complete study flow is illustrated in Figure 4.

To investigate whether CRP apheresis improves clinical outcome parameters after ischemic stroke, patients will undergo assessments according to standardized clinical scales, namely National Institute of Health Stroke Scale (NIHSS) score, Barthel ADL index (BI), modified Rankin scale (mRS) and measurements of infarct volume (via magnetic resonance imaging; MRI). In addition, immunological and neurodegenerative biomarkers (interleukin-6, serum amyloid A) will be evaluated to objectify a potential beneficial effect of CRP apheresis on inflammatory pathways. Measurements of primary and secondary outcome parameters will be performed at baseline (before first apheresis), daily during apheresis, and 90 days after stroke.

Immunoadsorption with the PentraSorb® CRP is performed with the ADAsorb apheresis device as described in detail in 3. CRP apheresis is performed for a maximum amount of three times (three days) or until CRP concentration is below 10 mg/L.

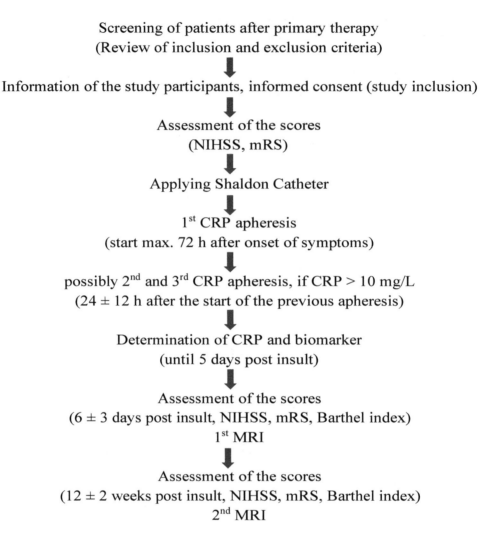

Screening of patients after primary therapy
(Review of inclusion and exclusion criteria)

Information of the study participants, informed consent (study inclusion)

Assessment of the scores
(NIHSS, mRS)

Applying Shaldon Catheter

1st CRP apheresis
(start max. 72 h after onset of symptoms)

possibly 2nd and 3rd CRP apheresis, if CRP > 10 mg/L
(24 ± 12 h after the start of the previous apheresis)

Determination of CRP and biomarker
(until 5 days post insult)

Assessment of the scores
(6 ± 3 days post insult, NIHSS, mRS, Barthel index)
1st MRI

Assessment of the scores
(12 ± 2 weeks post insult, NIHSS, mRS, Barthel index)
2nd MRI

Figure 4. Study flow of the CASTRO1 trial. MRI magnetic resonance imaging; NIHSS National Institute of Health Stroke Scale; mRs modified Rankin scale.

5. CRP Apheresis in Other Indications

Both AMI and ischemic stroke feature a common underlying pathophysiology and the therapeutic application and benefit after AMI has been already shown. However, reduction of dramatically high CRP concentrations in other indications which are not defined by an ischemic pathophysiology could also be beneficial. The overcompensating immune reaction which often triggers SIRS after surgery, causes detrimental deterioration during acute pancreatitis, or mediates a cytokine storm after infection, could be dampened with CRP apheresis. Therefore, clinical trials investigating the safety and efficacy of CRP apheresis during pancreatitis and after coronary bypass surgery are ongoing (CAPRI1-study DRKS00014265; CABY1-study DRKS00013012). Further, first patients suffering from Covid-19 have been treated with CRP apheresis in order to inhibit the CRP-mediated autoimmune response leading to respiratory failure and multi-organ failure [57,94].

6. Conclusions and Outlook

CRP has been established as a general biomarker of inflammation and infection in clinical practice. Recently, its role as a stable and highly useful prognostic factor for cardiovascular and cerebral disease in healthy individuals has been widely acknowledged and utilized [95,96]. However, the characterization of CRP as not only a biomarker but also a mediator or even trigger of immunological destruction of tissue is widely ignored [8,37,39].

Therapeutic CRP removal by immunoadsorption might present a logical and promising therapy for pathologies in which the extent of tissue damage is aggravated by inflammation and correlated with a worse clinical outcome, including ischemic events.

CRP apheresis has been applied successfully in a controlled multi-center trial in patients with myocardial infarction (CAMI-1 trial). It showed very few and only moderate side effects and managed to significantly reduce CRP levels, thereby positively affecting infarct size and left ventricular ejection fraction [44,45,55,56]. Applying CRP apheresis in ischemic stroke is the next plausible step. However, the immunological situation in the brain is different. Neurons have a low tolerance to oxidative stress, and the physiologically important blood-brain-barrier may impair the effectiveness of this method [97–99].

The CASTRO study will show whether CRP apheresis can be safely performed in patients with ischemic stroke and also provide preliminary results whether reducing the concentration of serum CRP levels facilitates reduction of tissue damage of the brain, consequently improving clinical outcome measures compared to the control group.

Other anti-inflammatory therapies have been investigated in AMI and ischemic stroke, such as colchicine [100], anti-CD18 agents [101] and agents targeting IL-1 or IL-6 [102–104]. CRP removal intends to stop the destruction of tissue already during the acute event. Furthermore, targeting specifically and selectively CRP may constitute a superior choice because it does not cause a pleiotropic effect. The maximum removal of CRP in patients was 79% by now. This leaves enough CRP for potential repair processes. Importantly, cardiac or neural repair is not impaired by the intervention as opposed to former pharmacological interventions like the methylprednisolone trial in myocardial infarction which resulted in a catastrophic outcome [105].

Preliminary evidence suggests that CRP apheresis induces very few side effects and features a low risk profile [45]. One drawback is that the procedure takes relatively long. Nevertheless, CRP apheresis fits well into the management of stroke patients because it does not collide with acute measures and may therefore complement methods aiming at reperfusion.

The acute inflammatory response has two facets. For one thing it plays a key role in initial host defense against infections. But on the downside, it can cause collateral damage of tissues. Especially in situations with an inciting sterile stimulus, the cost-benefit ratio is unfavorable.

CRP as an ancient protein of the innate immune system physiologically disposes cells and reacts to almost every disturbance of tissue homeostasis. Therefore, the span of potential indications for CRP apheresis is broad, and the ongoing clinical trials will illuminate whether this therapy is beneficial in these specific indications.

Author Contributions: Conceptualization, S.K., P.B. and A.S.; writing—original draft preparation, S.K., A.S. and P.B.; writing—review and editing, K.A., J.D. and A.S.; All authors have read and agreed to the published version of the manuscript.

Acknowledgments: We thank the CAMI1-study group for the realization of the CAMI-1 trial.

Conflicts of Interest: S.K. is an employee of Pentracor GmbH. J.D. received speaker honoraria and research fund from Fresenius Medical Care GmbH and Fresenius Medical Care Deutschland GmbH. A.S. is a founder, shareholder and managing director of Pentracor GmbH. P.B. and K.A. do not have any conflict of interest.

References

1. Netea, M.G.; Balkwill, F.; Chonchol, M.; Cominelli, F.; Donath, M.Y.; Giamarellos-Bourboulis, E.J.; Golenbock, U.; Gresnigt, M.S.; Heneka, M.T.; Hoffman, H.M.; et al. A guiding map for inflammation. *Nat. Immunol.* **2017**, *18*, 826–831. [CrossRef]

2. Eming, S.A.; Krieg, T.; Davidson, J.M. Inflammation in Wound Repair: Molecular and Cellular Mechanisms. *J. Investig. Dermatol.* **2007**, *127*, 514–525. [CrossRef] [PubMed]

3. Ong, S.-B.; Hernández-Reséndiz, S.; Crespo-Avilan, G.E.; Mukhametshina, R.T.; Kwek, X.-Y.; Cabrera-Fuentes, H.A.; Hausenloy, D.J. Inflammation following acute myocardial infarction: Multiple

players, dynamic roles, and novel therapeutic opportunities. *Pharmacol. Ther.* **2018**, *186*, 73–87. [CrossRef] [PubMed]

4.   Anzai, T. Inflammatory Mechanisms of Cardiovascular Remodeling. *Circ. J.* **2018**, *82*, 629–635. [CrossRef]

5.   Neher, M.D.; Weckbach, S.; Flierl, M.A.; Huber-Lang, M.; Stahel, P.F. Molecular mechanisms of inflammation and tissue injury after major trauma-is complement the "bad guy"? *J. Biomed. Sci.* **2011**, *18*, 90. [CrossRef]

6.   Day, J.; Taylor, K. The systemic inflammatory response syndrome and cardiopulmonary bypass. *Int. J. Surg.* **2005**, *3*, 129–140. [CrossRef] [PubMed]

7.   Tillett, W.S.; Francis, T. Serological Reactions in Pneumonia with a Non-Protein Somatic Fraction of Pneumococcus. *J. Exp. Med.* **1930**, *52*, 561–571. [CrossRef]

8.   Kunze, R. C-Reactive Protein: From Biomarker to Trigger of Cell Death? *Ther. Apher. Dial.* **2019**, *23*, 494–496. [CrossRef]

9.   Mortensen, R.F. C-Reactive Protein, Inflammation, and Innate Immunity. *Immunol. Res.* **2001**, *24*, 163–176. [CrossRef]

10. Du Clos, T.W. Pentraxins: Structure, Function, and Role in Inflammation. *ISRN Inflamm.* **2013**, *2013*, 1–22. [CrossRef]

11. Toniatti, C.; Arcone, R.; Majello, B.; Ganter, U.; Arpaia, G.; Ciliberto, G. Regulation of the human C-reactive protein gene, a major marker of inflammation and cancer. *Mol. Biol. Med.* **1990**, *7*, 199–212. [PubMed]

12. Zhang, D.; Sun, M.; Samols, D.; Kushner, I. STAT3 Participates in Transcriptional Activation of the C-reactive Protein Gene by Interleukin-6. *J. Biol. Chem.* **1996**, *271*, 9503–9509. [CrossRef] [PubMed]

13. Kramer, F.; Torzewski, J.; Kamenz, J.; Veit, K.; Hombach, V.; Dedio, J.; Ivashchenko, Y. Interleukin-1β stimulates acute phase response and C-reactive protein synthesis by inducing an NFκB- and C/EBPβ-dependent autocrine interleukin-6 loop. *Mol. Immunol.* **2008**, *45*, 2678–2689. [CrossRef] [PubMed]

14. Weinhold, B.; Bader, A.; Poli, V.; Rüther, U. Interleukin-6 is necessary, but not sufficient, for induction of the humanC-reactive protein gene in vivo. *Biochem. J.* **1997**, *325*, 617–621. [CrossRef] [PubMed]

15. Kushner, I.; Broder, M.L.; Karp, D. Control of the Acute Phase Response. *J. Clin. Investig.* **1978**, *61*, 235–242. [CrossRef] [PubMed]

16. Pietilä, K.; Harmoinen, A.; Hermens, W.; Simoons, M.L.; Van De Werf, F.; Verstraete, M. Serum C-reactive protein and infarct size in myocardial infarct patients with a closed versus an open infarct-related coronary artery after thrombolytic therapy. *Eur. Hear. J.* **1993**, *14*, 915–919. [CrossRef] [PubMed]

17. Dimitrijević, O.; Stojcevski, B.D.; Ignjatović, S.; Singh, N.M. Serial Measurements of C-Reactive Protein After Acute Myocardial Infarction in Predicting One-Year Outcome. *Int. Hear. J.* **2006**, *47*, 833–842. [CrossRef]

18. Gabriel, A.S.; Martinsson, A.; Wretlind, B.; Ahnve, S. IL-6 levels in acute and post myocardial infarction: Their relation to CRP levels, infarction size, left ventricular systolic function, and heart failure. *Eur. J. Intern. Med.* **2004**, *15*, 523–528. [CrossRef]

19. Szalai, A.J.; Briles, D.E.; Volanakis, J.E. Role of complement in C-reactive-protein-mediated protection of mice from Streptococcus pneumoniae. *Infect. Immun.* **1996**, *64*, 4850–4853. [CrossRef]

20. Mold, C.; Rodic-Polic, B.; Du Clos, T.W. Protection from Streptococcus pneumoniae Infection by C-Reactive Protein and Natural Antibody Requires Complement But Not Fcγ Receptors. *J. Immunol.* **2002**, *168*, 6375–6381. [CrossRef]

21. Chang, M.-K.; Binder, C.J.; Torzewski, M.; Witztum, J.L. C-reactive protein binds to both oxidized LDL and apoptotic cells through recognition of a common ligand: Phosphorylcholine of oxidized phospholipids. *Proc. Natl. Acad. Sci. USA* **2002**, *99*, 13043–13048. [CrossRef] [PubMed]

22. Li, Y.P.; Mold, C.; Du Clos, T.W. Sublytic complement attack exposes C-reactive protein binding sites on cell membranes. *J. Immunol.* **1994**, *152*, 2995–3005. [PubMed]

23. Sparkes, B.L.; Woods, K.; Roth, M.; Welti, R.; Fleming, S.D. Phospholipase A2 alters membrane lipid composition during ischemia/reperfusion (39.55). *J. Immunol.* **2009**, *182*, 39.55.

24. Yagami, T.; Yamamoto, Y.; Koma, H. The Role of Secretory Phospholipase A2 in the Central Nervous System and Neurological Diseases. *Mol. Neurobiol.* **2013**, *49*, 863–876. [CrossRef]

25. Murakami, M.; Taketomi, Y.; Sato, H.; Yamamoto, K. Secreted phospholipase A2 revisited. *J. Biochem.* **2011**, *150*, 233–255. [CrossRef] [PubMed]

26. Fujioka, D.; Kawabata, K.-I.; Ishimoto, Y.; Suzuki, N.; Hanasaki, K.; Sato, R.; Hasebe, H.; Kobayashi, T.; Saito, Y.; Kanazawa, M.; et al. Abstract 1435: Reduction in Myocardial Ischemia-reperfusion Injury in Group X Secretory Phospholipase A_2-deficient Mice. *Circulation* **2006**, *114*, II_275. [CrossRef]

27. Yano, T.; Fujioka, D.; Saito, Y.; Kobayashi, T.; Nakamura, T.; Obata, J.-E.; Kawabata, K.; Watanabe, K.; Watanabe, Y.; Mishina, H.; et al. Group V secretory phospholipase A2 plays a pathogenic role in myocardial ischaemia–reperfusion injury. *Cardiovasc. Res.* **2010**, *90*, 335–343. [CrossRef]

28. Nijmeijer, R.; Lagrand, W.K.; Baidoshvili, A.; Lubbers, Y.T.P.; Hermens, W.T.; Meijer, C.J.L.M.; Visser, C.A.; Hack, C.E.; Niessen, H.W.M. Secretory type II phospholipase A(2) binds to ischemic myocardium during myocardial infarction in humans. *Cardiovasc. Res.* **2002**, *53*, 138–146. [CrossRef]

29. Nijmeijer, R.; Willemsen, M.; Meijer, C.J.L.M.; Visser, C.A.; Verheijen, R.H.; Gottlieb, R.A.; Hack, C.E.; Niessen, H.W.M. Type II secretory phospholipase A2 binds to ischemic flip-flopped cardiomyocytes and subsequently induces cell death. *Am. J. Physiol. Circ. Physiol.* **2003**, *285*, H2218–H2224. [CrossRef]

30. Sproston, N.R.; Ashworth, J.J. Role of C-Reactive Protein at Sites of Inflammation and Infection. *Front. Immunol.* **2018**, *9*, 754. [CrossRef]

31. Goda, T.; Miyahara, Y. Calcium-independent binding of human C-reactive protein to lysophosphatidylcholine in supported planar phospholipid monolayers. *Acta Biomater.* **2017**, *48*, 206–214. [CrossRef] [PubMed]

32. Kushner, I.; Kaplan, M.H. Studies of acute phase protein: I. An Immunohistochemical method for the localization of cx-reactive protein in rabbits. Association with necrosis in local inflammatory lesions. *J. Exp. Med.* **1961**, *114*, 961–974. [CrossRef] [PubMed]

33. Narkates, A.J.; Volanakis, J.E. C-reactive protein binding specificities: Artificial and natural phospholipid bilayers. *Ann. N. Y. Acad. Sci.* **1982**, *389*, 172–182. [CrossRef] [PubMed]

34. Kushner, I.; Rakita, L.; Kaplan, M.H. Studies of acute-phase protein. II. Localization of Cx-reactive protein in heart in induced myocardial infarction in rabbits. *J. Clin. Investig.* **1963**, *42*, 286–292. [CrossRef] [PubMed]

35. Vogt, B.; Führnrohr, B.; Müller, R.; Sheriff, A. CRP and the disposal of dying cells: Consequences for systemic lupus erythematosus and rheumatoid arthritis. *Autoimmunity* **2007**, *40*, 295–298. [CrossRef]

36. Gaboriaud, C.; Juanhuix, J.; Gruez, A.; Lacroix, M.; Darnault, C.; Pignol, D.; Verger, D.; Fontecilla-Camps, J.C.; Arlaud, G.J. The Crystal Structure of the Globular Head of Complement Protein C1q Provides a Basis for Its Versatile Recognition Properties. *J. Biol. Chem.* **2003**, *278*, 46974–46982. [CrossRef] [PubMed]

37. Gill, R.; Kemp, J.A.; Sabin, C.; Pepys, M.B. Human C-Reactive Protein Increases Cerebral Infarct Size after Middle Cerebral Artery Occlusion in Adult Rats. *Br. J. Pharmacol.* **2004**, *24*, 1214–1218. [CrossRef]

38. Hack, C.; Wolbink, G.-J.; Schalkwijk, C.; Speijer, H.; Hermens, W.T.; Bosch, H.V.D. A role for secretory phospholipase A2 and C-reactive protein in the removal of injured cells. *Immunol. Today* **1997**, *18*, 111–115. [CrossRef]

39. Griselli, M.; Herbert, J.; Hutchinson, W.; Taylor, K.; Sohail, M.; Krausz, T.; Pepys, M.B. C-Reactive Protein and Complement Are Important Mediators of Tissue Damage in Acute Myocardial Infarction. *J. Exp. Med.* **1999**, *190*, 1733–1740. [CrossRef]

40. Nijmeijer, R.; Lagrand, W.K.; Lubbers, Y.T.P.; Visser, C.A.; Meijer, C.J.L.M.; Niessen, H.W.M.; Hack, C.E. C-Reactive Protein Activates Complement in Infarcted Human Myocardium. *Am. J. Pathol.* **2003**, *163*, 269–275. [CrossRef]

41. Sheriff, A.; Schindler, R.; Vogt, B.; Abdel-Aty, H.; Unger, J.K.; Bock, C.; Gebauer, F.; Slagman, A.; Jerichow, T.; Mans, D.; et al. Selective apheresis of C-reactive protein: A new therapeutic option in myocardial infarction? *J. Clin. Apher.* **2014**, *30*, 15–21. [CrossRef] [PubMed]

42. Slagman, A.; Bock, C.; Abdel-Aty, H.; Vogt, B.; Gebauer, F.; Janelt, G.; Wohlgemuth, F.; Morgenstern, R.; Yapici, G.; Puppe, A.; et al. Specific Removal of C-Reactive Protein by Apheresis in a Porcine Cardiac Infarction Model. *Blood Purif.* **2011**, *31*, 9–17. [CrossRef] [PubMed]

43. Pepys, M.B.; Hirschfield, G.M.; Tennent, G.A.; Gallimore, J.R.; Kahan, M.C.; Bellotti, V.; Hawkins, P.N.; Myers, R.M.; Smith, M.D.; Polara, A.; et al. Targeting C-reactive protein for the treatment of cardiovascular disease. *Nature* **2006**, *440*, 1217–1221. [CrossRef] [PubMed]

44. Ries, W.; Heigl, F.; Garlichs, C.; Sheriff, A.; Torzewski, J. *Die CRP-Apherese: Eine neue Therapiemöglichkeit bei Inflammation*; Nephro-News, Medicom VerlagsgmbH Bruck: Mur, Austria, 2019; pp. 23–27.

45. Ries, W.; Heigl, F.; Garlichs, C.; Sheriff, A.; Torzewski, J. Selective C-Reactive Protein-Apheresis in Patients. *Ther. Apher. Dial.* **2019**, *23*, 570–574. [CrossRef]

46. Braig, D.; Nero, T.L.; Koch, H.-G.; Kaiser, B.; Wang, X.; Thiele, J.R.; Morton, C.J.; Zeller, J.; Kiefer, J.; Potempa, L.A.; et al. Transitional changes in the CRP structure lead to the exposure of proinflammatory binding sites. *Nat. Commun.* **2017**, *8*, 14188. [CrossRef]

47. Thiele, J.R.; Habersberger, J.; Braig, D.; Schmidt, Y.; Goerendt, K.; Maurer, V.; Bannasch, H.; Scheichl, A.; Woollard, K.J.; Von Dobschütz, E.; et al. Dissociation of Pentameric to Monomeric C-Reactive Protein Localizes and Aggravates Inflammation. *Circulation* **2014**, *130*, 35–50. [CrossRef]

48. McFadyen, J.D.; Kiefer, J.; Braig, D.; Loseff-Silver, J.; Potempa, L.A.; Eisenhardt, S.U.; Peter, K. Dissociation of C-Reactive Protein Localizes and Amplifies Inflammation: Evidence for a Direct Biological Role of C-Reactive Protein and Its Conformational Changes. *Front. Immunol.* **2018**, *9*. [CrossRef]

49. Zhang, L.; Li, H.-Y.; Li, W.; Shen, Z.-Y.; Wang, Y.-D.; Ji, S.-R.; Wu, Y. An ELISA Assay for Quantifying Monomeric C-Reactive Protein in Plasma. *Front. Immunol.* **2018**, *9*, 9. [CrossRef]

50. Thiele, J.R.; Zeller, J.; Bannasch, H.; Stark, G.B.; Peter, K.; Eisenhardt, S.U. Targeting C-Reactive Protein in Inflammatory Disease by Preventing Conformational Changes. *Mediat. Inflamm.* **2015**, *2015*, 1–9. [CrossRef]

51. Caprio, V.; Badimon, L.; Di Napoli, M.; Fang, W.-H.; Ferris, G.R.; Guo, B.; Iemma, R.S.; Liu, D.; Zeinolabediny, Y.; Slevin, M. pCRP-mCRP Dissociation Mechanisms as Potential Targets for the Development of Small-Molecule Anti-Inflammatory Chemotherapeutics. *Front. Immunol.* **2018**, *9*. [CrossRef]

52. Frangogiannis, N.G.; Smith, C.W.; Entman, M.L. The inflammatory response in myocardial infarction. *Cardiovasc. Res.* **2002**, *53*, 31–47. [CrossRef]

53. Prasad, K. C-Reactive Protein (CRP)-Lowering Agents. *Cardiovasc. Drug Rev.* **2006**, *24*, 33–50. [CrossRef] [PubMed]

54. Mattecka, S.; Brunner, P.; Hähnel, B.; Kunze, R.; Vogt, B.; Sheriff, A. PentraSorb C-Reactive Protein: Characterization of the Selective C-Reactive Protein Adsorber Resin. *Ther. Apher. Dial.* **2019**, *23*, 474–481. [CrossRef] [PubMed]

55. Boljevic, D.; Nikolic, A.; Rusovic, S.; Lakcevic, J.; Bojic, M.; Balint, B. A Promising Innovative Treatment for ST-Elevation Myocardial Infarction: The Use of C-Reactive Protein Selective Apheresis: Case Report. *Blood Purif.* **2020**, 1–5. [CrossRef] [PubMed]

56. Ries, W.; Sheriff, A.; Heigl, F.; Zimmermann, O.; Garlichs, C.D.; Torzewski, J. "First in Man": Case Report of Selective C-Reactive Protein Apheresis in a Patient with Acute ST Segment Elevation Myocardial Infarction. *Case Rep. Cardiol.* **2018**, *2018*, 1–4. [CrossRef]

57. Torzewski, J.; Heigl, F.; Zimmermann, O.; Wagner, F.; Schumann, C.; Hettich, R.; Bock, C.; Kayser, S.; Sheriff, A. First-in-Man: Case Report of Selective C-Reactive Protein Apheresis in a Patient with SARS-CoV-2 Infection. *Am. J. Case Rep.* **2020**, *21*, e925020.

58. Xing, C.; Arai, K.; Lo, E.H.; Hommel, M. Pathophysiologic cascades in ischemic stroke. *Int. J. Stroke* **2012**, *7*, 378–385. [CrossRef]

59. Heusch, G.; Gersh, B.J. The pathophysiology of acute myocardial infarction and strategies of protection beyond reperfusion: A continual challenge. *Eur. Hear. J.* **2016**, *38*, 774–784. [CrossRef]

60. Kalogeris, T.; Baines, C.P.; Krenz, M.; Korthuis, R.J. Cell biology of ischemia/reperfusion injury. *Int. Rev. Cell Mol. Boil.* **2012**, *298*, 229–317. [CrossRef]

61. Yellon, D.M.; Hausenloy, D.J. Myocardial Reperfusion Injury. *N. Engl. J. Med.* **2007**, *357*, 1121–1135. [CrossRef]

62. Pegues, M.A.; McCrory, M.A.; Zarjou, A.; Szalai, A.J. C-reactive protein exacerbates renal ischemia-reperfusion injury. *Am. J. Physiol. Ren. Physiol.* **2013**, *304*, F1358–F1365. [CrossRef] [PubMed]

63. Valtchanova-Matchouganska, A.; Gondwe, M.; Nadar, A. The role of C-reactive protein in ischemia/reperfusion injury and preconditioning in a rat model of myocardial infarction. *Life Sci.* **2004**, *75*, 901–910. [CrossRef] [PubMed]

64. Stone, G.W.; Selker, H.P.; Thiele, H.; Patel, M.R.; Udelson, J.E.; Ohman, E.; Maehara, A.; Eitel, I.; Granger, C.B.; Jenkins, P.L.; et al. Relationship between Infarct Size and Outcomes Following Primary PCI. *J. Am. Coll. Cardiol.* **2016**, *67*, 1674–1683. [CrossRef]

65. De Waha, S.; Patel, M.R.; Granger, C.B.; Ohman, E.M.; Maehara, A.; Eitel, I.; Ben-Yehuda, O.; Jenkins, P.; Thiele, H.; Stone, G.W. Relationship between microvascular obstruction and adverse events following primary percutaneous coronary intervention for ST-segment elevation myocardial infarction: An individual patient data pooled analysis from seven randomized trials. *Eur. Hear. J.* **2017**, *38*, 3502–3510. [CrossRef]

66. Frangogiannis, N.G. Regulation of the Inflammatory Response in Cardiac Repair. *Circ. Res.* **2012**, *110*, 159–173. [CrossRef] [PubMed]

67. Danesh, J.; Wheeler, J.G.; Hirschfield, G.M.; Eda, S.; Eiriksdottir, G.; Rumley, A.; Lowe, G.D.O.; Pepys, M.B.; Gudnason, V. C-Reactive Protein and Other Circulating Markers of Inflammation in the Prediction of Coronary Heart Disease. *N. Engl. J. Med.* **2004**, *350*, 1387–1397. [CrossRef] [PubMed]

68. Koenig, W.; Sund, M.; Fröhlich, M.; Fischer, H.G.; Löwel, H.; Döring, A.; Hutchinson, W.L.; Pepys, M.B. C-Reactive protein, a sensitive marker of inflammation, predicts future risk of coronary heart disease in initially healthy middle-aged men: Results from the MONICA (Monitoring Trends and Determinants in Cardiovascular Disease) Augsburg Cohort Study, 1984 to 1992. *Circulation* **1999**, *99*, 237–242. [PubMed]

69. Verma, S.; Szmitko, P.E.; Ridker, P.M. C-reactive protein comes of age. *Nat. Clin. Pract. Neurol.* **2005**, *2*, 29–36. [CrossRef]

70. Beranek, J.T. C-reactive protein and complement in myocardial infarction and postinfarction heart failure. *Eur. Hear. J.* **1997**, *18*, 1834–1835. [CrossRef]

71. Liu, D.; Qi, X.; Li, Q.; Jia, W.; Wei, L.; Huang, A.; Liu, K.; Li, Z. Increased complements and high-sensitivity C-reactive protein predict heart failure in acute myocardial infarction. *Biomed. Rep.* **2016**, *5*, 761–765. [CrossRef]

72. Mani, P.; Puri, R.; Schwartz, G.G.; Nissen, S.E.; Shao, M.; Kastelein, J.J.P.; Menon, V.; Lincoff, A.M.; Nicholls, S.J. Association of Initial and Serial C-Reactive Protein Levels With Adverse Cardiovascular Events and Death After Acute Coronary Syndrome. *JAMA Cardiol.* **2019**, *4*, 314. [CrossRef] [PubMed]

73. Suleiman, M.; Khatib, R.; Agmon, Y.; Mahamid, R.; Boulos, M.; Kapeliovich, M.; Levy, Y.; Beyar, R.; Markiewicz, W.; Hammerman, H.; et al. Early Inflammation and Risk of Long-Term Development of Heart Failure and Mortality in Survivors of Acute Myocardial Infarction. *J. Am. Coll. Cardiol.* **2006**, *47*, 962–968. [CrossRef] [PubMed]

74. Stumpf, C.; Sheriff, A.; Zimmermann, S.; Schaefauer, L.; Schlundt, C.; Raaz, D.; Garlichs, C.D.; Achenbach, S. C-reactive protein levels predict systolic heart failure and outcome in patients with first ST-elevation myocardial infarction treated with coronary angioplasty. *Arch. Med. Sci.* **2017**, *5*, 1086–1093. [CrossRef]

75. Reindl, M.; Reinstadler, S.J.; Feistritzer, H.-J.; Klug, G.; Tiller, C.; Mair, J.; Mayr, A.; Jaschke, W.; Metzler, B. Relation of inflammatory markers with myocardial and microvascular injury in patients with reperfused ST-elevation myocardial infarction. *Eur. Hear. J. Acute Cardiovasc. Care* **2016**, *6*, 640–649. [CrossRef]

76. Mevorach, D.; Mascarenhas, J.O.; Gershov, D.; Elkon, K.B. Complement-dependent Clearance of Apoptotic Cells by Human Macrophages. *J. Exp. Med.* **1998**, *188*, 2313–2320. [CrossRef]

77. Lagrand, W.K.; Niessen, H.W.M.; Wolbink, G.-J.; Jaspars, L.H.; Visser, C.A.; Verheugt, F.W.; Meijer, C.J.; Hack, C.E. C-Reactive Protein Colocalizes With Complement in Human Hearts During Acute Myocardial Infarction. *Circulation* **1997**, *95*, 97–103. [CrossRef] [PubMed]

78. Barrett, T.D.; Hennan, J.K.; Marks, R.M.; Lucchesi, B.R. C-Reactive-Protein-Associated Increase in Myocardial Infarct Size after Ischemia/Reperfusion. *J. Pharmacol. Exp. Ther.* **2002**, *303*, 1007–1013. [CrossRef] [PubMed]

79. Krijnen, P.A.; Meischl, C.; Nijmeijer, R.; Visser, C.A.; Hack, C.E.; Niessen, H.W. Inhibition of sPLA2-IIA, C-reactive protein or complement: New therapy for patients with acute myocardial infarction? *Cardiovasc. Hematol. Disord. Drug Targets* **2006**, *6*, 113–123. [CrossRef]

80. Heinecke, J.W. Chemical knockout of C-reactive protein in cardiovascular disease. *Nat. Methods* **2006**, *2*, 300–301. [CrossRef]

81. Kitsis, R.N.; Jialal, I. Limiting Myocardial Damage during Acute Myocardial Infarction by Inhibiting C-Reactive Protein. *N. Engl. J. Med.* **2006**, *355*, 513–515. [CrossRef]

82. Virani, S.S.; Alonso, A.; Benjamin, E.J.; Bittencourt, M.S.; Callaway, C.W.; Carson, A.P.; Chamberlain, A.M.; Chang, A.R.; Cheng, S.; Delling, F.N.; et al. Heart Disease and Stroke Statistics—2020 Update: A Report From the American Heart Association. *Circulation* **2020**, *141*, e139–e596. [CrossRef]

83. Catanese, L.; Tarsia, J.; Fisher, M. Acute Ischemic Stroke Therapy Overview. *Circ. Res.* **2017**, *120*, 541–558. [CrossRef] [PubMed]

84. Anrather, J.; Iadecola, C. Inflammation and Stroke: An Overview. *Neurotherapeutics* **2016**, *13*, 661–670. [CrossRef] [PubMed]

85. Muir, K.W.; Tyrrell, P.; Sattar, N.; Warburton, E. Inflammation and ischaemic stroke. *Curr. Opin. Neurol.* **2007**, *20*, 334–342. [CrossRef] [PubMed]

86. Montaner, J.; Fernández-Cadenas, I.; Molina, C.A.; Ribo, M.; Huertas, R.; Rosell, A.; Penalba, A.; Ortega, L.; Chacoón, P.; Álvarez-Sabín, J. Poststroke C-Reactive Protein Is a Powerful Prognostic Tool Among Candidates for Thrombolysis. *Stroke* **2006**, *37*, 1205–1210. [CrossRef]

87. Winbeck, K.; Poppert, H.; Etgen, T.; Conrad, B.; Sander, D. Prognostic relevance of early serial C-reactive protein measurements after first ischemic stroke. *Stroke* **2002**, *33*, 2459–2464. [CrossRef]

88.   Arenillas, J.F.; Álvarez-Sabín, J.; Molina, C.A.; Chacoón, P.; Montaner, J.; Rovira, A.; Ibarra, B.; Quintana, M. C-Reactive Protein Predicts Further Ischemic Events in First-Ever Transient Ischemic Attack or Stroke Patients with Intracranial Large-Artery Occlusive Disease. *Stroke* **2003**, *34*, 2463–2468. [CrossRef]

89.   Di Napoli, M.; Papa, F.; Bocola, V. Prognostic Influence of Increased C-Reactive Protein and Fibrinogen Levels in Ischemic Stroke. *Stroke* **2001**, *32*, 133–138. [CrossRef]

90.   Elkind, M.S.V.; Tai, W.; Coates, K.; Paik, M.C.; Sacco, R.L. High-Sensitivity C-Reactive Protein, Lipoprotein-Associated Phospholipase A2, and Outcome After Ischemic Stroke. *Arch. Intern. Med.* **2006**, *166*, 2073–2080. [CrossRef]

91.   Woodward, M.; Lowe, G.D.; Campbell, D.J.; Colman, S.; Rumley, A.; Chalmers, J.P.; Neal, B.C.; Patel, A.; Jenkins, A.J.; E Kemp, B.; et al. Associations of Inflammatory and Hemostatic Variables with the Risk of Recurrent Stroke. *Stroke* **2005**, *36*, 2143–2147. [CrossRef]

92.   Muir, K.W.; Weir, C.J.; Alwan, W.; Squire, I.B.; Lees, K.R. C-reactive protein and outcome after ischemic stroke. *Stroke* **1999**, *30*, 981–985. [CrossRef] [PubMed]

93.   Ringleb, P.A.; Bousser, M.-G.; Ford, G.; Bath, P.; Brainin, M.; Caso, V.; Cervera, Á.; Chamorro, A.; Cordonnier, C.; Csiba, L.; et al. Ischaemic Stroke and Transient Ischaemic Attack. In *European Handbook of Neurological Management*; Wiley: Hoboken, NJ, USA, 2010; pp. 101–158.

94.   Kayser, S.; Kunze, R.; Sheriff, A. Selective C-reactive protein apheresis for Covid-19 patients suffering from organ damage. *Ther. Apher. Dial.* **2020**. [CrossRef] [PubMed]

95.   Di Napoli, M.; Schwaninger, M.; Cappelli, R.; Ceccarelli, E.; Di Gianfilippo, G.; Donati, C.; Emsley, H.; Forconi, S.; Hopkins, S.J.; Masotti, L.; et al. Evaluation of C-Reactive Protein Measurement for Assessing the Risk and Prognosis in Ischemic Stroke. *Stroke* **2005**, *36*, 1316–1329. [CrossRef] [PubMed]

96.   Peters, S.A.E.; Visseren, F.L.; Grobbee, D.E. Screening for C-reactive protein in CVD prediction. *Nat. Rev. Cardiol.* **2012**, *10*, 12–14. [CrossRef] [PubMed]

97.   Kuhlmann, C.R.; Librizzi, L.; Closhen, D.; Pflanzner, T.; Lessmann, V.; Pietrzik, C.U.; De Curtis, M.; Luhmann, H.J. Mechanisms of C-Reactive Protein-Induced Blood–Brain Barrier Disruption. *Stroke* **2009**, *40*, 1458–1466. [CrossRef]

98.   Elwood, E.; Lim, Z.; Naveed, H.; Galea, I. The effect of systemic inflammation on human brain barrier function. *Brain Behav. Immun.* **2017**, *62*, 35–40. [CrossRef]

99.   Lasek-Bal, A.; Jedrzejowska-Szypulka, H.; Student, S.; Warsz-Wianecka, A.; Zareba, K.; Puz, P.; Bal, W.; Pawletko, K.; Lewin-Kowalik, J. The importance of selected markers of inflammation and blood-brain barrier damage for short-term ischemic stroke prognosis. *J. Psysiol. Pharmacol.* **2019**, *70*, 209–217.

100. Khandkar, C.; Vaidya, K.; Patel, S. Colchicine for Stroke Prevention: A Systematic Review and Meta-analysis. *Clin. Ther.* **2019**, *41*, 582–590.e3. [CrossRef]

101. Dove, A. CD18 trials disappoint again. *Nat. Biotechnol.* **2000**, *18*, 817–818. [CrossRef]

102. Pawluk, H.; Woźniak, A.; Grześk, G.; Kołodziejska, R.; Kozakiewicz, M.; Kopkowska, E.; Grzechowiak, E.; Kozera, G. The Role of Selected Pro-Inflammatory Cytokines in Pathogenesis of Ischemic Stroke. *Clin. Interv. Aging* **2020**, *15*, 469–484. [CrossRef]

103. Mizuma, A.; Yenari, M.A. Anti-Inflammatory Targets for the Treatment of Reperfusion Injury in Stroke. *Front. Neurol.* **2017**, *8*, 467. [CrossRef] [PubMed]

104. Drieu, A.; Levard, D.; Vivien, D.; Rubio, M. Anti-inflammatory treatments for stroke: From bench to bedside. *Ther. Adv. Neurol. Disord.* **2018**, *11*, 1756286418789854. [CrossRef] [PubMed]

105. Roberts, R.; Demello, V.; Sobel, B.E. Deleterious effects of methylprednisolone in patients with myocardial infarction. *Circulation* **1976**, *53*, 204–206.

4

The Expanding Role of Ketogenic Diets in Adult Neurological Disorders

Tanya J. W. McDonald and Mackenzie C. Cervenka *

Department of Neurology, Johns Hopkins University School of Medicine, 600 North Wolfe Street, Meyer 2-147, Baltimore, MD 21287, USA; twill145@jhmi.edu
* Correspondence: mcerven1@jhmi.edu

Abstract: The current review highlights the evidence supporting the use of ketogenic diet therapies in the management of adult epilepsy, adult malignant glioma and Alzheimer's disease. An overview of the scientific literature, both preclinical and clinical, in each area is presented and management strategies for addressing adverse effects and compliance are discussed.

Keywords: modified Atkins diet; epilepsy; glioblastoma multiforme; malignant glioma; Alzheimer's disease

1. Introduction

The ketogenic diet (KD) was formally introduced into practice in the 1920s although the origins of ketogenic medicine may date back to ancient Greece [1]. This high-fat, low-carbohydrate diet induces ketone body production in the liver through fat metabolism with the goal of mimicking a starvation state without depriving the body of necessary calories to sustain growth and development [2,3]. The ketone bodies acetoacetate and β-hydroxybutyrate then enter the bloodstream and are taken up by organs including the brain where they are further metabolized in mitochondria to generate energy for cells within the nervous system. The ketone body acetone, produced by spontaneous decarboxylation of acetoacetate, is rapidly eliminated through the lungs and urine. The classic KD is typically composed of a macronutrient ratio of 4:1 (4 g of fat to every 1 g of protein plus carbohydrates combined), thus shifting the predominant caloric source from carbohydrate to fat. Lower ratios of 3:1, 2:1, or 1:1 (referred to as a modified ketogenic diet) can be used depending on age, individual tolerability, level of ketosis and protein requirements [4]. To increase flexibility and palatability, more 'relaxed' variants have been developed, including the modified Atkins diet (MAD), the low glycemic index treatment (LGIT) and the ketogenic diet combined with medium chain triglyceride oil (MCT). Introduced in 2003, the MAD typically employs a net 10–20 g/day carbohydrate limit which is roughly equivalent to a ratio of 1–2:1 of fat to protein plus carbohydrates [5,6]. The LGIT recommends 40–60 g daily of carbohydrates with the selection of foods with glycemic indices <50 and ~60% of dietary energy derived from fat and 20–30% from protein [7]. The primary goal of this diet, primarily used in children, is not to induce metabolic ketosis and will not be further explored in this review. The MCT variant KD uses medium-chain fatty acids provided in coconut and/or palm kernel oil as a diet supplement and allows for greater carbohydrate and protein intake than even a lower-ratio classic KD [8], which can improve compliance. While there is an extensive literature documenting the use of KDs for weight loss and epilepsy [9,10], these diets have garnered increased interest as potential treatments of other diet-sensitive neurological disorders. The aim of the current review is to describe the evidence, preclinical and clinical, supporting KD use in the management of adult epilepsy, adult malignant gliomas and Alzheimer's disease. Several randomized controlled trials support the use of KDs for the treatment of drug-resistant epilepsy and there is emerging evidence that these diets may also be effective in treating refractory status epilepticus, malignant glioma and Alzheimer's disease in adults.

2. KDs in the Management of Adult Epilepsy and Refractory Seizures

Despite being first recognized as an effective tool in the treatment of epilepsy in the 1920s [11,12], interest in diet therapy subsequently waned following the introduction of anti-epileptic drugs (AEDs) until the 1990s. Studies and clinical trials emerged demonstrating its efficacy in patients with drug-resistant epilepsy and particular pediatric epilepsy syndromes [11–13]. In the management of drug-resistant epilepsy (seizures resistant to two or more appropriate AEDs), adult patients have a less than 5% chance of seizure freedom with additional drugs added and may not be surgical candidates due to a generalized epilepsy, multifocal nature, or non-resectable seizure focus [14,15]. Seizures that evolve into status epilepticus (prolonged seizure lasting longer than 5 minutes or recurrent seizures without return to baseline between seizures) despite appropriate first- and second-line AEDs are classified as refractory status epilepticus (RSE). If status epilepticus continues or recurs 24 h or more after the initiation of treatment with anesthetic agents to induce burst- or seizure-suppression, patients are diagnosed with super-refractory status epilepticus (SRSE) [16]. Growing preclinical and clinical evidence suggests that KDs can offer seizure reduction and seizure freedom in patients with drug-resistant epilepsy and status epilepticus through a variety of potential mechanisms.

There has been controversy over whether the major ketone bodies produced by the liver are responsible for the anti-seizure effect of the KD primarily due to the clinical observation that blood ketone (i.e., β-hydroxybutyrate) levels inconsistently correlate with seizure control amongst studies [17–21], although findings may relate to diet heterogeneity and methodological differences between studies. In addition, ketone levels at the neuronal or synaptic level may be a more accurate reflection of ketone effects on excitability [22] as opposed to systemic concentrations. As recently reviewed [23], an increasing number of compelling experimental studies highlight pleiotropic anti-seizure and neuroprotective actions of ketones. Such effects include ketone-induced changes in neurotransmitter balance and release as well as changes in neural membrane polarity to dampen the increased neuronal excitability associated with seizures. In rat models of epilepsy, acetoacetate and β-hydroxybutyrate increased the accumulation of γ-aminobutyric acid (GABA) in presynaptic vessels [24]. Ketotic rats, moreover, exhibit lower levels of glutamate in neurons but stable amounts of GABA, suggesting a shift in the total balance of neurotransmitters towards inhibition [25]. Supporting these pre-clinical data, humans maintained on a KD showed increased GABA levels in the cerebrospinal fluid and in brain using magnetic resonance spectroscopy [26,27]. Ketones can slow spontaneous neuronal firing in cultured mouse hippocampal neurons by opening adenosine tri-phosphate (ATP)-sensitive potassium channels [28,29]. Medium chain fatty acids, like decanoic acid, have also exhibited efficacy in *in vitro* and *in vivo* models of seizure activity. Decanoic acid application blocked seizure-like activity in hippocampal slices treated with pentetrazol and increased seizure thresholds in animal models of acute seizures using both the 6 Hz stimulation test (a model of drug-resistant seizures) and the maximal electroshock test (a model of tonic-clonic seizures), potentially through a mechanism involving selective inhibition of AMPA receptors [30–32].

Moreover, there may also be an additional neuroprotective benefit of ketogenic therapies related to improved mitochondrial function due to increased energy reserves combined with decreased production of reactive oxygen species (ROS) [33]. For example, the KD has been shown to stimulate mitochondrial biogenesis, increase cerebral ATP concentrations, and result in lower ROS production in animal models [34,35]. Animal models have similarly demonstrated that the KD may influence seizures associated with the mammalian target of rapamycin (mTOR) pathway, as rats fed a KD showed reduced insulin levels and reduced phosphorylation of Akt and S6, suggesting decreased mTOR activation and increased AMP-activated protein kinase signaling [36,37]. Ketone reduction of oxidative stress may occur via genomic effects, as ketone application in *in vitro* models inhibits histone deactylases (HDACs) resulting in increased transcriptional activity of peroxisome proliferator-activated receptor (PPAR) γ and upregulation of genes including the antioxidants catalase, mitochondrial superoxide dismutase and metallothionein 2 [38,39]. Lastly, there is emerging evidence that ketone bodies exhibit protective anti-inflammatory effects [40]. In animal models, KD treatment reduces microglial activation, expression of pro-inflammatory cytokines and pain and inflammation after thermal nociception [41–43]. Similar experimental work in non-epilepsy models suggested that ketone body anti-inflammatory effects may be mediated by hydroxy-carboxylic acid receptor 2 (HCA2) and/or inhibition of the innate immune sensor NOD-like receptor 3 (NLRP3) inflammasome [23,43,44]. These anti-inflammatory properties may explain the observed benefit of KD in treating patients with SRSE secondary to auto-immune and presumed auto-immune encephalitis such as those with new-onset refractory status epilepticus (NORSE) and febrile infection-related epilepsy syndrome (FIRES) [45].

In contrast to the aforementioned studies highlighting mechanisms mediated largely by ketones, recent preclinical work suggests the anti-seizure properties bestowed by KDs may instead relate to modulation of gut microbiota. The KD has been shown to alter the composition of gut microbiota in mice and ketosis is associated with altered gut microbiota in humans [46–49]. Studies using two mouse models of epilepsy (6 Hz stimulation test and mice harboring a null mutation in the alpha subunit of voltage-gated potassium channel Kv1.1) demonstrate that KD induced changes in gut microbiota, produced by feeding or fecal transplant, are necessary and sufficient to confer seizure protection. The effect appears to be mediated by select microbial interactions that reduce bacterial gamma-glutamylation activity, decrease peripheral gamma-glutamylated-amino acids and elevate bulk hippocampal GABA/glutamate ratios [50]. As rodent studies have shown different taxonomic shifts in response to KD therapy, the gut microbiota induced by KDs will depend on host genetics and baseline metabolic profiles [46,50]. Further research is needed to determine effects of the KD on microbiome profiles in adults with drug-resistant epilepsy and whether particular taxonomic changes in gut microbiota correlate with seizure severity and response to therapy.

A surge of clinical studies since the turn of the century support KD use in the management of chronic epilepsy in adults, with most reporting efficacy defined by the proportion of patients achieving ≥50% seizure reduction (defined as responders). A 2011 review pooled data from seven studies of the classic KD to show that 49% of 206 patients had ≥50% seizure reduction and, of these, 13% were seizure-free [51]. A 2015 meta-analysis reviewing ketogenic dietary treatments in adults from 12 studies of the classic KD, the MAD and the classic KD in combination with MCT found efficacy rates of KDs in drug-resistant epilepsy ranged from 13–70% with a combined efficacy rate of 52% for the classic KD and 34% for the MAD [52]. In the largest observational study of 101 adult patients naïve to diet therapy who subsequently started the MAD, 39% had ≥50% seizure reduction and 22% became seizure-free following 3 months of treatment [53]. Based on intention-to-treat (ITT) data from observational studies to date, the classic KD reduces seizures by ≥50% in 22–70% of patients while the MAD reduces seizures by ≥50% in 12–67% of patients [52,54,55], with some suggestion that dietary intervention may be more effective in patients with generalized rather than focal epilepsy [56,57].

Two randomized controlled trials (RCTs) evaluating MAD efficacy in adults with drug-resistant epilepsy have been reported recently. The first RCT in Iran compared the proportion of patients with focal or generalized epilepsy achieving ≥50% seizure reduction between 34 patients randomized to MAD use for 2 months (of whom 22 completed the study) compared to 32 control patients and found 35.5% (12/34) efficacy in the MAD group (ITT analysis) at 2 months compared to 0% in the control group [58]. These findings are in line with reports from meta-analyses of observational studies using MAD in adults [52]. The second RCT in Norway compared the change in seizure frequency following intervention in patients with drug-resistant (who had tried ≥3 AEDs) focal or multifocal epilepsy randomized to either 12 weeks of MAD (37 patients, of whom 28 received the intervention and 24 completed the study) or their habitual diet (38 patients, of whom 34 received the intervention and 32 completed the study) [59]. While they found no statistically significant difference in seizure frequency nor in 50% responder rate between the two groups following the intervention, a significant reduction in seizure frequency in the diet group compared to controls was observed among patients who completed the study but only for moderate benefit (25–50% seizure reduction). Importantly, compared to the patient population in the Iranian RCT with roughly half generalized and focal epilepsy patients (length of epilepsy 14–17 years on average, 6–9 mean seizures per month and had tried on average 3–4 AEDs), the Norwegian study investigated MAD treatment in adults with solely focal epilepsy who were particularly drug-resistant (length of epilepsy more than 20 years on average, with a median of 15 seizures per month and had tried on average 9–10 AEDs) and did note an improvement in overall seizure severity in the diet group, as measured by the Liverpool Seizure Severity Scale [58,59]. Additional RCTs of larger sample size are warranted to investigate MAD efficacy in different subpopulations of adult epilepsy patients.

Several case reports and case series have also demonstrated the successful use of KD therapy for management of RSE and SRSE [60–64]. For example, a case series of 10 adults with SRSE of median duration 21.5 days treated with a KD (either 4:1 or 3:1 ratio KD) showed successful cessation of status epilepticus in 100% of patients who achieved ketosis (9 out of 10 adults) at a median of 3 days (range 1–31 days) [65]. In the largest phase I/II clinical trial of 15 adult patients treated with a 4:1 ratio KD (14 of whom completed therapy) after a median of 10 days of SRSE, 11 (79% of patients who completed KD therapy, 73% of all patients enrolled) achieved resolution of seizures in a median of 5 days (range 0–10 days) [66]. As both RSE and SRSE carry high rates of morbidity and mortality [67], KDs offer a needed adjunctive strategy for management. KDs have the potential advantages of working rapidly and synergistically with other concurrent treatments; are relatively easy to start, monitor and maintain in the controlled intensive care unit setting with close follow up; do not contribute to hemodynamic instability seen with anesthetic agents and could potentially reduce the need for prolonged use of anesthetic drugs.

3. KDs in the Management of Adult Malignant Gliomas

Malignant gliomas are a highly heterogeneous tumor, refractory to treatment and the most frequently diagnosed primary brain tumor. Glioblastoma multiforme (GBM), the most aggressive type of glioma, carries an exceptionally poor prognosis with a median overall survival duration between 12 and 15 months from time of diagnosis and a 5-year survival rate of less than 5% [68,69]. The current standard of care for treating patients with GBM consists of maximal safe resection, followed by radiotherapy and concurrent chemotherapy with temozolomide [69]. Additional therapeutic strategies include glucocorticoid management of peritumoral edema and anti-angiogenic treatment with bevacicumab (Avastin); however therapeutic progress, particularly in regard to overall survival, remains poor [70]. Emerging research efforts over the past two decades seek to exploit a known cancer hallmark of abnormal energy metabolism in tumor cells named the "Warburg effect" following the discovery of physician, biochemist and Nobel laureate Otto Warburg that tumors exhibit high rates of aerobic glycolysis followed by predominant fermentation of pyruvate to lactate despite sufficient oxygen availability [71,72]. This metabolic phenotype confers several potential advantages to the cancer cell that include (1) more efficient generation of carbon equivalents for macromolecular synthesis; (2) bypassed mitochondrial oxidative metabolism and its concurrent production of reactive oxygen species and (3) acidification of the tumor site to facilitate invasion and progression [73]. As a result of this metabolic alteration, malignant glioma cells critically depend on glucose as the main energy source to survive and sustain their aggressive proliferative properties [74]. Moreover, clinical findings have identified hyperglycemia as a negative predictor of overall survival and a marker of poor prognosis in patients with GBM [75–78]. These findings have prompted nutritional strategies to target glycemic modulation using KDs, caloric restriction, intermittent fasting and combinatorial diet protocols broadly classified as ketogenic metabolic therapy.

Numerous preclinical studies have investigated KDs and/or exogenous supplementation of ketones or ketogenic agents in the treatment of malignant glioma. In the CT-2A malignant mouse astrocytoma model, a calorie-restricted KD decreased plasma glucose, plasma insulin-like growth factor and tumor weight when administered as a stand-alone therapy and elicited potent synergistic anti-cancer effects when administered in combination with glycolytic inhibitor 2-deoxy-D-glucose (2-DG) [79,80]. In the GL-261 malignant glioma model, KD fed mice had reduced peritumoral edema and tumor microvasculature, 20–30% increased median survival time and achieved complete and long-term remission when used concomitantly with radiation therapy [81–83]. A similar synergistic effect was observed between KD and temozolomide in the GL-261 model [84]. Comparable effects of KDs on tumor growth and survival time have also been shown in glioma derived mouse models of metastatic cancer and in patient-derived GBM subcutaneous and orthotopic implantation models [85,86]. These and other studies suggest that KDs induce a metabolic shift in malignant brain tissue towards a pro-apoptotic, anti-angiogenic, anti-invasive and anti-inflammatory state accompanied by a marked reduction in tumor growth in vivo [70] via mechanisms that include:

(1)   Reduction in blood glucose and insulin growth factor-1 levels [79];
(2)   Attenuated insulin activated Akt/mTOR and Ras/mitogen-activated protein kinase (MAPK) signaling pathways [87,88];
(3)   Induction of genes involved in oxidative stress protection and elimination of ROS through histone deactylase inhibition and altered expression of genes related to angiogenesis, vascular remodeling, invasion potential and the hypoxic response [38,82,84];
(4)   Enhanced cytotoxic T cell anti-tumor immunity [89]; and
(5)   Reduced inflammation via ketone body inhibition of the NLRP3 inflammasome and a reduction in other circulating inflammatory markers [43,90].

The first published case report in 2010 of an adult female patient with newly diagnosed GBM treated with a calorie restricted KD concomitant with standard care (radiation plus chemotherapy) following partial surgical resection demonstrated no tumor detection using fluorodeoxyglucose positron emission tomography (FDG-PET) and magnetic resonance imaging (MRI) after two months of treatment. However, after discontinuing diet therapy, tumor recurrence was detected 10 weeks later [91]. Subsequently a retrospective review reported 6 adult patients with newly diagnosed GBM treated with a KD, 4 of whom were alive at a median follow-up of 14 months and demonstrated reduced mean glucose compared to patients on a regular diet but only one patient was without evidence of disease for 12 months at the time of publication [92]. In another case report of 2 adult patients with recurrent GBM treated with a 3:1 calorie-restricted KD, both patients showed evidence of tumor progression by 12 weeks [93]. In the largest pilot trial, of 20 adult patients with recurrent GBM treated with a ≤60 g/day carbohydrate restricted diet, 3 discontinued because of poor tolerability, 3 had stable disease after 6 weeks that lasted 11–13 weeks and 1 had a minor response, with an overall trend towards an increase in progression-free survival in patients with stable ketosis [94]. A more recent case report documented an adult patient with newly diagnosed GBM who continued to experience significant tumor regression 24 months following combined treatment with subtotal resection, calorie restricted KD, hyperbaric oxygen and other targeted metabolic therapies [95]. These early observational, pilot studies and case reports principally provide evidence of feasibility and short-term safety as no serious adverse events were reported. Although they suggest a role for KDs in the management of GBM substantiated by an array of preclinical studies, given study design heterogeneity particularly in regard to diet formulation and calorie restriction, paucity of control groups and differences in endpoints, no conclusive statistical analysis of the clinical impact of KDs on adult GBM patient outcomes can be made. Consequently, a growing scientific interest has led to an increased number of registered clinical trials, including 4 randomized controlled trials (NCT02302235, NCT01754350, NCT01865162 and NCT03075514) of KDs (compared to a standard diet or between two KD types) in the management of adult GBM, 2 of which also include caloric restriction and a primary outcome of overall survival or progression-free survival [70,96].

4. KDs in the Management of Alzheimer's Disease

In Alzheimer's disease (AD), the most common form of progressive dementia, loss of recent memory and cognitive deficits are associated with extracellular deposition of amyloid-β peptide, intracellular tau protein neurofibrillary tangles and hippocampal neuronal death. Theories vary regarding the etiology of the overall disease process but mitochondrial dysfunction and glucose hypometabolism are recognized biochemical hallmarks [97]. Defects in mitochondrial function and a decline in respiratory chain function alter amyloid precursor protein (APP) processing to favor the production of the pathogenic amyloid-β fragment [98]. Reduced uptake and metabolism of glucose have been strongly linked to progressive cognitive degeneration, as neurons starve due to inefficient glycolysis [99]. Moreover, FDG-PET studies find asymptomatic individuals with genetic risk for AD or a positive family history show less prefrontal cortex, posterior cingulate, entorhinal cortex and hippocampal glucose uptake than normal-risk individuals. This reduction is associated with downregulation of the glucose transporter GLUT1 in the brain of individuals with AD [40,100]. Increasing evidence has demonstrated an association between high-glycemic diet and greater cerebral amyloid burden in humans [101] and that increased insulin resistance contributes to the development of sporadic AD [102,103], suggesting diet as a potential modifiable behavior to prevent cerebral amyloid accumulation and reduce AD risk.

Preclinical work supports the role of ketogenic therapies to prevent or ameliorate histological and biochemical changes related to Alzheimer's disease pathology. *In vitro* studies showed attenuation of deleterious amyloid-β induced effects on rat cortical neurons by pre-treatment with coconut oil (containing high concentrations of MCT) or medium chain fatty acids via activation of Akt and extracellular-signal-regulated kinase (ERK) signaling pathways [104]. Similarly, preclinical studies using animal models of dementia demonstrated reduced brain amyloid-β levels, protection from amyloid-β toxicity and better mitochondrial function following administration of the KD, ketones and MCT [105–108]. Importantly, ketone body suppression of mitochondrial amyloid entry has been further shown to improve learning and memory ability in a symptomatic mouse model of AD [109]. In aged rats, a KD administered for 3 weeks improved learning and memory and was associated with increased angiogenesis and capillary density suggesting the KD may support cognition through improved vascular function [110]. In summary, these preclinical observations provide insight into potential mechanisms through which KDs and ketones may influence AD risk and pathology and lay the foundation for subsequent studies in humans.

In the first randomized controlled trial in humans, 20 patients with AD or mild cognitive impairment (MCI) received a single oral dose of either MCT or placebo on separate days and demonstrated expected elevations in serum ketone level following ingestion but only patients without the Apolipoprotein E (APOE) ε4 allele showed enhanced short-term cognitive performance on a brief screening tool measuring cognitive domains that included attention, memory, language and praxis [111]. This study was later replicated with similar improvements in working memory, visual attention and task switching seen in 19 elderly patients without dementia who received the MCT supplement [112]. Another RCT in adults with MCI treated with either a very low (5–10%) or high (50%) carbohydrate diet over 6 weeks showed an improvement in verbal memory performance that correlated with ketone levels in the ketogenic diet group [113]. A 2015 case report suggested that regular ketone monoester ((R)-3-hydroxybutyl (R)-3-hydroxybutyrate) supplementation, rather than a change to habitual diet, produced repeated diurnal elevations in circulating serum β-hydroxybutyrate levels and improved cognitive and daily activity performance over a 20-month period [114]. A single-arm pilot trial in 15 patients with mild-moderate AD using an MCT-supplemented ≥ 1:1 ratio KD for 3 months showed an improved Alzheimer's disease Assessment Scale –cognitive subscale score in 9 out of 10 patients who completed the study and achieved ketosis (as measured by elevated serum β-hydroxybutyrate levels at follow-up) [115]. Three additional studies in patients with MCI or mild-moderate AD using at least 3-month treatment protocols (2 randomized studies of MCT or a ketogenic product compared to placebo for 3–6 months and 1 observational study administering a ketogenic meal over 3 months) reported that the cognitive benefit of ketogenic therapies was greatest in patients who did not have the APOE ε4 allele [116,117] and, in the observational study, was limited to APOE ε4 negative patients with mild AD [118]. A recent study of patients with mild-moderate AD treated with 1 month of MCT supplements demonstrated increased ketone consumption, quantified by brain ^{11}C-acetoacetate PET imaging before and after administration, suggesting ketones from MCT can compensate for the brain glucose deficit observed in AD [119]. The clinical evidence lends support for the use of KDs and/or supplements to improve cognitive outcomes in patients with AD, however results indicate that stage/level of disease progression and APOE ε4 genotype may affect response to dietary treatment. Ongoing registered randomized clinical trials sponsored by Johns Hopkins University (NCT02521818), Wake Forest University (NCT03130036, NCT03472664 and NCT02984540), Université de Sherbrooke (NCT02709356) and the University of British Columbia (NCT02912936) are underway (active, recruiting, or completed) in individuals with subjective memory impairment, mild AD, and/or healthy controls to evaluate the impact of:

(1) 6–18 weeks of a modified Ketogenic-Mediterranean diet compared to a low-fat diet;
(2) 12 weeks of MAD compared to a recommended diet for seniors to achieve a healthy eating index;
(3) 1 month treatment with two different MCT oil emulsions (60–40 oil or C8 oil); or
(4) 10 days, twice a day, supplementation with a lactose-free skim milk drink containing either 10–50 g/day of MCT oil or 10–50 g/day of placebo (high-oleic sunflower oil)

On primary outcomes that include brain acetoacetate/glucose metabolism using PET, AD biomarkers, level of serum ketones, safety and feasibility as well as secondary outcomes that include cognition, function and examining key treatment response variables such as APOE genotype, amyloid positivity and metabolic status that could inform precision medicine approaches to dietary prescription.

5. Management of Adverse Effects and Poor Compliance in Adults

The most commonly reported adverse effects associated with KD use in adults with epilepsy and long-term diet use in children with epilepsy are gastrointestinal effects, weight loss and a transient increase in lipids [120,121]. Similar side effects have been reported in clinical studies of KD use in malignant glioma and AD, although a true assessment of risk in these populations is difficult due to the small number of trials, short duration of follow up and heterogeneity in KD therapy applied [70,122]. The gastrointestinal side effects which include constipation, diarrhea and occasional nausea and vomiting are typically mild, improve with time, can often be managed with diet adjustments with the guidance of a dietitian or nutritionist and infrequently require medical intervention. Smaller meals, increased fiber intake, exercise and increased sodium and fluid intake can often prevent or alleviate these complaints. Weight loss may be an intended positive effect in patients who are overweight but for those who want to maintain or gain weight, adjustments in caloric intake are recommended. This is of particular importance in patients with malignant glioma as the development of cachexia, due to weight loss principally affecting skeletal muscle mass, is associated with decreased cancer therapy tolerance and impaired respiratory function, leading to lower survival rates [123]. Increases in serum lipids have been shown to normalize with continued diet therapy (after 1 year) or return to normal after cessation of diet therapy in adult epilepsy patients [57,124,125]. In addition, very low carbohydrate diets that induce ketosis have been shown to lead to reductions in serum triglycerides, low-density lipoprotein and total cholesterol and increased levels of high-density lipoprotein cholesterol in adults [9]. Other potential side effects can result from vitamin and mineral deficiencies secondary to restricting carbohydrates and prolonged ketonemia, including osteopenia and osteoporosis [3,126,127], although the precise mechanism remains unclear. The standard practice of supplementing a recommended daily allowance of multivitamin and mineral supplements can reduce the risk of such deficiencies.

Diet adherence and compliance remain significant barriers to successful implementation and an adequate assessment of KD efficacy. Common methodologies to assess and document KD adherence in adults beyond patient self-report include frequent measurements of serum β-hydroxybutyrate or urine acetoacetate concentrations during the first few weeks on the diet and/or collection of dietary food records [57,121,128]. As examples, daily urine ketone assessments are traditionally used in adults with epilepsy during MAD initiation until moderate to large levels of ketosis are reached and serum ketone assessments using drops of blood from a finger stick have been used to guide short-term KD therapy in patients with GBM [53,128]. Still, the majority of studies traditionally report adherence based on patient self-report. A combined adherence rate of 45% for all KD types, 38% for the classic KD and 56% for the MAD, has been reported in a review of the epilepsy literature [52]. In the largest observational study of 139 adult epilepsy patients treated with KDs, 48% (67/139) discontinued the diet (39%) or were lost after initial follow up (9%) with approximately half of patients citing difficulty with compliance or restrictiveness as the reason for stopping [53]. The literature of adherence rates in adult GBM and AD is sparse but growing, with the largest GBM study reporting 15% (3/20) drop-out after 2–3 weeks due to subjectively decreased quality of life [94] and a recent 3 month single-arm AD pilot trial of a MCT-supplemented KD reporting 33% (5/15) attrition due to caregiver burden [115]. Often the provision of food recipes and resources to patients and families during initial diet training and subsequent visits can emphasize the variety of food choices and ease of use rather than perceived restrictiveness. Additional methods to improve adherence and compliance, as well as access for patients who live distant from a KD center, include scheduled telephone calls or electronic communication with the supervising dietitian or nutritionist, provision of ketogenic supplements and use of electronic applications like KetoDietCalculator^{TM} (The Charlie Foundation for Ketogenic Therapies, Santa Monica, CA, USA) to prevent drop-out and emphasize progress and success [6,129].

6. Conclusions

Although the neurological conditions discussed in this review-epilepsy, malignant glioma and Alzheimer's disease—have distinct disease processes, each exhibit disrupted energy metabolism, increased oxidative stress and neuro-inflammation. As each of these pathophysiologic factors can be influenced through diet manipulation, it is logical and reasonable that diet could alter the course and outcomes of these and other neurologic disorders that share common pathways. Extensive preclinical work supports the use of KDs and/or ketone bodies to thwart or ameliorate histological and biochemical changes leading to neurologic dysfunction and disease. Demonstrated and hypothesized mechanisms by which ketogenic therapies influence epilepsy, malignant glioma and Alzheimer's disease include metabolic regulation, neurotransmission modulation, reduced oxidative stress and anti-inflammatory and genomic effects that were highlighted in this review and summarized in Table 1. In some instances, an understanding of the mechanisms by which the KD and ketones exert their effects has led to novel therapeutic targets and work to develop new pharmaceutical drugs [130]. For many disorders, the clinical literature is still growing and limited by the conditions that make dietary interventions difficult to evaluate. For example, evaluation of whole diet changes cannot be performed under blinded circumstances as the participant will be aware of the diet changes made and/or the content of their meals. Other methodological constraints relate to limitations in inter-study comparison due to the heterogeneity of diet intervention used and reduced statistical power to detect significant effects when baseline levels of nutrient intake and individual variability are appropriately controlled. There are also challenges in monitoring diet compliance in the ambulatory setting as adherence to a prescribed diet can be more difficult to achieve than with a traditional pharmaceutical intervention. However, dietary interventions have the advantage of being non-invasive, relatively low risk and generally without serious adverse effects in the appropriate clinical context and may be particularly useful as an adjunctive therapy that synergizes with other pharmacologic and non-pharmacologic approaches. The scientific evidence collected from clinical studies in humans to date has supported KD therapy use in adult epilepsy, adult malignant glioma and Alzheimer's disease, although overall assessment of efficacy remains limited due to study heterogeneity and indications that particular patient subpopulations may achieve disparate levels of benefit. Further clinical investigation using more standardized KD protocols and in patient subpopulations is warranted.

Table 1. Hypothesized mechanisms through which ketogenic therapies influence neurological disease.

Ketogenic Mechanisms	Epilepsy	Malignant Glioma	Alzheimer's Disease
Metabolic Regulation			
↓Glucose uptake & glycolysis	+	+	
↓Insulin, IGF1 signaling		+	+
↑Ketones/ketone metabolism	+		+
Altered gut microbiota	+		
Neurotransmission			
Altered balance of excitatory/inhibitory neurotransmitters	+		
Inhibition of AMPA receptors	+		
↓mTOR activation & signaling	+	+	
Modulation of ATP-sensitive potassium channels	+		
Oxidative Stress			
↓Production of reactive oxygen species	+	+	
↑Mitochondrial biogenesis/function	+		+
Inflammation/Neuroprotection			
↓Inflammatory cytokines	+	+	
NLRP3 inflammasome inhibition	+	+	
↑cytotoxic T cell function		+	
↓peritumoral edema		+	
↓amyloid-β levels			+
Genomic Effects			
Inhibition of HDACs	+	+	
↑PPARγ	+		
↓Expression of angiogenic factors in tumor cells		+	

AMPA—α-amino-3-hydroxyl-5-methyl-4-isoxazolepropionic acid; IGF1—insulin-like growth factor 1; HDACs—histone deacetylases; mTOR—mammalian target of rapamycin; NLRP3—NOD-like receptor protein 3; PPAR—peroxisome proliferator-activated receptor. ↓—decreased; ↑—increased; +—mechanism shown in *in vitro* or *in vivo* studies.

Acknowledgments: We would like to acknowledge the multidisciplinary team at the Johns Hopkins Adult Epilepsy Diet Center-Eric Kossoff, Rebecca Fisher, Joanne Barnett, Bobbie Henry-Barron and Diane Vizthum-as well as our patients and their families.

Conflicts of Interest: Mackenzie C. Cervenka has received grant support from Nutricia North America, Vitaflo, Army Research Laboratory, The William and Ella Owens Medical Research Foundation and BrightFocus Foundation. She receives speaking honoraria from LivaNova, Nutricia North America and the Glut1 Deficiency Foundation and performs consulting with Nutricia North America and Sage Therapeutics and Royalties from Demos Health.

References

1. Hippocrates. On the Sacred Disease. Available online: http://classics.mit.edu/Hippocrates/sacred.html (accessed on 16 May 2017).

2. McNally, M.A.; Hartman, A.L. Ketone bodies in epilepsy. *J. Neurochem.* **2012**, *121*, 28–35. [CrossRef] [PubMed]

3. Cervenka, M.C.; Kossoff, E.H. Dietary treatment of intractable epilepsy. *Continuum (Minneap Minn.)* **2013**, *19*, 756–766. [CrossRef] [PubMed]

4. Zupec-Kania, B.A; Spellman, E. An overview of the ketogenic diet for pediatric epilepsy. *Nutr. Clin. Pract.* **1998**, *23*, 589–596. [CrossRef] [PubMed]

5. Kossoff, E.H.; Rowley, H.; Sinha, S.R.; Vining, E.P.G. A prospective study of the modified Atkins diet for intractable epilepsy in adults. *Epilepsia* **2008**, *49*, 316–319. [CrossRef] [PubMed]

6. Cervenka, M.C.; Terao, N.N.; Bosarge, J.L.; Henry, B.J.; Klees, A.A.; Morrison, P.F.; Kossoff, E.H. E-mail management of the modified Atkins diet for adults with epilepsy is feasible and effective. *Epilepsia* **2012**, *53*, 728–732. [CrossRef] [PubMed]

7.   Muzykewicz, D.A.; Lyczkowski, D.A.; Memon, N.; Conant, K.D.; Pfeifer, H.H.; Thiele, E.A. Efficacy, safety and tolerability of the low glycemic index treatment in pediatric epilepsy. *Epilepsia* **2009**, *50*, 1118–1126. [CrossRef] [PubMed]

8.   Neal, E.G.; Cross, J.H. Efficacy of dietary treatments for epilepsy. *J. Hum. Nutr. Diet.* **2010**, *23*, 113–119. [CrossRef] [PubMed]

9.   Paoli, A.; Rubini, A.; Volek, J.S.; Grimaldi, K.A. Beyond weight loss: A review of the therapeutic uses of very-low-carbohydrate (ketogenic) diets. *Eur. J. Clin. Nutr.* **2013**, *67*, 789–796. [CrossRef] [PubMed]

10. McDonald, T.J.W.; Cervenka, M.C. Ketogenic diets for adults with highly refractory epilepsy. *Epilepsy Curr.* **2017**, *17*. [CrossRef] [PubMed]

11. Barborka, C.J. Ketogenic diet treatment of epilepsy in adults. *JAMA* **1928**, *9*, 73–78. [CrossRef]

12. Barborka, C.J. Epilepsy in adults: Results of treatment by ketogenic diet in one hundred cases. *Arch. Neurol. Psych.* **1930**, *23*, 904–914. [CrossRef]

13. Martin, K.; Jackson, C.F.; Levy, R.G.; Cooper, P.N. Ketogenic diet and other dietary treatments for epilepsy. *Cochrane Database Syst. Rev.* **2016**. [CrossRef] [PubMed]

14. Brodie, M.J.; Barry, S.J.E.; Bamagous, G.A.; Norrie, J.D.; Kwan, P. Patterns of treatment response in newly diagnosed epilepsy. *Neurology* **2012**, *78*, 1548–1554. [CrossRef] [PubMed]

15. Chen, Z.; Brodie, M.J.; Liew, D.; Kwan, P. Treatment outcomes in patients with newly diagnosed epilepsy treated with established and new antiepileptic drugs a 30-year longitudinal cohort study. *JAMA Neurol.* **2018**, *75*, 279–286. [CrossRef] [PubMed]

16. Hocker, S.E.; Britton, J.W.; Mandrekar, J.N.; Wijdicks, E.F.M.; Rabinstein, A.A. Predictors of outcome in refractory status epilepticus. *JAMA Neurol.* **2013**, *70*, 72–77. [CrossRef] [PubMed]

17. Gilbert, D.L.; Pyzik, P.L.; Freeman, J.M. The ketogenic diet: Seizure control correlates better with serum beta-hydroxybutyrate than with urine ketones. *J. Child Neurol.* **2000**, *15*, 787–790. [CrossRef] [PubMed]

18. Van Delft, R.; Lambrechts, D.; Verschuure, P.; Hulsman, J.; Majoie, M. Blood beta-hydroxybutyrate correlates better with seizure reduction due to ketogenic diet than do ketones in the urine. *Seizure* **2010**, *19*, 36–39. [CrossRef] [PubMed]

19. Kossoff, E.H.; Zupec-Kania, B.A.; Amark, P.E.; Ballaban-Gil, K.R.; Christina Bergqvist, A.G.; Blackford, R.; Buchhalter, J.R.; Caraballo, R.H.; Helen Cross, J.; Dahlin, M.G.; et al. Optimal clinical management of children receiving the ketogenic diet: Recommendations of the International Ketogenic Diet Study Group. *Epilepsia* **2009**, *50*, 304–317. [CrossRef] [PubMed]

20. Kossoff, E.H.; Rho, J.M. Ketogenic diets: Evidence for short- and long-term efficacy. *Neurotherapeutics* **2009**, *6*, 406–414. [CrossRef] [PubMed]

21. Buchhalter, J.R.; D'Alfonso, S.; Connolly, M.; Fung, E.; Michoulas, A.; Sinasac, D.; Singer, R.; Smith, J.; Singh, N.; Rho, J.M. The relationship between d-beta-hydroxybutyrate blood concentrations and seizure control in children treated with the ketogenic diet for medically intractable epilepsy. *Epilepsia Open* **2017**, *2*, 317–321. [CrossRef] [PubMed]

22. Stafstrom, C.E. Dietary Approaches to Epilepsy Treatment: Old and New Options on the Menu. *Epilepsy Curr.* **2004**, *4*, 215–222. [CrossRef] [PubMed]

23. Simeone, T.A.; Simeone, K.A.; Stafstrom, C.E.; Rho, J.M. Do ketone bodies mediate the anti-seizure effects of the ketogenic diet? *Neuropharmacology* **2018**, *133*, 233–241. [CrossRef] [PubMed]

24. Erecińska, M.; Nelson, D.; Daikhin, Y.; Yudkoff, M. Regulation of GABA level in rat brain synaptosomes: Fluxes through enzymes of the GABA shunt and effects of glutamate, calcium and ketone bodies. *J. Neurochem.* **1996**, *67*, 2325–2334. [CrossRef] [PubMed]

25. Melø, T.M.; Nehlig, A.; Sonnewald, U. Neuronal-glial interactions in rats fed a ketogenic diet. *Neurochem. Int.* **2006**, *48*, 498–507. [CrossRef] [PubMed]

26. Wang, Z.J.; Bergqvist, C.; Hunter, J.V.; Jin, D.; Wang, D.J.; Wehrli, S.; Zimmerman, R.A. In vivo measurement of brain metabolites using two-dimensional double-quantum MR spectroscopy-Exploration of GABA levels in a ketogenic diet. *Magn. Reson. Med.* **2003**, *49*, 615–619. [CrossRef] [PubMed]

27. Dahlin, M.; Elfving, Å.; Ungerstedt, U.; Åmark, P. The ketogenic diet influences the levels of excitatory and inhibitory amino acids in the CSF in children with refractory epilepsy. *Epilepsy Res.* **2005**, *64*, 115–125. [CrossRef] [PubMed]

28. Tanner, G.R.; Lutas, A.; Martinez-Francois, J.R.; Yellen, G. Single KATP Channel Opening in Response to Action Potential Firing in Mouse Dentate Granule Neurons. *J. Neurosci.* **2011**, *31*, 8689–8696. [CrossRef] [PubMed]

29. Ma, W.; Berg, J.; Yellen, G. Ketogenic Diet Metabolites Reduce Firing in Central Neurons by Opening KATP Channels. *J. Neurosci.* **2007**, *27*, 3618–3625. [CrossRef] [PubMed]

30. Tan, K.N.; Carrasco-Pozo, C.; McDonald, T.S.; Puchowicz, M.; Borges, K. Tridecanoin is anticonvulsant, antioxidant and improves mitochondrial function. *J. Cereb. Blood Flow Metab.* **2017**, *37*, 2035–2048. [CrossRef] [PubMed]

31. Wlaź, P.; Socała, K.; Nieoczym, D.; Zarnowski, T.; Zarnowska, I.; Czuczwar, S.J.; Gasior, M. Acute anticonvulsant effects of capric acid in seizure tests in mice. *Prog. Neuropsychopharmacol. Biol. Psychiatry* **2015**, *57*, 110–116. [CrossRef] [PubMed]

32. Chang, P.; Augustin, K.; Boddum, K.; Williams, S.; Sun, M.; Terschak, J.A.; Hardege, J.D.; Chen, P.E.; Walker, M.C.; Williams, R.S.B. Seizure control by decanoic acid through direct AMPA receptor inhibition. *Brain* **2016**, *139*, 431–443. [CrossRef] [PubMed]

33. Maalouf, M.; Rho, J.M.; Mattson, M.P. The neuroprotective properties of calorie restriction, the ketogenic diet and ketone bodies. *Brain Res. Rev.* **2009**, *59*, 293–315. [CrossRef] [PubMed]

34. Sullivan, P.G.; Rippy, N.A.; Dorenbos, K.; Concepcion, R.C.; Agarwal, A.K.; Rho, J.M. The Ketogenic Diet Increases Mitochondrial Uncoupling Protein Levels and Activity. *Ann. Neurol.* **2004**, *55*, 576–580. [CrossRef] [PubMed]

35. Bough, K.J.; Wetherington, J.; Hassel, B.; Pare, J.F.; Gawryluk, J.W.; Greene, J.G.; Shaw, R.; Smith, Y.; Geiger, J.D.; Dingledine, R.J. Mitochondrial Biogenesis in the Anticonvulsant Mechanism of the Ketogenic Diet. *Ann. Neurol.* **2006**, *60*, 223–235. [CrossRef] [PubMed]

36. Yamada, K.A. Calorie restriction and glucose regulation. *Epilepsia* **2008**, *49*, 94–96. [CrossRef] [PubMed]

37. McDaniel, S.S.; Rensing, N.R.; Thio, L.L.; Yamada, K.A.; Wong, M. The ketogenic diet inhibits the mammalian target of rapamycin (mTOR) pathway. *Epilepsia* **2011**, *52*, 7–11. [CrossRef] [PubMed]

38. Shimazu, T.; Hirschey, M.; Newman, J.; He, W.; Shirakawa, K.; Moan, N.L.; Grueter, C.A.; Lim, H.; Saunders, L.R.; Stevens, R.D.; et al. Suppression of Oxidative Stress by β-Hydroxybutyrate, an Endogenous Histone Deacetylase Inhibitor. *Science* **2013**, *339*, 211–214. [CrossRef] [PubMed]

39. Jeong, E.A.; Jeon, B.T.; Shin, H.J.; Kim, N.; Lee, D.H.; Kim, H.J.; Kang, S.S.; Cho, G.J.; Choi, W.S.; Roh, G.S. Ketogenic diet-induced peroxisome proliferator-activated receptor-γ activation decreases neuroinflammation in the mouse hippocampus after kainic acid-induced seizures. *Exp. Neurol.* **2011**, *232*, 195–202. [CrossRef] [PubMed]

40. Koppel, S.J.; Swerdlow, R.H. Neurochemistry International Neuroketotherapeutics: A modern review of a century-old therapy. *Neurochem. Int.* **2017**. [CrossRef]

41. Ruskin, D.N.; Kawamura, M.; Masino, S.A. Reduced Pain and Inflammation in Juvenile and Adult Rats Fed a Ketogenic Diet. *PLoS ONE* **2009**, *4*, 1–6. [CrossRef] [PubMed]

42. Yang, X.; Cheng, B. Neuroprotective and Anti-inflammatory Activities of Ketogenic Diet on MPTP-induced Neurotoxicity. *J. Mol. Neurosci.* **2010**, 145–153. [CrossRef] [PubMed]

43. Youm, Y.; Nguyen, K.Y.; Grant, R.W.; Goldberg, E.L.; Bodogai, M.; Kim, D.; Agostino, D.D.; Planavsky, N.; Lupfer, C.; Kanneganti, T.D.; et al. The ketone metabolite β-hydroxybutyrate blocks NLRP3 inflammasome–mediated inflammatory disease. *Nat. Med.* **2015**, *21*, 263–269. [CrossRef] [PubMed]

44. Rahman, M.; Muhammad, S.; Khan, M.A.; Chen, H.; Ridder, D.A.; Müller-Fielitz, H.; Pokorná, B.; Vollbrandt, T.; Stölting, I.; Nadrowitz, R.; et al. The β-hydroxybutyrate receptor HCA 2 activates a neuroprotective subset of macrophages. *Nat. Commun.* **2014**, *5*, 1–11. [CrossRef] [PubMed]

45. Gaspard, N.; Hirsch, L.J.; Sculier, C.; Loddenkemper, T.; Van Baalen, A.; Lancrenon, J.; Emmery, M.; Specchio, N.; Farias-Moeller, R.; Wong, N.; et al. New-onset refractory status epilepticus (NORSE) and febrile infection–related epilepsy syndrome (FIRES): State of the art and perspectives. *Epilepsia* **2018**, *59*, 745–752. [CrossRef] [PubMed]

46. Klein, M.S.; Newell, C.; Bomhof, M.R.; Reimer, R.A.; Hittel, D.S.; Rho, J.M.; Vogel, H.J.; Shearer, J. Metabolomic Modeling to Monitor Host Responsiveness to Gut Microbiota Manipulation in the BTBR T+tf/j Mouse. *J. Proteome Res.* **2016**, *15*, 1143–1150. [CrossRef] [PubMed]

47. Newell, C.; Bomhof, M.R.; Reimer, R.A.; Hittel, D.S.; Rho, J.M.; Shearer, J. Ketogenic diet modifies the gut microbiota in a murine model of autism spectrum disorder. *Mol. Autism.* **2016**, *7*, 1–6. [CrossRef] [PubMed]

48. Duncan, S.H.; Lobley, G.E.; Holtrop, G.; Ince, J.; Johnstone, A.M.; Louis, P.; Flint, H.J. Human colonic microbiota associated with diet, obesity and weight loss. *Int. J. Obes.* **2008**, *32*, 1720–1724. [CrossRef] [PubMed]

49. David, L.A.; Maurice, C.F.; Carmody, R.N.; Gootenberg, D.B.; Button, J.E.; Wolfe, B.E.; Ling, A.V.; Devlin, A.S.; Varma, Y.; Fischbach, M.A.; et al. Diet rapidly and reproducibly alters the human gut microbiome. *Nature* **2014**, *505*, 559–563. [CrossRef] [PubMed]

50. Olson, C.A.; Vuong, H.E.; Yano, J.M.; Liang, QY.; Nusbaum, D.J.; Hsiao, E.Y. The Gut Microbiota Mediates the Anti-Seizure Effects of the Ketogenic Diet. *Cell* **2018**, *173*, 1728–1741. [CrossRef] [PubMed]

51. Payne, N.E.; Cross, J.H.; Sander, J.W.; Sisodiya, S.M. The ketogenic and related diets in adolescents and adults-A review. *Epilepsia* **2011**, *52*, 1941–1948. [CrossRef] [PubMed]

52. Ye, F.; Li, X.J.; Jiang, W.L.; Sun, H.B.; Liu, J. Efficacy of and patient compliance with a ketogenic diet in adults with intractable epilepsy: A meta-analysis. *J. Clin. Neurol.* **2015**, *11*, 26–31. [CrossRef] [PubMed]

53. Cervenka, M.C.; Henry, B.J.; Felton, E.A.; Patton, K.; Kossoff, E.H. Establishing an Adult Epilepsy Diet Center: Experience, efficacy and challenges. *Epilepsy Behav.* **2016**, *58*, 61–68. [CrossRef] [PubMed]

54. Williams, T.; Cervenka, M.C. The role for ketogenic diets in epilepsy and status epilepticus in adults. *Clin. Neurophysiol. Pract.* **2017**, *2*, 154–160. [CrossRef]

55. Liu, H.; Yang, Y.; Wang, Y.; Tang, H.; Zhang, F.; Zhang, Y.; Zhao, Y. Ketogenic diet for treatment of intractable epilepsy in adults: A meta-analysis of observational studies. *Epilepsia Open* **2018**, *3*, 9–17. [CrossRef] [PubMed]

56. Kverneland, M.; Selmer, K.K.; Nakken, K.O.; Iversen, P.O.; Taubøll, E. A prospective study of the modified Atkins diet for adults with idiopathic generalized epilepsy. *Epilepsy Behav.* **2015**, *53*, 197–201. [CrossRef] [PubMed]

57. Klein, P.; Janousek, J.; Barber, A.; Weissberger, R. Ketogenic diet treatment in adults with refractory epilepsy. *Epilepsy Behav.* **2010**, *19*, 575–579. [CrossRef] [PubMed]

58. Zare, M.; Okhovat, A.A.; Esmaillzadeh, A.; Mehvari, J.; Najafi, M.R.; Saadatnia, M. Modified atkins diet in adult patients with refractory epilepsy: A controlled randomized clinical trial. *Iran. J. Neurol.* **2017**, *16*, 72–77. [CrossRef]

59. Kverneland, M.; Molteberg, E.; Iversen, P.O.; Veierød, M.B.; Taubøll, E.; Selmer, K.K.; Nakken, K.O. Effect of modified Atkins diet in adults with drug-resistant focal epilepsy: A randomized clinical trial. *Epilepsia* **2018**, 1–10. [CrossRef] [PubMed]

60. Bodenant, M.; Moreau, C.; Sejourné, C.; Auvin, S.; Delval, A.; Cuisset, J.M.; Derambure, P.; Destée, A.; Defebvre, L. Interest of the ketogenic diet in a refractory status epilepticus in adults. *Rev. Neurol.* **2008**, *164*, 194–199. [CrossRef] [PubMed]

61. Wusthoff, C.J.; Kranick, S.M.; Morley, J.F.; Bergqvist, A.G.C. The ketogenic diet in treatment of two adults with prolonged nonconvulsive status epilepticus. *Epilepsia* **2010**, *51*, 1083–1085. [CrossRef] [PubMed]

62. Martikainen, M.H.; Paivarinta, M.; Jaaskelainen, S.; Majamaa, K. Successful treatment of POLG-related mitochondrial epilepsy. *Epileptic Disord.* **2012**, *14*, 438–441. [PubMed]

63. Nam, S.H.; Lee, B.L.; Lee, C.G.; Yu, H.J.; Joo, E.Y.; Lee, J.; Lee, M. The role of ketogenic diet in the treatment of refractory status epilepticus. *Epilepsia* **2011**, *52*, e181–e184. [CrossRef] [PubMed]

64. Strzelczyk, A.; Reif, P.S.; Bauer, S.; Belke, M.; Oertel, W.H.; Knake, S.; Rosenow, F. Intravenous initiation and maintenance of ketogenic diet: Proof of concept in super-refractory status epilepticus. *Seizure* **2013**, *22*, 581–583. [CrossRef] [PubMed]

65. Thakur, K.T.; Probasco, J.C.; Hocker, S.E.; Roehl, K.; Henry, B.; Kossoff, E.H.; Kaplan, P.W.; Geocadin, R.G.; Hartman, A.L.; Venkatesan, A.; et al. Ketogenic diet for adults in super-refractory status epilepticus. *Neurology* **2014**, *82*, 665–670. [CrossRef] [PubMed]

66. Cervenka, M.C.; Hocker, S.E.; Koenig, M.; Bar, B.; Henry-Barron, B.; Kossoff, E.H.; Hartman, A.L.; Probasco, J.C.; Benavides, D.R.; Venkatesan, A.; et al. Phase I/II multicenter ketogenic diet study for adult superrefractory status epilepticus. *Neurology* **2017**, *88*, 938–943. [CrossRef] [PubMed]

67. Shorvon, S.; Ferlisi, M. The outcome of therapies in refractory and super-refractory convulsive status epilepticus and recommendations for therapy. *Brain* **2012**, *135*, 2314–2328. [CrossRef] [PubMed]

68. Wen, P.; Kesari, S. Malignant Gliomas in Adults. *N. Engl. J. Med.* **2008**, *359*, 492–507. [CrossRef] [PubMed]

69. Carlsson, S.K.; Brothers, S.P.; Wahlestedt, C. Emerging treatment strategies for glioblastoma multiforme. *EMBO Mol. Med.* **2014**, *6*, 1359–1370. [CrossRef] [PubMed]

70. Winter, S.F.; Loebel, F.; Dietrich, J. Role of ketogenic metabolic therapy in malignant glioma: A systematic review. *Crit. Rev. Oncol. Hematol.* **2017**, *112*, 41–58. [CrossRef] [PubMed]

71. Warburg, O. On the origin of cancer cells. *Science* **1956**, *123*, 309–314. [CrossRef] [PubMed]

72. Seyfried, T.N.; Flores, R.E.; Poff, A.M.; D'Agostino, D.P. Cancer as a metabolic disease: Implications for novel therapeutics. *Carcinogenesis* **2014**, *35*, 515–527. [CrossRef] [PubMed]

73. Branco, A.F.; Ferreira, A.; Simões, R.F.; Magalhães-Novais, S.; Zehowski, C.; Cope, E.; Silva, A.M.; Pereira, D.; Sardão, V.A.; Cunha-Oliveira, T. Ketogenic diets: From cancer to mitochondrial diseases and beyond. *Eur. J. Clin. Invest.* **2016**, *46*, 285–298. [CrossRef] [PubMed]

74. Jelluma, N. Glucose Withdrawal Induces Oxidative Stress followed by Apoptosis in Glioblastoma Cells but not in Normal Human Astrocytes. *Mol. Cancer Res.* **2006**, *4*, 319–330. [CrossRef] [PubMed]

75. Derr, R.L.; Ye, X.; Islas, M.U.; Desideri, S.; Saudek, C.D.; Grossman, S.A. Association between hyperglycemia and survival in patients with newly diagnosed glioblastoma. *J. Clin. Oncol.* **2009**, *27*, 1082–1086. [CrossRef] [PubMed]

76. McGirt, M.J.; Chaichana, K.L.; Gathinji, M.; Attenello, F.; Than, K.; Ruiz, A.J.; Olivi, A.; Quiñones-Hinojosa, A. Persistent outpatient hyperglycemia is independently associated with decreased survival after primary resection of malignant brain astrocytomas. *Neurosurgery* **2008**, *63*, 286–291. [CrossRef] [PubMed]

77. Mayer, A.; Vaupel, P.; Struss, H.G.; Giese, A.; Stockinger, M.; Schmidberger, H. Ausgeprägt negativer prognostischer Einfluss von hyperglykämischen Episoden während der adjuvanten Radiochemotherapie des Glioblastoma multiforme. *Strahlenther. Onkol.* **2014**, *190*, 933–938. (In German) [CrossRef] [PubMed]

78. Adeberg, S.; Bernhardt, D.; Foerster, R.; Bostel, T.; Koerber, S.A.; Mohr, A.; Koelsche, C.; Rieken, S.; Debus, J. The influence of hyperglycemia during radiotherapy on survival in patients with primary glioblastoma. *Acta Oncol.* **2016**, *55*, 201–207. [CrossRef] [PubMed]

79. Seyfried, T.N.; Sanderson, T.M.; El-Abbadi, M.M.; McGowan, R.; Mukherjee, P. Role of glucose and ketone bodies in the metabolic control of experimental brain cancer. *Br. J. Cancer* **2003**, *89*, 1375–1382. [CrossRef] [PubMed]

80. Marsh, J.; Mukherjee, P.; Seyfried, T.N. Drug/diet synergy for managing malignant astrocytoma in mice: 2-deoxy-D-glucose and the restricted ketogenic diet. *Nutr. Metab.* **2008**, *5*, 1–5. [CrossRef] [PubMed]

81. Abdelwahab, M.G.; Fenton, K.E.; Preul, M.C.; Rho, J.M.; Lynch, A.; Stafford, P.; Scheck, A.C. The ketogenic diet is an effective adjuvant to radiation therapy for the treatment of malignant glioma. *PLoS ONE* **2012**, *7*, 1–7. [CrossRef] [PubMed]

82. Woolf, E.C.; Curley, K.L.; Liu, Q.; Turner, G.H.; Charlton, J.A.; Preul, M.C.; Scheck, A.C. The ketogenic diet alters the hypoxic response and affects expression of proteins associated with angiogenesis, invasive potential and vascular permeability in a mouse glioma model. *PLoS ONE* **2015**, *10*, 1–18. [CrossRef] [PubMed]

83. Woolf, E.C.; Syed, N.; Scheck, A.C. Tumor Metabolism, the Ketogenic Diet and β-Hydroxybutyrate: Novel Approaches to Adjuvant Brain Tumor Therapy. *Front. Mol. Neurosci.* **2016**, *9*, 1–11. [CrossRef] [PubMed]

84. Poff, A.; Koutnik, A.P.; Egan, K.M.; Sahebjam, S.; D'Agostino, D.; Kumar, N.B. Targeting the Warburg effect for cancer treatment: Ketogenic diets for management of glioma. *Semin. Cancer Biol.* **2018**. [CrossRef] [PubMed]

85. Martuscello, R.T.; Vedam-Mai, V.; McCarthy, D.J.; Schmoll, M.E.; Jundi, M.A.; Louviere, C.D.; Griffith, B.G.; Skinner, C.L.; Suslov, O.; Deleyrolle, L.P.; et al. A supplemented high-fat low-carbohydrate diet for the treatment of glioblastoma. *Clin. Cancer Res.* **2016**, *22*, 2482–2495. [CrossRef] [PubMed]

86. Poff, A.M.; Ari, C.; Seyfried, T.N.; D'Agostino, D.P. The Ketogenic Diet and Hyperbaric Oxygen Therapy Prolong Survival in Mice with Systemic Metastatic Cancer. *PLoS ONE* **2013**, *8*. [CrossRef] [PubMed]

87. Cairns, R.A.; Harris, I.S.; Mak, T.W. Regulation of cancer cell metabolism. *Nat. Rev. Cancer* **2011**, *11*, 85–95. [CrossRef] [PubMed]

88. Bowers, L.W.; Rossi, E.L.; O'Flanagan, C.H.; De Graffenried, L.A.; Hursting, S.D. The role of the insulin/IGF system in cancer: Lessons learned from clinical trials and the energy balance-cancer link. *Front. Endocrinol.* **2015**, *6*, 1–16. [CrossRef] [PubMed]

89. Lussier, D.M.; Woolf, E.C.; Johnson, J.L.; Brooks, K.S.; Blattman, J.N.; Scheck, A.C. Enhanced immunity in a mouse model of malignant glioma is mediated by a therapeutic ketogenic diet. *BMC Cancer* **2016**, *16*, 1–10. [CrossRef] [PubMed]

90. Forsythe, C.E.; Phinney, S.D.; Fernandez, M.L.; Quann, E.E.; Wood, R.J.; Bibus, D.M.; Kraemer, W.J.; Feinman, R.D.; Volek, J.S. Comparison of low fat and low carbohydrate diets on circulating fatty acid composition and markers of inflammation. *Lipids* **2008**, *43*, 65–77. [CrossRef] [PubMed]

91. Zuccoli, G.; Marcello, N.; Pisanello, A.; Servadei, F.; Vaccaro, S.; Mukherjee, P.; Seyfried, T.N. Metabolic management of glioblastoma multiforme using standard therapy together with a restricted ketogenic diet: Case Report. *Nutr. Metab.* **2010**, *7*, 1–7. [CrossRef] [PubMed]

92. Champ, C.E.; Palmer, J.D.; Volek, J.S.; Werner-Wasik, M.; Andrews, D.W.; Evans, J.J.; Glass, J.; Kim, L.; Shi, W. Targeting metabolism with a ketogenic diet during the treatment of glioblastoma multiforme. *J. Neurooncol.* **2014**, *117*, 125–131. [CrossRef] [PubMed]

93. Schwartz, K.; Chang, H.T.; Nikolai, M.; Pernicone, J.; Rhee, S.; Olson, K.; Kurniali, P.C.; Hord, N.G.; Noel, M. Treatment of glioma patients with ketogenic diets: Report of two cases treated with an IRB-approved energy-restricted ketogenic diet protocol and review of the literature. *Cancer Metab.* **2015**, *3*, 3. [CrossRef] [PubMed]

94. Rieger, J.; Bähr, O.; Maurer, G.D.; Hattingen, E.; Franz, K.; Brucker, D.; Walenta, S.; Kämmerer, U.; Coy, J.F.; Weller, M.; et al. ERGO: A pilot study of ketogenic diet in recurrent glioblastoma. *Int. J. Oncol.* **2014**, *45*, 1843–1852. [CrossRef] [PubMed]

95. Elsakka, A.M.A.; Bary, M.A.; Abdelzaher, E.; Elnaggar, M.; Kalamian, M.; Mukherjee, P.; Seyfried, T.N. Management of Glioblastoma Multiforme in a Patient Treated With Ketogenic Metabolic Therapy and Modified Standard of Care: A 24-Month Follow-Up. *Front. Nutr.* **2018**, *5*, 1–11. [CrossRef] [PubMed]

96. Martin-McGill, K.J.; Marson, A.G.; Tudur Smith, C.; Jenkinson, M.D. Ketogenic diets as an adjuvant therapy in glioblastoma (the KEATING trial): Study protocol for a randomised pilot study. *Pilot Feasibility Stud.* **2017**, *3*, 1–11. [CrossRef] [PubMed]

97. Swerdlow, R.H. Brain aging, Alzheimer's disease and mitochondria. *Biochim. Biophys. Acta-Mol. Basis Dis.* **2011**, *1812*, 1630–1639. [CrossRef] [PubMed]

98. Wilkins, H.M.; Swerdlow, R.H. Amyloid precursor protein processing and bioenergetics. *Brain Res. Bull.* **2017**, *133*, 71–79. [CrossRef] [PubMed]

99. Castellano, C.A.; Nugent, S.; Paquet, N.; Tremblay, S.; Bocti, C.; Lacombe, G.; Imbeault, H.; Turcotte, E.; Fulop, T.; Cunnane, S. Lower brain 18F-fluorodeoxyglucose uptake but normal 11C-acetoacetate metabolism in mild Alzheimer's disease dementia. *J. Alzheimer's Dis.* **2015**, *43*, 1343–1353. [CrossRef] [PubMed]

100. Winkler, E.A.; Nishida, Y.; Sagare, A.P.; Rege, S.V.; Bell, R.D.; Perlmutter, D.; Sengillo, J.D.; Hillman, S.; Kong, P.; Nelson, A.R.; et al. GLUT1 reductions exacerbate Alzheimer's disease vasculo-neuronal dysfunction and degeneration. *Nat. Neurosci.* **2015**, *18*, 521–530. [CrossRef] [PubMed]

101. Taylor, M.K.; Sullivan, D.K.; Swerdlow, R.H.; Vidoni, E.D.; Morris, J.K.; Mahnken, J.D.; Burns, J.M. A high-glycemic diet is associated with cerebral amyloid burden in cognitively normal older adults. *Am. J. Clin. Nutr.* **2017**, *106*, 1463–1470. [CrossRef] [PubMed]

102. De la Monte, S.M. Insulin Resistance and Neurodegeneration: Progress Towards the Development of New Therapeutics for Alzheimer's Disease. *Drugs* **2017**, *77*, 47–65. [CrossRef] [PubMed]

103. Gaspar, J.M.; Baptista, F.I.; MacEdo, M.P.; Ambrósio, A.F. Inside the Diabetic Brain: Role of Different Players Involved in Cognitive Decline. *ACS Chem. Neurosci.* **2016**, *7*, 131–142. [CrossRef] [PubMed]

104. Nafar, F.; Clarke, J.P.; Mearow, K.M. Coconut oil protects cortical neurons from amyloid beta toxicity by enhancing signaling of cell survival pathways. *Neurochem. Int.* **2017**, *105*, 64–79. [CrossRef] [PubMed]

105. Kashiwaya, Y.; Bergman, C.; Lee, J.H.; Wan, R.; King, M.T.; Mughal, M.R.; Okun, E.; Clarke, K.; Mattson, M.P.; Veech, R.L. A ketone ester diet exhibits anxiolytic and cognition-sparing properties and lessens amyloid and tau pathologies in a mouse model of Alzheimer's disease. *Neurobiol. Aging* **2013**, *34*, 1530–1539. [CrossRef] [PubMed]

106. Studzinski, C.M.; MacKay, W.A.; Beckett, T.L.; Henderson, S.T.; Murphy, M.P.; Sullivan, P.G.; Burnham, W.M.I. Induction of ketosis may improve mitochondrial function and decrease steady-state amyloid-β precursor protein (APP) levels in the aged dog. *Brain Res.* **2008**, *1226*, 209–217. [CrossRef] [PubMed]

107. Kashiwaya, Y.; Takeshima, T.; Mori, N.; Nakashima, K.; Clarke, K.; Veech, R.L. D-b-Hydroxybutyrate protects neurons in models of Alzheimer's and Parkinson's disease. *Proc. Natl. Acad. Sci. USA* **2000**, *97*, 5440–5444. [CrossRef] [PubMed]

108. Van Der Auwera, I.; Wera, S.; Van Leuven, F.; Henderson, S.T. A ketogenic diet reduces amyloid beta 40 and 42 in a mouse model of Alzheimer's disease. *Nutr. Metab.* **2005**, *2*, 1–8. [CrossRef] [PubMed]

109. Yin, J.X.; Maalouf, M.; Han, P.; Zhao, M.; Gao, M.; Dharshaun, T.; Ryan, C.; Whitelegge, J.; Wu, J.; Eisenberg, D.; et al. Ketones block amyloid entry and improve cognition in an Alzheimer's model. *Neurobiol. Aging* **2016**, *39*, 25–37. [CrossRef] [PubMed]

110. Xu, K.; Sun, X.Y.; Eroku, B.O.; Tsipis, C.P.; Puchowicz, M.A.; Lamanna, J.C. Diet-induced ketosis improves cognitive performance in aged rats. In *Oxygen Transport to Tissue XXXI*; Springer: Boston, MA, USA, 2010; Volume 662, pp. 71–75.

111. Reger, M.A.; Henderson, S.T.; Hale, C.; Cholerton, B.; Baker, L.D.; Watson, G.S.; Hyde, K.; Chapman, D.; Craft, S. Effects of β-hydroxybutyrate on cognition in memory-impaired adults. *Neurobiol. Aging* **2004**, *25*, 311–314. [CrossRef]

112. Ota, M.; Matsuo, J.; Ishida, I.; Hattori, K.; Teraishi, T.; Tonouchi, H.; Ashida, K.; Takahashi, T.; Kunugi, H. Effect of a ketogenic meal on cognitive function in elderly adults: Potential for cognitive enhancement. *Psychopharmacology* **2016**, *233*, 3797–3802. [CrossRef] [PubMed]

113. Krikorian, R.; Shidler, M.D.; Dangelo, K.; Couch, S.C.; Benoit, S.C.; Clegg, D.J. Dietary ketosis enhances memory in mild cognitive impairment. *Neurobiol. Aging* **2012**, *33*, 425-e19. [CrossRef] [PubMed]

114. Newport, M.T.; Vanitallie, T.B.; Kashiwaya, Y.; King, M.T.; Veech, R.L. A new way to produce hyperketonemia: Use of ketone ester in a case of Alzheimer's disease. *Alzheimer's Dement.* **2015**, *11*, 99–103. [CrossRef] [PubMed]

115. Taylor, M.K.; Sullivan, D.K.; Mahnken, J.D.; Burns, J.M.; Swerdlow, R.H. Feasibility and efficacy data from a ketogenic diet intervention in Alzheimer's disease. *Alzheimer's Dement. Transl. Res. Clin. Interv.* **2018**, *4*, 28–36. [CrossRef] [PubMed]

116. Henderson, S.T.; Vogel, J.L.; Barr, L.J.; Garvin, F.; Jones, J.J.; Costantini, L.C. Study of the ketogenic agent AC-1202 in mild to moderate Alzheimer's disease: A randomized, double-blind, placebo-controlled, multicenter trial. *Nutr. Metab.* **2009**, *6*, 31. [CrossRef] [PubMed]

117. Rebello, C.J.; Keller, J.N.; Liu, A.G.; Johnson, W.D.; Greenway, F.L. Pilot feasibility and safety study examining the effect of medium chain triglyceride supplementation in subjects with mild cognitive impairment: A randomized controlled trial. *BBA Clin.* **2015**, *3*, 123–125. [CrossRef] [PubMed]

118. Ohnuma, T.; Toda, A.; Kimoto, A.; Takebayashi, Y.; Higashiyama, R.; Tagata, Y.; Ito, M.; Ota, T.; Shibata, N.; Arai, H. Benefits of use and tolerance of, medium-chain triglyceride medical food in the management of Japanese patients with Alzheimer's disease: A prospective, open-label pilot study. *Clin. Interv. Aging* **2016**, *11*, 29–36. [CrossRef] [PubMed]

119. Croteau, E.; Castellano, C.A.; Richard, M.A.; Fortier, M.; Nugent, S.; Lepage, M.; Duchesne, S.; Whittingstall, K.; Turcotte, E.E.; Bocti, C.; et al. Ketogenic Medium Chain Triglycerides Increase Brain Energy Metabolism in Alzheimer's Disease. *J. Alzheimers. Dis.* **2018**, 1–2. [CrossRef] [PubMed]

120. Patel, A.; Pyzik, P.L.; Turner, Z.; Rubenstein, J.E.; Kossoff, E.H. Long-term outcomes of children treated with the ketogenic diet in the past. *Epilepsia* **2010**, *51*, 1277–1282. [CrossRef] [PubMed]

121. Schoeler, N.E.; Cross, J.H. Ketogenic dietary therapies in adults with epilepsy: A practical guide. *Pract. Neurol.* **2016**, *16*, 208–214. [CrossRef] [PubMed]

122. Pinto, A.; Bonucci, A.; Maggi, E.; Corsi, M.; Businaro, R. Anti-Oxidant and Anti-Inflammatory Activity of Ketogenic Diet: New Perspectives for Neuroprotection in Alzheimer's Disease. *Antioxidants* **2018**, *7*, 63. [CrossRef] [PubMed]

123. Tisdale, M. Mechanisms of cancer cachexia. *Physiol. Rev.* **2009**, *89*, 381–410. [CrossRef] [PubMed]

124. Mosek, A.; Natour, H.; Neufeld, M.Y.; Shiff, Y.; Vaisman, N. Ketogenic diet treatment in adults with refractory epilepsy: A prospective pilot study. *Seizure* **2009**, *18*, 30–33. [CrossRef] [PubMed]

125. Cervenka, M.C.; Patton, K.; Eloyan, A.; Henry, B.; Kossoff, E.H. The impact of the modified Atkins diet on lipid profiles in adults with epilepsy. *Nutr. Neurosci.* **2016**, *19*, 131–137. [CrossRef] [PubMed]

126. Mackay, M.T.; Bicknell-Royle, J.; Nation, J.; Humphrey, M.; Harvey, A.S. The ketogenic diet in refractory childhood epilepsy. *J. Paediatr. Child Health* **2005**, *41*, 353–357. [CrossRef] [PubMed]

127. Bergqvist, A.G.C.; Schall, J.I.; Stallings, V.A.; Zemel, B.S. Progressive bone mineral content loss in children with intractable epilepsy treated with the ketogenic diet. *Am. J. Clin. Nutr.* **2008**, *88*, 1678–1684. [CrossRef] [PubMed]

128. Schwartz, K.A.; Noel, M.; Nikolai, M.; Chang, H.T. Investigating the Ketogenic Diet As Treatment for Primary Aggressive Brain Cancer: Challenges and Lessons Learned. *Front. Nutr.* **2018**, *5*. [CrossRef] [PubMed]

129. Mcdonald, T.J.W.; Henry-barron, B.J.; Felton, E.A.; Gutierrez, E.G.; Barnett, J.; Fisher, R.; Lwin, M.; Jan, A.; Vizthum, D.; Kossoff, E.H.; et al. Improving compliance in adults with epilepsy on a modified Atkins diet: A randomized trial. *Seizure Eur. J. Epilepsy* **2018**, *60*, 132–138. [CrossRef] [PubMed]

130. Youngson, N.A.; Morris, M.J.; Ballard, B. The mechanisms mediating the antiepileptic effects of the ketogenic diet and potential opportunities for improvement with metabolism-altering drugs. *Seizure* **2017**, *52*, 15–19. [CrossRef] [PubMed]

Turning Analysis during Standardized Test Using On-Shoe Wearable Sensors in Parkinson's Disease

Nooshin Haji Ghassemi [1,*], Julius Hannink [1], Nils Roth [1], Heiko Gaßner [2], Franz Marxreiter [2], Jochen Klucken [2] and Björn M. Eskofier [1]

[1] Machine Learning and Data Analytics Lab, Department of Computer Science, Friedrich-Alexander-University Erlangen-Nürnberg (FAU), Carl-Thiersch-Strasse 2b, D-91052 Erlangen, Germany

[2] Department of Molecular Neurology, University Hospital Erlangen, Schwabachanlage 6, D-91054 Erlangen, Germany

* Correspondence: nooshin.haji@fau.de

Abstract: Mobile gait analysis systems using wearable sensors have the potential to analyze and monitor pathological gait in a finer scale than ever before. A closer look at gait in Parkinson's disease (PD) reveals that turning has its own characteristics and requires its own analysis. The goal of this paper is to present a system with on-shoe wearable sensors in order to analyze the abnormalities of turning in a standardized gait test for PD. We investigated turning abnormalities in a large cohort of 108 PD patients and 42 age-matched controls. We quantified turning through several spatio-temporal parameters. Analysis of turn-derived parameters revealed differences of turn-related gait impairment in relation to different disease stages and motor impairment. Our findings confirm and extend the results from previous studies and show the applicability of our system in turning analysis. Our system can provide insight into the turning in PD and be used as a complement for physicians' gait assessment and to monitor patients in their daily environment.

Keywords: Parkinson's disease; pathological gait; turning analysis; wearable sensors; mobile gait analysis

1. Introduction

Gait is an important part of mobility that is impaired in neurodegenerative diseases like Parkinson's disease (PD). As the disease progresses, gait fluctuations become more severe. Different locomotor patterns in gait, such as straight walking and turning, require different levels of functioning and coordination. For a person with impaired mobility caused, for example, by PD, turning is challenging and potentially risky, even more than straight walking [1,2]. There have been attempts to identify and characterize turning abnormalities in order to complement the physicians' assessment of pathological gait.

Studies showed that turning deficits are manifested in mild PD even when there are no signs of impairment in straight walking [3]. Difficulty while turning may lead to posture instability and, potentially, even falls [4,5]. Risk of falling is higher during turning compared with straight walking [4,5]. Furthermore, deterioration of motor function during turning can cause progressive episodes of freezing of gait (FoG) [6–8].

Some studies have attempted to utilize the definition of disease stages and motor impairments by UPDRS-III [9] and H&Y [10] clinical scores and objectively assess turning deficits [11–15]. Studies on spatio-temporal parameters quantifying turning have demonstrated decreased speed, longer duration of turning, and a larger number of strides as the disease progresses [3,16–18]. Postural stability also decreases during turning for PD patients in comparison to healthy controls, particularly during fast walking [19].

Outside the clinics and in the majority of standardized clinical tests, a gait sequence includes both straight walking and turning. In order to differentiate between them during the course of a gait, different definitions of turning have been presented in the literature. For example, turning was defined as the movement between two pre-defined points that indicated the initiation and termination of turning [5]. Salarian et al. [17] used mathematical modeling in order to isolate turns from the whole gait sequence. Spatio-temporal parameters extracted from individual strides are different in straight walking compared to turning. Many studies used characteristics and statistics of spatio-temporal gait parameters to define turning [3,6,20]. Without a standard turning definition, studies then presented some clinical validations to support their definitions—for example, they showed that turning parameters were correlated to the established clinical scores [3,6,20].

Gait and turning can be measured by a variety of systems—from accurate but stationary motion capture systems [19] to small wearable sensors [3,17]. The focus of this study is on wearable sensors, since they give the opportunity to perform long-term monitoring of PD patients. Sensor placement plays a crucial factor in designing wearable systems. Many turning studies place the sensors on the upper extremity [3,6,20]. One advantage is that turning is easily detectable in the sensor signals [17]. However, gait disturbances such as FoG cannot be detected clearly from sensors on the upper extremity. Such systems still need additional sensors on the lower extremity in order to quantify turning in terms of spatio-temporal parameters [3,17]. In contrast, sensors on the lower extremity and, in particular, on the shoe provide higher biomechanical resolutions. Panebianco et al. [21] examined different sensor locations and showed that as sensors get closer to the foot, higher accuracy for gait events and parameters can be obtained. Moreover, for long-term monitoring of patients, sensors integrated in the footwear are less obtrusive and stigmatizing.

In order to measure gait, we used wearable sensors mounted on the lateral side of the shoe. In order to isolate turning from gait, we used the statistics of spatio-temporal parameters. The goal of this study is to show the applicability of the system in the objective analysis of turning and to evaluate whether it confirms the findings of other studies. To this end, we first introduce our novel turning isolation algorithm targeting data from a standardized 4×10 m gait test measured with wearable sensors placed on the shoe. Then, we quantify the isolated turnings through several spatio-temporal parameters that proved to be effective in detecting pathological gait [22–24]. Through meticulous statistical analysis, we evaluate the turning abnormalities in a large PD cohort. The value of this objective turning assessment was clinically validated by the correlation of the turn-derived parameters to clinical scores, including motor impairment and disease stages in PD.

2. Methods

2.1. Wearable Measurement System

For our experiments, data was recorded with a Shimmer 2R/3 Inertial measurement unit (IMU) (Shimmer Sensing, Dublin, Ireland), measuring acceleration and angular velocity at 102.4 Hz. Each unit consisted of a tri-axial accelerometer (range Shimmer 2R: ±6 g, Shimmer 3: ±8 g) and a tri-axial gyroscope (range Shimmer 2R: $\pm500°$/s, Shimmer 3: $\pm 1000°$/s). The sensor units were mounted laterally on each shoe below the patient's ankle. The measurements from both feet were included in the experiments. Figure 1 shows the sensor placement on the shoe and the axes definition.

2.2. Study Population

We recruited 108 PD patients during their regular visit in the movement disorder outpatient center at the University Hospital Erlangen. Sporadic PD was defined according to the guidelines of the German Association for Neurology (DGN), which are similar to the UK PD Society Brain Bank criteria [25]. Patients had to be able to walk independently (H&Y < 4, UPDRS gait item < 3) [10,26]. All PD patients were clinically (UPDRS-III) and biomechanically (gait analysis) investigated in stable ON medication without the presence of clinically relevant motor fluctuations during the assessments.

We had an exclusion criterion for a severe cognitive impairment. To obtain quantitative gait data from controls, we recruited 42 age-matched controls with no signs of PD and/or other motor impairments. With respect to age, height, and body-mass-index (BMI), PD and control cohorts were matched (see Table 1). Data regarding laterality of the disease can be found in Table 1, where the UPDRS sub-items of rigidity lower and upper extremities were reported. This data shows that patients affected on the right and left sides are almost equally represented in our cohort. Written informed consent was obtained from all participants (IRB-approval-No. 4208, 21.04.2010, IRB, Medical Faculty, Friedrich-Alexander University Erlangen-Nürnberg, Germany).

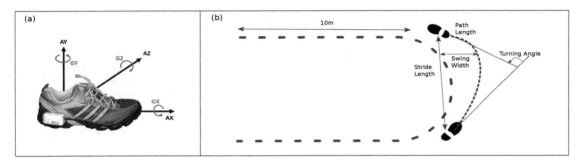

Figure 1. (a) Shimmer sensor placement and axes definition. (b) Definition of turning angle, stride length, path length, and swing width.

Table 1. Clinical characteristics of patients with Parkinson's disease (PD) and healthy controls.

	PD (N = 108)	Control (N = 42)
Age (years)	57.61 ± 10.42 [36–85]	58.78 ± 11.14 [41–84]
Sex (Male/Female)	74/34	25/17
Height (m)	1.74 ± 0.1	1.73 ± 0.07
BMI	25.81 ± 3.71	26.48 ± 3.76
Hoehn and Yahr stage	2.06 ± 0.84	
I ($<$1)	28	
II (1-2]	34	
III (2$<$)	46	
UPDRS-III total	18.24 ± 9.8 [2–50]	
Low [0–12]	36	
[13–22]	38	
High [23$<$)	34	
Laterality based on Rigidity item (upper and lower extremity)		
No rigidity or both sides	22%	
Right side	42%	
Left side	36%	
Gait item		
0 [0]	34	
1 (0–1]	62	
2 (1–2]	12	
Postural stability item		
0 [0]	46	
1 (0–1]	49	
2 (1–2]	13	

Participants walked freely at a comfortable, self-chosen speed in an obstacle-free and flat environment for 4 × 10 m. After each 10 m of straight walking, participants were instructed to turn 180° at a preferred direction.

2.3. Turning Isolation

The standardized 4 × 10 m walking included four straight gait bouts and three turnings in between each two straight bouts. The goal was to isolate the three turnings from the whole gait sequence. To this end, the gait sequence was segmented to individual strides semi-automatically [27,28]. These strides should then be categorized as straight walking, turning, and transitions between straight walking and turning. In order to differentiate between these categories, we used statistics of spatio-temporal parameters.

The change of azimuth between two successive mid-stances was defined as the turning angle between consecutive strides (see Figure 1). The absolute values of turning angles were considered since the sign of values only showed the direction of the turnings, which is not of importance in our analysis. Similarly to Mariani et al. [20], strides with turning angles larger than 20° were classified as turning.

In order to identify transition strides in a gait sequence [20], again, statistics over turning angles were used, since this parameter is the best indicator of spatial foot movement during turning (see Figure 1). The turning strides with angles larger than 20° were eliminated from the sequence. A gamma distribution was then fitted to the tuning angels from the rest of the strides. We chose gamma distribution due to the fact that the distribution is one-hand tailed, in a way that strides from straight walking mainly centers on the mean. The highest 10% of the distribution was classified as the transition if the strides were adjacent to the turning strides. In fact, the strides in the highest 10% of the distribution were considered as anomalies in the distribution of straight strides. For turning analysis, we only considered turning and transition strides.

2.4. Turning Parameters

After the turning isolation, we had three sets of strides related to three turns in the standardized test. We extracted spatio-temporal parameters from these strides based on the algorithms in previous works [20,22]. The algorithms for obtaining parameters from our wearable sensor-based system were validated previously using a gold standard, such as an optical motion capture system or instrumented walkway. To quantify turning, two sets of parameters were computed for each turning—per-stride parameters and global parameters per-turn.

For the first group, a set of parameters was extracted from each stride: stride time, path length (normalized on patient's height), stride length (normalized on patient's height), stride velocity, and swing width. In turning, it is very likely that a stride has a curved trajectory, rather than a straight line. In such cases, length of movement in the straight line between the beginning and end of a stride is measured as stride length. In addition, path length was introduced to measure curve length between the beginning and end of a stride (see Figure 1). All these parameters were calculated from mid-stance of a stride to the successive mid-stance.

For the global parameters, we calculated the number of strides and total duration per turn. This set of parameters measures characteristics of the whole turn.

2.5. Statistical Analysis

In order to determine whether parameters can distinguish between different groups (controls and three stages of disease (see Table 1)), we applied the one-way analysis of variance (ANOVA). When a significant difference was found, a post hoc analysis was performed using Bonferroni's test to obtain a pairwise comparison between the groups. The significance level was set at $p < 0.05$. For measuring effect sizes, η^2 was defined as the ratio of variability between groups to the total variation in the data that was used. Cutoff values for small, medium, and large effect sizes were set at 0.01, 0.06, and 0.14, respectively, according to Cohen [29]. Statistical analysis and parameter computations were performed using MATLAB R2015a.

3. Results

As the disease progresses, gait impairment associated with deteriorated mobility becomes more prevalent. In this section, we examined whether spatio-temporal parameters that characterize turning were able to reflect gait impairments.

Figures 2 and 3 show spatio-temporal parameters that are characteristic of turning for global and per-stride parameters, respectively. Clinical scores in PD studies determine the severity of gait impairment and disease stages: the H&Y, UPDRS-III score, and the UPDRS-III sub-items for gait and postural instability. Patients with different levels of disease severity (see Table 1) and controls were statistically compared using ANOVA, followed by Bonferroni's post hoc test.

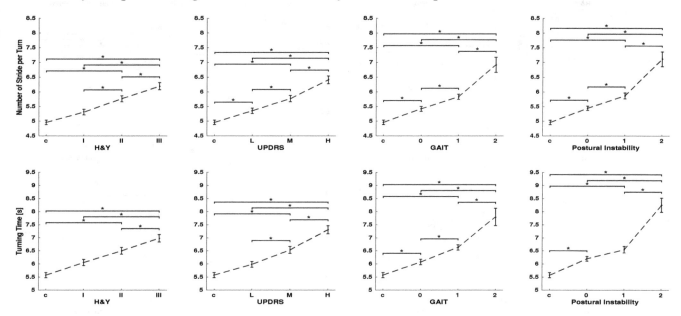

Figure 2. Global parameters characterizing turning: number of strides per-turn and turning time were calculated for controls and PD patients grouped according to H&Y disease stage, UPDRS-III total score, and the single items, gait and postural instability of the UPDRS-III. Group data are displayed as mean ± SEM and were compared using one-way ANOVA followed by Bonferroni's post hoc test, where * indicates $p < 0.05$.

As the disease progresses, stride velocity, path length, stride length, and swing width (per-stride parameters) decreases, and as a result, patients need more strides and time (global parameters) to complete a turn. This can be observed for all clinical scores, although the two sub-items of gait and postural instability are showing larger differences between stages of the disease. Stride time shows no clear change between different groups.

Global parameters showed that PD patients, in contrast to controls, need significantly more time and a larger number of strides to complete a turn (see Figure 2). Number of strides per turn, in particular, shows a significant difference between the control and even early stage of the disease for the UPDRS-III score and its two sub-items. Moreover, there are significant differences between stages of the disease in most comparisons. Per-stride parameters, except stride time, show a significant difference between the controls, mild, and severe stages of the disease for all clinical scores. Stride velocity, stride length, path length, and swing width are able to differentiate disease severity by means of all tested clinical scores (see Figure 3).

To quantify effect sizes, η^2 is reported in Table 2. The effect sizes range from small to large. The largest effect sizes are obtained consistently over all clinical scores with $p < 0.001$ by the global parameters, number of strides per turn, and turning time. Path length showed consistently higher effect sizes than stride length, which suggests that it is a more meaningful parameter for estimation of spatial foot displacement in turning. The effect sizes of per-stride duration are very small.

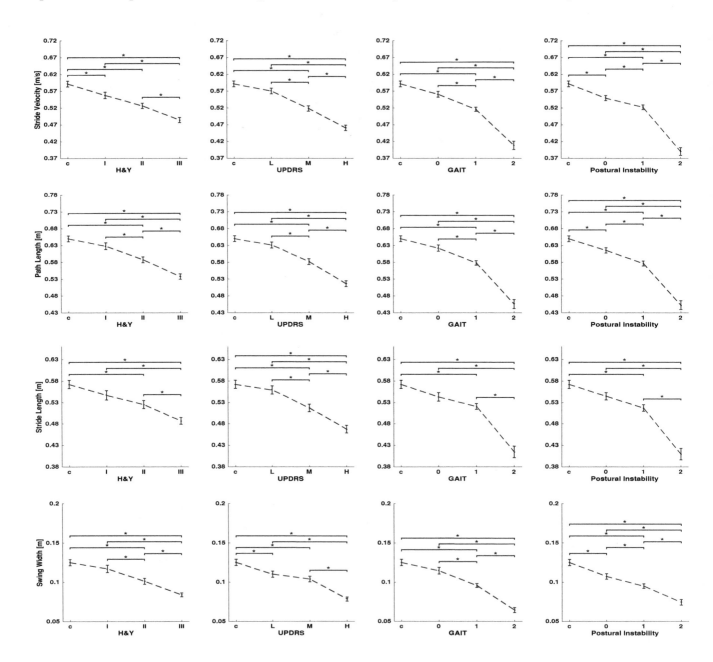

Figure 3. Per-stride parameters characterizing turning: stride velocity, path length, stride length, and swing width were calculated for controls and PD patients who were grouped according to the H&Y disease stage, UPDRS-III score, and the single items, gait and postural instability, of the UPDRS-III. Group data are displayed as mean ± SEM and were compared using one-way ANOVA, followed by Bonferroni's post hoc test, where * indicates $p < 0.05$.

Table 2. ANOVA test: η^2 values for different parameters and clinical scores. Values with * correspond to $p < 0.001$. Bold font indicates values with strong effect sizes.

Parameters	H&Y	UPDRS	Gait	Postural Instability
Number of Strides per-Turn	**0.172 ***	**0.2 ***	**0.202 ***	**0.232 ***
Turning Time	**0.149 ***	**0.199 ***	**0.187 ***	**0.228 ***
Stride Velocity	0.054 *	0.057 *	0.06 *	0.069 *
Path Length	0.054 *	0.054 *	0.06 *	0.063 *
Stride Length	0.03 *	0.03 *	0.034 *	0.038 *
Mid Swing	0.034 *	0.035 *	0.039 *	0.029 *
Stride Time	0.003	0.003	0.002	0.007 *

4. Discussion

The aim of the present study was to investigate whether an on-shoe, sensor-based gait analysis system reflected turning abnormalities and whether it could objectively complement physicians' gait assessments. To this end, we recruited 108 PD patients and 42 age-matched controls, and measured their gait during a 4 × 10 m walk by using our system. We then isolated the turnings from the whole gait sequence and quantified them using several spatio-temporal parameters. The parameters extracted using an on-shoe wearable system were previously validated against gold-standard systems, such as an optical motion capturing system [30] or instrumented walkway [22], and results indicated their technical validity. The clinical validation that followed turn quantification showed that turning parameters extracted using our measurement system and the turn isolation algorithm can effectively reflect gait abnormalities and be successfully used for the objective assessment of turning.

There have been many studies regarding turning analysis in PD [3,17,20]; yet, there is no unique way to define turning. Turning has been defined using mathematical modeling [17], statistics of spatio-temporal parameters [20], or the path between two pre-defined points [5]. One reason for these diverse turning definitions is that, basically, there is no standard way to determine the start and end of the turning. Common gold standards, such as motion-capture systems or videos, cannot provide a ground truth for turning. Since transitions between straight walking and turning happen gradually, it is inherently difficult to determine a specific start- and end-point for turning. A technical validation seems impractical with the usual gold standards. Nevertheless, a specific definition of turning, supported by some clinical validations that show its usability, can be an asset in objective gait assessment [3,17,20].

Turns can have different lengths, angles, and bases of support. We can expect that different types of turning require different levels of coordination [19]. In this study, we analyzed 180° during the 4 × 10 m walk test. Turnings with 180° were also analyzed in other standardized tests, like Timed Up and Go (TUG) [16,31,32]. We studied a 4 × 10 m walk because it includes three turns, which makes it statistically more meaningful to draw any general conclusions from the experiments. Regardless of the type of the turns, the underlying concepts that were used in this study are valid, although the turning isolation algorithm may need some adjustments to distinguish between straight walking and turning in an optimal way.

The findings of this study confirm the results from other studies [11–15], showing that spatio-temporal parameters can manifest gait deficits even in early stages of the disease. Results show that as the total duration of a turn increases, the stride length and velocity decreases and more strides are needed to complete a turn in the PD population. Such changes in parameters were scaled with PD severity. Global parameters of turning, such as the number of strides per turn and the total duration of the turn, can distinguish different groups. This is an important finding for PD studies, because gait problems are difficult to detect by physicians in early stages of the disease, whereas sensor signals can capture subtle differences between a healthy and abnormal gait in the early stages of the disease.

The large effect sizes for global parameters further emphasized the efficiency of these parameters for yielding statistical differences between different groups. Previous studies showed similar results for such global turning parameters [3,16,17]. Per-stride parameters of stride velocity, path length, stride length, and swing width can distinguish the majority of groups, although to a lesser extent in contrast to global parameters. For example, the distinction between controls and early-stage PD patients is more effective in global parameters. Furthermore, the effect sizes for per-stride parameters are in the range of small to medium (see Table 2), which again proves to be less effective than global parameters.

The total duration of turns showed a clear correlation with clinical scores, but such a correlation has not been obtained for per-stride timing. We may be able to explain this by considering two kinds of compensatory actions taken by patients in order to complete the turning. One compensatory action is to take smaller strides, and the other one is having longer pauses in a mid-stance phase in order to secure balance. While the first compensatory action decreases the per-stride time, the latter increases it. These compensatory actions may be different from patient to patient, and a patient may take both of these actions to safely complete a turn. Hence, overall, we cannot see any clear increase or decrease in the per-stride duration; however, the total turn duration did increase, because we may have a decrease of time per stride but patients take more strides that compensate for the decrease in time per stride. Having a long pause at mid-stance phases did not have any effect on stride and path length. These parameters decrease as the disease progresses.

Established clinical scores have no sub-item to assess specific characteristics of turning. Turning is evaluated as part of the gait in general; yet, our findings show that clinical scores reveal turning deficits at different levels. Parameters consistently show a higher correlation with gait and postural instability sub-items than with H&Y and UPDRS-III global scores, both in terms of p-values and effect sizes. Postural instability and gait sub-items are widely used for assessing gait, balance, and risk of falling in PD patients [23]. These two sub-items effectively demonstrate turning abnormalities, even at early stages of the disease (see Figure 2).

Despite the importance, there has not been a study to objectively compare straight walking and turning parameters in order to understand which set of parameters reflects gait abnormalities better. However, parameters quantifying straight walking differentiate between controls and PD patients in more moderate stages of the disease or higher levels of motor impairment [23]. Spatio-temporal parameters characterizing gait abnormalities have been widely used in data-driven applications, from PD diagnosis to disease monitoring [20,33]. However, most of such studies focus only on analyzing straight walking. Our results suggest that turning analysis may improve the performance of data-driven methods in medical applications.

One of the key goals of mobile gait analysis is to monitor patients outside of the clinics. Long-term monitoring of patients during the course of a day can provide better insight into their disease condition, in contrast to time-limited examinations inside the clinics [3]. Moreover, continuous monitoring of patients can be supplemented with preventative strategies for falling and FoG. The fact that turning during standardized tests demonstrates clear signs of deficiency emphasizes that turning analysis needs to be integrated into the long-term gait analysis. Turning isolation during long-term monitoring is even more challenging than in a standardized test, since the strides can be highly variable and different types of turning may happen within the course of a day. Some studies successfully addressed turning analysis in long-term monitoring [3,6], although they did not use on-shoe sensor systems. More research is needed to understand how findings of the current study can be transferred using an on-shoe sensor system to long-term monitoring.

Laterality of PD is another important factor in turning analysis, since turning to the direction of the most affected side is more challenging for patients. However, analyzing the laterality of the disease was beyond the scope of this study—here, the patients were instructed to turn at a convenient speed and preferred direction.

A limitation of our study is that we were, at this stage, not able to analyze the asymmetry between the left and right foot, since the sensors were not synchronized. Even better results may be obtained by an experiment design that takes into account the specific characteristics of PD patients and assessments during OFF medication.

5. Conclusions

Mobile gait analysis using wearable sensors offers elaborate assessments of pathological gait, leading to deeper insight into the motor deficits of PD. A high level of deficiency has been frequently reported for turning in PD. We investigated the feasibility of turning analysis during standardized gait tests using on-shoe wearable sensors. Turning measurements in our experiments clearly demonstrated turning deficits in Parkinson's patients. However, global parameters proved more effective than per-stride parameters. This should be taken into account in designing gait analysis systems, and has an important implication for PD clinical examinations, since physicians can readily assess global parameters. The current result is in alignment with other studies of turning in Parkinson's patients, which proves the feasibility of turning analysis using on-shoe sensor systems. The results of the current study can be applied to studies evaluating turning inside the clinic, and provide useful insight into long-term monitoring outside the clinic.

Author Contributions: Conceptualization, H.G., F.M., N.H.G., J.K. and B.M.E.; Formal analysis, N.H.G.; Funding acquisition, J.K. and B.M.E.; Methodology, H.G., N.H.G.; Resources, H.G. and J.K.; Software, J.H. and N.R., N.H.G.; Supervision, H.G., J.K. and B.M.E.; Writing—original draft, N.H.G.; Writing—review & editing, J.H., N.R., H.G., F.M., J.K. and B.M.E.

Acknowledgments: N. Haji Ghassemi acknowledges financial support from the Bavarian Research Foundation (BFS) and Federal Ministry of Education and Research (BMBF). This work was in part supported by the FAU Emerging Fields Initiative (EFIMoves), Bavarian Ministry for Economy, Regional Development & Energy via the Medical Valley Award 2017 (FallRiskPD Project) and EIT Health innovation project. F. Marxreiter is supported by the interdisciplinary center for clinical research Erlangen (IZKF), clinician scientist program. Björn M. Eskofier gratefully acknowledges the support of the German Research Foundation (DFG) within the framework of the Heisenberg professorship program (grant number ES 434/8-1).

References

1.   Stack, E.; Ashburn, A. Dysfunctional turning in Parkinson's disease. *Disabil. Rehabil.* **2008**, *30*, 1222–1229. [CrossRef] [PubMed]
2.   Crenna, P.; Carpinella, I.; Rabuffetti, M.; Calabrese, E.; Mazzoleni, P.; Nemni, R.; Ferrarin, M. The association between impaired turning and normal straight walking in Parkinson's disease. *Gait Posture* **2007**, *26*, 172–178. [CrossRef] [PubMed]
3.   El-Gohary, M.; Pearson, S.; McNames, J.; Mancini, M.; Horak, F.; Mellone, S.; Chiari, L. Continuous monitoring of turning in patients with movement disability. *Sensors* **2014**, *14*, 356–369. [CrossRef] [PubMed]
4.   Pickering, R.M.; Grimbergen, Y.A.; Rigney, U.; Ashburn, A.; Mazibrada, G.; Wood, B.; Gray, P.; Kerr, G.; Bloem, B.R. A meta-analysis of six prospective studies of falling in Parkinson's disease. *Mov. Disord.* **2007**, *22*, 1892–1900. [CrossRef] [PubMed]
5.   Stack, E.; Jupp, K.; Ashburn, A. Developing methods to evaluate how people with Parkinson's disease turn 180°: An activity frequently associated with falls. *Disabil. Rehabil.* **2004**, *26*, 478–484. [CrossRef] [PubMed]
6.   Mancini, M.; Weiss, A.; Herman, T.; Hausdorff, J.M. Turn Around Freezing: Community-Living Turning Behavior in People with Parkinson's Disease. *Front. Neurol.* **2018**, *9*, 18. [CrossRef] [PubMed]
7.   Moore, O.; Peretz, C.; Giladi, N. Freezing of gait affects quality of life of peoples with Parkinson's disease beyond its relationships with mobility and gait. *Mov. Disord.* **2007**, *22*, 219–2195. [CrossRef]
8.   Bachlin, M.; Plotnik, M.; Roggen, D.; Maidan, I.; Hausdorff, J.M.; Giladi, N.; Troster, G. Wearable assistant for Parkinson's disease patients with the freezing of gait symptom. *IEEE Trans. Inf. Technol. Biomed.* **2010**, *14*, 436–446. [CrossRef]
9.   Goetz, C.G.; Tilley, B.C.; Shaftman, S.R.; Stebbins, G.T.; Fahn, S.; Martinez-Martin, P.; Poewe, W.; Sampaio, C.; Stern, M.B.; Dodel, R.; et al. Movement Disorder Society-sponsored revision of the Unified Parkinson's Disease Rating Scale (MDS-UPDRS): Scale presentation and clinimetric testing results. *Mov. Disord.* **2008**, *23*, 2129–2170. [CrossRef]

10. Hoehn, M.M.; Yahr, M.D. Parkinsonism: Onset, progression and mortality. *Neurology* **1967**, *17*, 427–442. [CrossRef]

11. Stack, E.L.; Ashburn, A.A.; Jupp, K.E. Strategies used by people with Parkinson's disease who report difficulty turning. *Park. Rel. Disord.* **2006**, *12*, 87–92. [CrossRef] [PubMed]

12. Mak, M.; Patle, A.; Hui-Chan, C. Sudden turn during walking is impaired in people with Parkinson's disease. *Exp. Brain Res.* **2008**, *190*, 43–51. [CrossRef] [PubMed]

13. Huxham, F.; Baker, R.; Morris, M.E.; Iansek, R. Footstep adjustments used to turn during walking in Parkinson's disease. *Mov. Disord.* **2008**, *23*, 817–823. [CrossRef] [PubMed]

14. Hong, M.; Perlmutter, J.; Earhart, G.A. kinematic and electromyographic analysis of turning in people with Parkinson disease. *Neurorehabil. Neural Repair* **2009**, *23*, 166–176. [CrossRef] [PubMed]

15. Hong, M.; Earhart, G.M. Effects of medication on turning deficits in individuals with Parkinson's disease. *J. Neurol. Phys. Ther.* **2010**, *34*, 11–16. [CrossRef]

16. King, L.; Mancini, M.; Priest, K.; Salarian, A.; Rodrigues-de Paula, F.; Horak, F. Do clinical scales of balance reflect turning abnormalities in people with Parkinson's disease? *J. Neurol. Phys. Ther.* **2012**, *36*, 25–31. [CrossRef] [PubMed]

17. Salarian, A.; Zampieri, C.; Horak, F.; Carlson-Kuhta, P.; Nutt, J.; Aminian, K. Analyzing 180 Degrees Turns Using an Inertial System Reveals Early Signs of Progression of Parkinson's Disease. In Proceedings of the 2009 IEEE Engineering in Medicine and Biology Society, Minneapolis, MN, USA, 3–6 September 2009; pp. 224–227.

18. Huxham, F.; Baker, R.; Morris, M.E.; Iansek, R. Head and trunk rotation during walking turns in Parkinson's disease. *Mov. Disord.* **2008**, *23*, 1391–1397. [CrossRef]

19. Mellone, S.; Mancini, M.; King, L.A.; Horak, F.B.; Chiari, L. The quality of turning in Parkinson's disease: A compensatory strategy to prevent postural instability? *J. Neuroeng. Rehabil.* **2016**, *13*, 39. [CrossRef]

20. Mariani, B.; Jimenez, M.; Vingerhoets, F.; Aminian, K. On-shoe wearable sensors for gait and turning assessment of patients with Parkinson's disease. *IEEE Trans. Biomed. Eng.* **2013**, *60*, 155–158. [CrossRef]

21. Panebianco, G.P.; Bisi, M.C.; Stagni, R.; Fantozzi, S. Analysis of the performance of 17 algorithms from a systematic review: Influence of sensor position, analysed variable and computational approach in gait timing estimation from IMU measurements. *Gait Posture* **2018**, *66*, 76–82. [CrossRef]

22. Rampp, A.; Barth; J., Schülein, S.; Gassmann; K. G.; Klucken, J.; Eskofier, B. M. Inertial sensor-based stride parameter calculation from gait sequences in geriatric patients. *IEEE Trans. Biomed. Eng.* **2014**, *62*, 1089–1097. [CrossRef] [PubMed]

23. Schlachetzki, J.C.; Barth, J.; Marxreiter, F.; Gossler, J.; Kohl, Z.; Reinfelder, S.; Gassner, H.; Aminian, K.; Eskofier, B.M.; Winkler, J.; et al. Wearable sensors objectively measure gait parameters in Parkinson's disease. *PLoS ONE* **2017**, *12*, e0183989. [CrossRef] [PubMed]

24. Gassner, H.; Raccagni, C.; Eskofier, B.M.; Klucken, J.; Wenning, G.K. The diagnostic scope of sensor-based gait analysis in atypical Parkinsonism: Further observations. *Front. Neurol.* **2019**, *10*, 5. [CrossRef] [PubMed]

25. Hughes, A.J.; Daniel, S.E.; Kilford, L.; Lees, A.J. Accuracy of clinical diagnosis of idiopathic parkinson's disease: A clinico-pathological study of 100 cases. *J. Neurol. Neurosurg. Psychiatry* **1992**, *55*, 181–184. [CrossRef] [PubMed]

26. Parkinson, J. *An Essay on the Shaking Palsy*; Neely & Jones: London, UK, 1817.

27. Haji Ghassemi, N.; Hannink, J.; Martindale, C.F.; Gassner, H.; Müller, M.; Klucken, J.; Eskofier, B.M. Segmentation of Gait Sequences in Sensor-Based Movement Analysis: A Comparison of Methods in Parkinson's Disease. *Sensors* **2018**, *18*, 145. [CrossRef]

28. Barth, J.; Oberndorfer, C.; Pasluosta, C.; Schülein, S.; Gassner, H.; Reinfelder, S.; Kugler, P.; Schuldhaus, D.; Winkler, J.; Klucken, J.; et al. Stride segmentation during free walk movements using multi-dimensional subsequence dynamic time warping on inertial sensor data. *Sensors* **2015**, *15*, 6419–6440. [CrossRef]

29. Cohen, J. *Statistical Power Analysis for the Behavioral Sciences*, 2nd ed.; Lawrence Erlbaum Associates: Hillsdale, NJ, USA, 1988.

30. Kanzler, C.M.; Barth, J.; Klucken, J.; Eskofier, B.M. Inertial sensor based gait analysis discriminates subjects with and without visual impairment caused by simulated macular degeneration. *Conf. Proc. IEEE Eng. Med. Biol. Soc.* **2016**, *2016*, 4979–4982.

31. Salarian, A.; Horak, F.B.; Carlson-Kuhta, P.; Nutt, J.; Zampieri, C.; Aminian, K. iTUG, a Sensitive and Reliable

Measure of Mobility. *IEEE Trans. Neural Syst. Rehabil. Eng.* **2010**, *18*, 303–310. [CrossRef]

32. Herman, T.; Giladi, N.; Hausdorff, J.M. Properties of the 'timed up and go' test: More than meets the eye. *Gerontology* **2011**, *57*, 203–210.

33. Klucken, J.; Barth, J.; Kugler, P.; Schlachetzki, J.; Henze, T.; Marxreiter, F.; Kohl, Z.; Steidl, R.; Hornegger, J.; Eskofier, B.; et al. Unbiased and Mobile Gait Analysis Detects Motor Impairment in Parkinson's Disease. *PLoS ONE* **2013**, *8*, e56956. [CrossRef]

6

Exploring Risk of Falls and Dynamic Unbalance in Cerebellar Ataxia by Inertial Sensor Assessment

Pietro Caliandro [1], Carmela Conte [2], Chiara Iacovelli [2,*], Antonella Tatarelli [3], Stefano Filippo Castiglia [4], Giuseppe Reale [5] and Mariano Serrao [4,6]

[1]   Unità Operativa Complessa Neurologia, Fondazione Policlinico Universitario A. Gemelli IRCCS, Largo A. Gemelli, 8, 00168 Rome, Italy; pietro.caliandro@policlinicogemelli.it

[2]   IRCCS Fondazione Don Carlo Gnocchi, Piazzale Morandi, 6, 20121 Milan, Italy; cconte@dongnocchi.it

[3]   Department of Occupational and Environmental Medicine, Epidemiology and Hygiene, INAIL, via Fontana Candida, 1, 00078 Monte Porzio Catone, Italy; antonellatatarelli@gmail.com

[4]   Department of Medical and Surgical Sciences and Biotechnologies, Sapienza University of Rome, Piazzale Aldo Moro, 5, 00185 Rome, Italy; stefanofilippo.castiglia@uniroma1.it (S.F.C.); mariano.serrao@uniroma1.it (M.S.)

[5]   Department of Neurosciences, Università Cattolica del Sacro Cuore, Largo F. Vito, 1, 00168 Rome, Italy; giureale@yahoo.it

[6]   Policlinico Italia, Movement Analysis Laboratory, Piazza del Campidano, 6, 00162 Rome, Italy

*   Correspondence: ciacovelli@dongnocchi.it

Abstract: Background. Patients suffering from cerebellar ataxia have extremely variable gait kinematic features. We investigated whether and how wearable inertial sensors can describe the gait kinematic features among ataxic patients. Methods. We enrolled 17 patients and 16 matched control subjects. We acquired data by means of an inertial sensor attached to an ergonomic belt around pelvis, which was connected to a portable computer via Bluetooth. Recordings of all the patients were obtained during overground walking. From the accelerometric data, we obtained the harmonic ratio (HR), i.e., a measure of the acceleration patterns, smoothness and rhythm, and the step length coefficient of variation (CV), which evaluates the variability of the gait cycle. Results. Compared to controls, patients had a lower HR, meaning a less harmonic and rhythmic acceleration pattern of the trunk, and a higher step length CV, indicating a more variable step length. Both HR and step length CV showed a high effect size in distinguishing patients and controls ($p < 0.001$ and $p = 0.011$, respectively). A positive correlation was found between the step length CV and both the number of falls ($R = 0.672$; $p = 0.003$) and the clinical severity (ICARS: $R = 0.494$; $p = 0.044$; SARA: $R = 0.680$; $p = 0.003$). Conclusion. These findings demonstrate that the use of inertial sensors is effective in evaluating gait and balance impairment among ataxic patients.

Keywords: inertial sensors; cerebellar ataxia; movement analysis; gait analysis; balance; personalized medicine; rehabilitation

1. Introduction

Patients suffering from cerebellar ataxia exhibit peculiar spatiotemporal and kinematic features that contribute to an unstable gait [1–5]. The gait impairment typically worsens over time, in parallel with the functional decline associated to the neurodegenerative process [6,7]. While stable gait is characterized by repeatable walking patterns [8], steadiness in the case of perturbations [9–13], and effectiveness in maintaining upright balance [14,15], ataxic gait is extremely variable over gait cycles [1] and exhibits inefficient coordination between upper and lower segments of body, even in the absence of external perturbations [16]. Taking into account such conditions, it is reasonable to hypothesize that when perturbation occurs in ataxic patients, the consequent fall risk increases, and the gait pattern can be defined as unstable [6,7].

The evaluation of gait instability and fall risk is, therefore, pivotal in the study of ataxic gait to prevent further disabilities, and in order to maximize and optimize the information we gather from such evaluation, it should be performed in a real-life environment outside the motion analysis laboratory for a long period of time. In this context, wearable magnetic and inertial measurement units (MIMUs), consisting of a three-axial accelerometer, a gyroscope, and a magnetometer, represent a self-contained alternative to conventional laboratory-based motion capture systems [17–19]. This technology estimates the three-dimensional (3D) orientation of MIMUs with respect to a global coordinate system by specific sensor fusion algorithms, using angular velocity, gravity and magnetic field vectors.

A series of biomechanical stability measures based on MIMU evaluations have been proposed in several studies on neurological gait disorders with dynamic unbalance [3,20–22]. The maximum Lyapunov exponent (λmax) is an available method to evaluate gait instability [4] and fall risk [3] in ataxic patients, but the relationship between λmax and clinical severity has not been definitively established, since it has been demonstrated to be both positively [4] and negatively [3] correlated to International Cooperative Ataxia Rating Scale (ICARS) scores. A possible explanation could be found in the heterogeneous etiologies of the study samples, respectively acquired cerebellar lesions after tumor resection [4], and neurodegenerative ataxia [3]. Another important issue is that λmax properly explores the nonlinear dynamic local stability of the trunk during locomotion when at least 150 continuous strides are recorded [15]. However, such stride numbers are often not practically feasible in ataxic patients, and this could have influenced the correlation analysis between λmax and clinical severity.

To the best of our knowledge, no other studies in the literature have used additional indexes of stability, like harmonic ratio (HR) and the coefficients of variation (CV) based on MIMU data to detect the instability of ataxic patients. Therefore, the aim of this study is to evaluate these indexes of stability and, in particular, examine the ability of each index to detect the instability of ataxic patients compared to healthy controls and determine the fall risk. HR was chosen to evaluate the trunk acceleration patterns, a key feature in determining the severity of the ataxic gait [5,16], while CV was chosen to evaluate the variability of step length, an important compensatory mechanism in ataxic patients.

2. Materials and Methods

2.1. Participants

Seventeen patients affected by primary degenerative cerebellar ataxia were enrolled in the study. Table 1 summarizes the patients' clinical features and genotype.

The complete neurological assessment included (1) cognitive evaluation according to mini-mental state examination (MMSE) scale, (2) cranial nerve evaluation, (3) muscle tone evaluation, (4) muscle strength evaluation, (5) joint coordination evaluation, (6) sensory examination, (7) tendon reflex elicitation, and (8) disease severity measured by International Cooperative Ataxia Rating Scale (ICARS) and Scale for the Assessment and Rating of Ataxia (SARA) [23,24]. We excluded patients with gait impairment due to extracerebellar symptoms or orthopedic disorders. Regarding the extracerebellar disorders affecting gait, we excluded patients with spasticity, polyneuropathy, cognitive deficits, and extrapyramidal disorders. Of the recruited patients, no one presented with signs of spasticity, hyposthenia, hypoesthesia, and/or cognitive impairment (MMSE > 24). All patients were able to walk alone without any kind of assistance or aid, and were receiving physical therapy, including active and passive exercises for upper and lower limbs as well as balance and gait re-education. Furthermore, no patient had significant visual deficits according to the Snellen visual acuity test. Almost all of the patients had non-disabling oculomotor abnormalities, such as nystagmus or square wave jerks pursuit movements, because of the underlying disorder. A brain MRI showed that all patients had cerebellar atrophy. Regarding the fall risk assessment, all patients had to complete a specific questionnaire designed to evaluate the number of falls in the previous year, the characteristics of such falls (side, associated injury), and the circumstances in which they occurred. The number of falls in the last year was used for correlation analysis. Sixteen age-matched healthy adults (age, ataxic patients 53.53 ± 12.12 years, healthy controls, 50.94 ± 8.79 years, p > 0.05) were enrolled as the control group. We obtained informed consent from each patient and healthy subject, which complied with the Helsinki Declaration and was approved by the local ethics committee.

Table 1. Ataxic patients' clinical and anthropometric characteristics.

	Number/Total	%	Mean (SD)
Male	9/17	52.9	-
Female	8/17	47.1	-
Age (years)	-	-	53.53 (12.12)
Height (m)	-	-	1.65 (0.09)
Weight (kg)	-	-	71.03 (12.74)
ICARS	-	-	24.70 (10.80)
SARA	-	-	12.20 (4.25)
Disease duration (years)	-	-	12.11 (4.52)
Diagnosis			
SAOA	9/17	52.9	-
SCA1	2/17	11.8	-
SCA2	3/17	17.6	-
SCA3	1/17	5.9	-
SCA8	1/17	5.9	-
FRDA	1/17	5.9	-

SAOA: sporadic adult onset ataxia of unknown etiology; SCA: spinocerebellar ataxia; FRDA: Friedreich's ataxia.

2.2. Gait Analysis

We acquired data with an inertial sensor (BTS GWALK, BTS, Milan, Italy), attached to an ergonomic belt placed around the pelvis at the level of the L5 vertebra, connected to a portable computer via Bluetooth. The sampling rate was 100 Hz, and the sensor, endowed with a tri-axial accelerometer (16 bit/axes), a tri-axial magnetometer (13 bit), and a tri-axial gyroscope (16 bit/axes), measured the linear trunk accelerations and the trunk angular velocities in three space directions (i.e., AR: anterior-posterior; ML: mediolateral; VT: vertical direction).

2.3. Task Description

Before starting the experimental session, participants were asked to walk along a predetermined route in order to familiarize themselves with the procedure. Recordings of all the patients were obtained during overground walking. We asked participants to walk along a corridor (3 m wide and 20 m long) at their preferred speed. Control subjects were asked to walk at a low speed in order to match the two groups for speed (ataxic patients, 0.939 ± 0.195 m/s; controls, 0.924 ± 0.239 m/s; p > 0.05).

2.4. Inertial Sensor Data Processing

The 'walking protocol' of the inertial sensor (G-STUDIO, BTS, Milan, Italy) was used to detect: (1) trunk acceleration patterns, (2) right and left heel strikes, and (3) toe-off. The HR and the CV were calculated using MATLAB software (MATLAB 7.4.0, MAthWorks, Natick, MA, USA).

Harmonic ratio. The harmonic ratio (HR), initially described by Gage [25] and later modified by Smidt et al. [26], provides an indication of the acceleration patterns, smoothness, and rhythm. Since the unit of measurement from a continuous walking trial is a stride (two steps), a stable, rhythmic gait pattern should be characterized by multiples of two repeated acceleration patterns within any given stride. Accelerations patterns that do not repeat in multiples of two generate out of phase accelerations, reflecting irregular accelerations during a walking trial and, therefore, an unstable gait pattern. The harmonic content of the acceleration signals can be analyzed in each spatial direction using stride frequency as the fundamental frequency component. Based on each stride time, 20 harmonics were calculated. Trunk accelerations of each stride were broken down into individual sinusoidal waveforms using discrete Fourier transform (DFT).

Since a stable smooth gait pattern is characterized by acceleration signals in VT and AP directions that repeat in multiples of two during a single stride, HRs in the VT and AP directions were calculated as the ratio of the sum of the amplitudes of the first 10 even harmonics divided by the sum of the amplitudes of the first 10 odd harmonics. In the ML direction, acceleration signals were repeated once for any given stride, so HRs in the ML direction were calculated as the sum of the amplitudes of the odd harmonics divided by the sum of the amplitudes of the even harmonics. We used a high-pass filter with cutoff at 20 Hz to eliminate noise signals.

HRs per stride were determined and averaged across a steady walk, resulting in a mean HR. HR in AP and VT, and in the ML direction, were calculated as below [19]:

HR in anterior–posterior and vertical directions

$$HR = \frac{\sum_{i=1}^{10} A_{2i}}{\sum_{i=1}^{10} A_{2i-1}}$$

HR in the medio-lateral direction

$$HR = \frac{\sum_{i=1}^{10} A_{2i-1}}{\sum_{i=1}^{10} A_{2i}}$$

where A_{2i} denotes the amplitude of the first 20 even harmonics and A_{2i-1} indicates the amplitude of the first 20 odd harmonics. The higher the HR value, the smoother the walking pattern.

Coefficient of variation. In order to compute the step length CV, the step length was estimated using the upward and downward movements of the trunk, as proposed by Zijlstra and Hof [27]. Assuming a compass gait type, the body's center of mass (CoM) movements in the sagittal plane follow a circular trajectory during each single support phase. In this inverted pendulum model, changes in height of CoM depend on step length [27]. Thus, step length can be deduced by known height changes and predicted from geometrical characteristics as follows: step length $= 2\sqrt{2lh - h^2}$.

In this equation, h is equal to the change in height of the CoM, and l represents the pendulum length. Changes in vertical position were calculated by a double integration of the vertical acceleration. A high-pass filter (fourth-order zero-lag Butterworth filter at 0.1 Hz) was used in order to avoid integration drift. The difference between highest and lowest position during a step cycle was used to determine the amplitude of changes in the vertical position (h). Leg length was considered as pendulum length (l). Step length was calculated as the mean of step lengths observed during seven subsequent steps of each subject.

Then, the step length coefficient of variation (CV) was computed as follows: $CV = 100\frac{SD}{mean}$ where mean is the mean step length and SD is the standard deviation over the entire step length for each subject [1]. The CV is a measure of the variability of a data set; the closer to 0 the CV is, the less variable the data are.

2.5. Statistical Analysis

We used the SPSS 17.0 software (SPSS Inc. Chicago, IL, USA) for statistical analysis. All data were expressed as mean ± standard deviation; $p < 0.05$ was considered statistically significant. We assessed the normality of distributions using the Shapiro-Wilk test.

Mean and standard deviation within subjects were computed for speed and stability indexes. We used the independent-samples t test to look for differences between the stability indexes of ataxic patients vs. controls. Cohen's d index was used to assess the effect size of the stability indexes in the three spatial directions [28,29]. We used the Pearson's test to investigate any correlation We used the Pearson test to investigate any correlation of acceleration HR and step length CV with (1) age, (2) height, (3) weight, (4) disease duration, (5) total ICARS and SARA scores and (6) number of falls in the last year.

3. Results

Looking at the low scores of ICARS and SARA, the recruited patients mainly showed cerebellar symptoms (see Table 1).

HR in all three directions and step length CV were all significantly different when compared to the controls (Table 2). Briefly, the HR of patients was lower than the HR of healthy subjects, meaning a less harmonic and rhythmic acceleration pattern of the trunk, while the CV of step length was greater in patients than in the controls, indicating a more variable step length in ataxic patients. Both HR and CV of step length showed a high effect size in distinguishing patients and controls, but HR in all three directions showed a higher effect size score when compared to the CV (Table 2).

Table 2. Comparisons of the stability indexes between 17 ataxic patients and 16 controls at matched gait speed.

Parameter	Patients	Controls	t	p	Cohen's d
HR-AP	1.665 ± 0.300	2.414 ± 0.540	4.964	<0.001	1.714
HR-ML	1.639 ± 0.282	2.347 ± 0.559	4.631	<0.001	1.599
HR-VT	1.694 ± 0.304	2.549 ± 0.715	4.519	<0.001	1.556
Step length CV (%)	21.249 ± 10.293	13.205 ± 6.004	−2.720	0.011	0.955
Step length (m)	0.499 ± 0.087	0.569 ± 0.067	−2.382	0.024	0.112
Speed (m/s)	0.939 ± 0.195	0.924 ± 0.239	−0.207	0.838	0.069

Mean ± standard deviation values, the results of the independent samples t-test and Cohen's d are reported. Values of p lower than 0.05 were considered statistically significant. HR-AP: harmonic ratio in the anterior–posterior direction; HR-ML: harmonic ratio in the mediolateral direction; and HR-VT: harmonic ratio in the vertical direction.

Surprisingly, no correlation was found between HR in all directions, falls/year, and clinical severity (ICARS and SARA scores) (Table 3), while a significant positive correlation was found between the CV of step length and the falls/years and ICARS and SARA scores (Figure 1).

Table 3. Correlation analysis between HR in all directions and ICARS, SARA, and falls/year.

Parameter	ICARS (R, p)	SARA (R, p)	falls/year (R, p)
HR-AP	−0.35, 0.24	−0.35, 0.13	−0.10, 0.66
HR-ML	−0.47, 0.10	−0.36, 0.11	0.02, 0.92
HR-VT	−0.41, 0.88	−0.43, 0.06	−0.01, 0.99

The reported values represent Pearson correlation value (R) and statistical significance value (p). HR-AP: harmonic ratio in the anterior–posterior direction; HR-ML: harmonic ratio in the mediolateral direction; and HR-VT: harmonic ratio in the vertical direction.

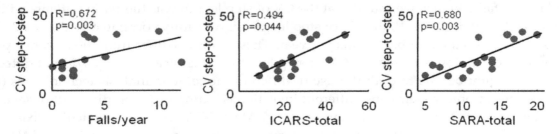

Figure 1. Correlations between the maximum step-to-step coefficient of variation and the falls/year, ICARS-total, and SARA-total scores in 17 ataxic patients. Pearson's R coefficient (R) and significance (p) are reported.

4. Discussion

In the present study, we found that trunk acceleration smoothness, as described by HR values, and the variability of step length, as described by the CV, may provide insights about gait stability in subjects with degenerative ataxia. Furthermore, the variability of step length correlated with both clinical severity and fall risk.

Regarding the acceleration patterns of the trunk, the HR of patients significantly differed from that of healthy controls in all three spatial planes. Moreover, it showed a high effect size, according to Cohen's d index (Table 2). This means that ataxic patients, compared to healthy subjects, exhibit a substantial reduction of trunk movement smoothness. When discussing these findings, we should bear in mind that the trunk has a great functional importance in minimizing the magnitude of linear and angular displacement of the head, ensuring clear vision [30,31], facilitating the integration of vestibular information [32], contributing to the maintenance of balance [5,6,16,33,34], and acting as a driving force for locomotion [35]. Consequently, investigating upper body stability in patients with degenerative cerebellar ataxia is essential, since the lack of motor control [5] and coordination [16] makes the trunk itself generate perturbations in a sort of vicious circle in parallel to the clinical decline [2]. In this context, trunk acceleration smoothness, as described by the HR values, provides a deeper insight into gait disturbances [14,36]. From the literature, we know that trunk acceleration smoothness during walking is predictive of gait dysfunction [37,38] and fall risk in older people [14,39]. Moreover, HR has already been found to be abnormal in patients who have suffered a stroke, Parkinson's disease, or multiple sclerosis [19,20,22,40].

Overall, these findings suggest that HR can substantially describe trunk accelerative behavior abnormalities among patients with degenerative ataxia [41]. On the other hand, we did not find any correlation between HR, the number of falls, and clinical severity. This last result is apparently in contrast with previous studies that found a relationship between clinical severity, increased range of motion of trunk [5] and trunk–thigh coordination deficit [16]. Considering the small sample size of our study, we cannot exclude a type II error. Nevertheless, another possible explanation might come from the different implemented technologies and protocols. In fact, previous studies assessed the kinematic patterns of the upper segment of the head and the trunk via optoelectronic systems [5,16]. This means that the body markers were located on body segments (i.e., the head and upper trunk) whose range of movements was wider than the lumbar one, as investigated by a BTS GWALK device located on L5 vertebra. Further studies will assess such differences, evaluating the role of the ergonomic belt placed around the thorax just underneath the axilla, and will validate inertial sensor findings against optoelectronic systems.

The other parameter we considered was the CV of step length, which has been reported to be significantly different in subjects with cerebellar ataxia when compared to healthy subjects [42]. During the progression of the disease (i.e., >4 years from the onset, as in our sample), subjects with degenerative ataxia tend to lose the ability to both enlarge their step width and fasten their walking speed and—maintaining the same step width and speed—they shorten their step length in order to reduce their single support time [43], with a significant increase in step length CV that can lead to an increased risk of falls. In fact, we found that the CV of step length was higher in patients with ataxia than the controls and, unlike HR, the CV of step length significantly correlated with the ICARS and SARA scores and with the number of falls per year. These findings differ from those from a previous study, where a correlation between the CV of step length and clinical severity was not detected [1]. This difference might be due to both the use of different movement analysis technologies (inertial sensor vs. optoelectronic system) and different investigated samples (sporadic adult onset ataxia of unknown etiology (SAOA)/ spinocerebellar ataxia (SCA) vs. SCA/SAOA/Friedreich's ataxia (FRDA)). Since a camera-based optoelectronic system can capture a smaller change of gait than MIMUs, our data should be interpreted with caution. However, the investigation of a large number of patients with FRDA in Serrao et al. [1] might explain, at least in part, such discrepant results. In this view, patients with FRDA and those with SCA and SAOA may show a different relationship between clinical features and gait stability; further studies are needed to explore this issue. However, our aim was not to obtain an alternative measure of step length, but to detect the relationship between the multifactorial gait impairment [5,6,16,33,34], clinical severity, and the fall risk. Because the MIMU-measured CV of step length is influenced by movements of the trunk [27], and trunk–thigh coordination is impaired in ataxic patients [16], our MIMU-measured CV might reflect trunk–thigh coordination variability. In this respect, the aforementioned limitation might come in handy, being such a multifactorial parameter able to summarize factors that, put together, explain gait instability in ataxic patients.

Finally, our results cannot be generalized as representative of the ataxic population because they refer to patients with a disease duration of at least 8 years, preserved walking ability, and without extracerebellar symptoms as disabling oculomotor abnormalities. Moreover, our findings highlight the need to investigate the relationship between each MIMU-measured index and the corresponding ones measured by traditional optoelectronic systems in order to have proper validation.

5. Conclusions

In conclusion, the present study highlighted that both HR and CV differed between ataxic patients and healthy subjects. However, when considering the correlation with clinical severity and fall risk, only MIMU-measured CV of step length was able to describe the burden of ataxic symptoms and to draw clinical attention towards a possible increased fall risk. These MIMU-based parameters might provide real-world information on patients' disabilities and falls, since they are obtained through wearable and comfortable devices.

Author Contributions: Conceptualization, P.C., M.S., C.I., C.C. and A.T. Methodology, P.C., C.C., M.S. and C.I.; Investigation, C.C., S.F.C., C.I.; Data Curation, C.I., C.C. and S.F.C. Writing—Original Draft Preparation, P.C., C.I., C.C. and S.F.C. Writing—Review & Editing: M.S. and G.R. Supervision: M.S.

Acknowledgments: Thanks to Matteo Gratta for language editing.

References

1.   Serrao, M.; Pierelli, F.; Ranavolo, A.; Draicchio, F.; Conte, C.; Don, R.; Di Fabio, R.; LeRose, M.; Padua, L.; Sandrini, G.; et al. Gait pattern in inherited cerebellar ataxias. *Cerebellum Lond. Engl.* **2012**, *11*, 194–211. [CrossRef] [PubMed]

2.   Serrao, M.; Ranavolo, A.; Casali, C. Neurophysiology of gait. *Handb. Clin. Neurol.* **2018**, *154*, 299–303. [PubMed]

3.   Chini, G.; Ranavolo, A.; Draicchio, F.; Casali, C.; Conte, C.; Martino, G.; Leonardi, L.; Padua, L.; Coppola, G.; Pierelli, F.; et al. Local Stability of the Trunk in Patients with Degenerative Cerebellar Ataxia During Walking. *Cerebellum Lond. Engl.* **2017**, *16*, 26–33. [CrossRef] [PubMed]

4.   Hoogkamer, W.; Bruijn, S.M.; Sunaert, S.; Swinnen, S.P.; Van Calenbergh, F.; Duysens, J. Toward new sensitive measures to evaluate gait stability in focal cerebellar lesion patients. *Gait Posture* **2015**, *41*, 592–596. [CrossRef]

5. Conte, C.; Pierelli, F.; Casali, C.; Ranavolo, A.; Draicchio, F.; Martino, G.; Harfoush, M.; Padua, L.; Coppola, G.; Sandrini, G.; et al. Upper body kinematics in patients with cerebellar ataxia. *Cerebellum Lond. Engl.* **2014**, *13*, 689–697. [CrossRef]

6. Schniepp, R.; Wuehr, M.; Schlick, C.; Huth, S.; Pradhan, C.; Dieterich, M.; Brandt, T.; Jahn, K. Increased gait variability is associated with the history of falls in patients with cerebellar ataxia. *J. Neurol.* **2014**, *261*, 213–223. [CrossRef]

7. Schniepp, R.; Schlick, C.; Pradhan, C.; Dieterich, M.; Brandt, T.; Jahn, K.; Wuehr, M. The interrelationship between disease severity, dynamic stability, and falls in cerebellar ataxia. *J. Neurol.* **2016**, *263*, 1409–1417. [CrossRef]

8. Dingwell, J.B.; Marin, L.C. Kinematic variability and local dynamic stability of upper body motions when walking at different speeds. *J. Biomech.* **2006**, *39*, 444–452. [CrossRef]

9. Terrier, P.; Dériaz, O. Kinematic variability, fractal dynamics and local dynamic stability of treadmill walking. *J. Neuroeng. Rehabil.* **2011**, *8*, 12. [CrossRef]

10. England, S.A.; Granata, K.P. The influence of gait speed on local dynamic stability of walking. *Gait Posture* **2007**, *25*, 172–178. [CrossRef]

11. Kobayashi, M.; Nomura, T.; Sato, S. Phase-dependent response during human locomotion to impulsive perturbation and its interpretation based on neural mechanism. *Jpn. J. Med. Electron. Biol. Eng.* **2000**, *38*, 20–32.

12. Nessler, J.A.; Spargo, T.; Craig-Jones, A.; Milton, J.G. Phase resetting behavior in human gait is influenced by treadmill walking speed. *Gait Posture* **2016**, *43*, 187–191. [CrossRef] [PubMed]

13. Nomura, T.; Kawa, K.; Suzuki, Y.; Nakanishi, M.; Yamasaki, T. Dynamic stability and phase resetting during biped gait. *Chaos Woodbury N* **2009**, *19*, 026103. [CrossRef] [PubMed]

14. Menz, H.B.; Lord, S.R.; Fitzpatrick, R.C. Acceleration patterns of the head and pelvis when walking on level and irregular surfaces. *Gait Posture* **2003**, *18*, 35–46. [CrossRef]

15. Bruijn, S.M.; Meijer, O.G.; van Dieën, J.H.; Kingma, I.; Lamoth, C.J.C. Coordination of leg swing, thorax rotations, and pelvis rotations during gait: The organisation of total body angular momentum. *Gait Posture* **2008**, *27*, 455–462. [CrossRef]

16. Caliandro, P.; Iacovelli, C.; Conte, C.; Simbolotti, C.; Rossini, P.M.; Padua, L.; Casali, C.; Pierelli, F.; Reale, G.; Serrao, M. Trunk-lower limb coordination pattern during gait in patients with ataxia. *Gait Posture* **2017**, *57*, 252–257. [CrossRef]

17. Filippeschi, A.; Schmitz, N.; Miezal, M.; Bleser, G.; Ruffaldi, E.; Stricker, D. Survey of Motion Tracking Methods Based on Inertial Sensors: A Focus on Upper Limb Human Motion. *Sensors* **2017**, *17*, 1257. [CrossRef]

18. Picerno, P. 25 years of lower limb joint kinematics by using inertial and magnetic sensors: A review of methodological approaches. *Gait Posture* **2017**, *51*, 239–246. [CrossRef]

19. Iosa, M.; Picerno, P.; Paolucci, S.; Morone, G. Wearable inertial sensors for human movement analysis. *Expert Rev. Med. Devices* **2016**, *13*, 641–659. [CrossRef]

20. Buckley, C.; Galna, B.; Rochester, L.; Mazzà, C. Upper body accelerations as a biomarker of gait impairment in the early stages of Parkinson's disease. *Gait Posture* **2019**, *71*, 289–295. [CrossRef]

21. Beck, Y.; Herman, T.; Brozgol, M.; Giladi, N.; Mirelman, A.; Hausdorff, J.M. SPARC: A new approach to quantifying gait smoothness in patients with Parkinson's disease. *J. Neuroeng. Rehabil.* **2018**, *15*, 49. [CrossRef] [PubMed]

22. Pau, M.; Mandaresu, S.; Pilloni, G.; Porta, M.; Coghe, G.; Marrosu, M.G.; Cocco, E. Smoothness of gait detects early alterations of walking in persons with multiple sclerosis without disability. *Gait Posture* **2017**, *58*, 307–309. [CrossRef] [PubMed]

23. Schmitz-Hübsch, T.; du Montcel, S.T.; Baliko, L.; Berciano, J.; Boesch, S.; Depondt, C.; Giunti, P.; Globas, C.; Infante, J.; Kang, J.-S.; et al. Scale for the assessment and rating of ataxia: Development of a new clinical scale. *Neurology* **2006**, *66*, 1717–1720. [CrossRef] [PubMed]

24. Trouillas, P.; Takayanagi, T.; Hallett, M.; Currier, R.D.; Subramony, S.H.; Wessel, K.; Bryer, A.; Diener, H.C.; Massaquoi, S.; Gomez, C.M.; et al. International Cooperative Ataxia Rating Scale for pharmacological assessment of the cerebellar syndrome. The Ataxia Neuropharmacology Committee of the World Federation of Neurology. *J. Neurol. Sci.* **1997**, *145*, 205–211. [CrossRef]

25.   Gage, H. *Accelerographic Analysis of Human Gait*; American Society for Mechanical Engineers: Washington, DC, USA, 1964.

26.   Smidt, G.L. Methods of studying gait. *Phys. Ther.* **1974**, *54*, 13–17. [CrossRef] [PubMed]

27.   Zijlstra, W. Assessment of spatio-temporal parameters during unconstrained walking. *Eur. J. Appl. Physiol.* **2004**, *92*, 39–44. [CrossRef] [PubMed]

28.   Lang, T. Statistical Analyses and Methods in the Published Literature: The SAMPL Guidelines. In *Guidelines for Reporting Health Research: A Users' Manual*, 1st ed.; Moher, D., Altman, D., Schulz, K., Simera, I., Wager, L., Eds.; John Wiley & Sons, Ltd.: The Atrium, Southern Gate, Chichester, PO19 8SQ, UK, 2014.

29.   Sullivan, G.M.; Feinn, R. Using Effect Size-or Why the P Value Is Not Enough. *J. Grad. Med. Educ.* **2012**, *4*, 279–282. [CrossRef]

30.   Grossman, G.E.; Leigh, R.J.; Abel, L.A.; Lanska, D.J.; Thurston, S.E. Frequency and velocity of rotational head perturbations during locomotion. *Exp. Brain Res.* **1988**, *70*, 470–476. [CrossRef]

31.   Hirasaki, E.; Moore, S.T.; Raphan, T.; Cohen, B. Effects of walking velocity on vertical head and body movements during locomotion. *Exp. Brain Res.* **1999**, *127*, 117–130. [CrossRef]

32.   Pozzo, T.; Berthoz, A.; Lefort, L. Head stabilization during various locomotor tasks in humans. *Exp. Brain Res.* **1990**, *82*, 97–106. [CrossRef]

33.   Prince, F.; Winter, D.; Stergiou, P.; Walt, S. Anticipatory control of upper body balance during human locomotion. *Gait Posture* **1994**, *2*, 19–25. [CrossRef]

34.   Winter, D.A.; Mcfadyen, B.J.; Dickey, J.P. Adaptability of the CNS in Human Walking. *Adv. Psychol.* **1991**, *78*, 127–144.

35.   Gracovetsky, S. An hypothesis for the role of the spine in human locomotion: A challenge to current thinking. *J. Biomed. Eng.* **1985**, *7*, 205–216. [CrossRef]

36.   Lowry, K.A.; Lokenvitz, N.; Smiley-Oyen, A.L. Age- and speed-related differences in harmonic ratios during walking. *Gait Posture* **2012**, *35*, 272–276. [CrossRef]

37.   Latt, M.D.; Menz, H.B.; Fung, V.S.; Lord, S.R. Walking speed, cadence and step length are selected to optimize the stability of head and pelvis accelerations. *Exp. Brain Res.* **2008**, *184*, 201–209. [CrossRef]

38.   Latt, M.D.; Menz, H.B.; Fung, V.S.; Lord, S.R. Acceleration patterns of the head and pelvis during gait in older people with Parkinson's disease: A comparison of fallers and nonfallers. *J. Gerontol. A Biol. Sci. Med. Sci.* **2009**, *64*, 700–706. [CrossRef]

39.   Doi, T.; Hirata, S.; Ono, R.; Tsutsumimoto, K.; Misu, S.; Ando, H. The harmonic ratio of trunk acceleration predicts falling among older people: Results of a 1-year prospective study. *J. Neuroeng. Rehabil.* **2013**, *10*, 7. [CrossRef]

40.   Conway, Z.J.; Blackmore, T.; Silburn, P.A.; Cole, M.H. Dynamic balance control during stair negotiation for older adults and people with Parkinson disease. *Hum. Mov. Sci.* **2018**, *59*, 30–36. [CrossRef]

41.   Kelley, K.; Preacher, K.J. On effect size. *Psychol. Methods* **2012**, *17*, 137–152. [CrossRef]

42.   Mari, S.; Serrao, M.; Casali, C.; Conte, C.; Martino, G.; Ranavolo, A.; Coppola, G.; Draicchio, F.; Padua, L.; Sandrini, G.; et al. Lower limb antagonist muscle co-activation and its relationship with gait parameters in cerebellar ataxia. *Cerebellum Lond. Engl.* **2014**, *13*, 226–236. [CrossRef]

43.   Serrao, M.; Chini, G.; Casali, C.; Conte, C.; Rinaldi, M.; Ranavolo, A.; Marcotulli, C.; Leonardi, L.; Fragiotta, G.; Bini, F.; et al. Progression of Gait Ataxia in Patients with Degenerative Cerebellar Disorders: A 4-Year Follow-Up Study. *Cerebellum Lond. Engl.* **2017**, *16*, 629–637. [CrossRef] [PubMed]

7

Effects of Transpulmonary Administration of Caffeine on Brain Activity in Healthy Men

Kazutaka Ueda * and Masayuki Nakao

Department of Mechanical Engineering, Graduate School of Engineering, The University of Tokyo, 7-3-1 Hongo, Bunkyo-ku, Tokyo 113-8656, Japan
* Correspondence: ueda@design-i.t.u-tokyo.ac.jp

Abstract: The present study aimed to examine the effect of transpulmonary administration of caffeine on working memory and related brain functions by electroencephalography measurement. The participants performed working memory tasks before and after vaporizer-assisted aspiration with inhalation of caffeinated- and non-caffeinated liquids in the caffeine and sham conditions, respectively. Transpulmonary administration of caffeine tended to increase the rate of correct answers. Moreover, our findings suggest that transpulmonary administration of caffeine increases the theta-band activity in the right prefrontal, central, and temporal areas during the task assigned post-aspiration. Our results may indicate an efficient and fast means of eliciting the stimulatory effects of transpulmonary administration of caffeine.

Keywords: caffeine; transpulmonary administration; working memory; electroencephalography; prefrontal cortex

1. Introduction

In recent years, vaporizers have been widely used to gain exhilaration and improve cognitive function. The vaporizer is a device that atomizes liquid by the heat generated from the heating element and performs transpulmonary aspiration of caffeine and herbs, besides nicotine. Oral consumption of caffeine has been reported to improve vigilance [1,2], attention [3,4], memory function [5], and mood [6]. On the contrary, little is known about the effects of transpulmonary administration of caffeine on cognitive function. When administered orally, the peak blood level of caffeine is achieved in 30 to 120 min [7], whereas transpulmonary administration achieves the same in a few seconds [8]. Moreover, caffeine is known to pass through the brain-blood barrier [9]. Based on these facts, transpulmonary administration of caffeine can be expected to have an immediate effect in improving cognitive and related brain functions.

The purpose of this study was to investigate the effects of transpulmonary administration of caffeine on cognitive and related brain functions. We performed electroencephalography (EEG) measurements of participants performing a working memory task before and after the transpulmonary administration of caffeine. We analyzed brain activity in the theta band [10], which is suggested to be related to working memory functions.

2. Materials and Methods

2.1. Participants

Nine healthy male participants (mean age ± standard deviation: 22.8 ± 1.4 years) with normal or corrected-to-normal vision participated in the experiments. None of them had a history of neurological or psychiatric illness. All participants reported being low caffeine consumers (mean consumption = 75 mg/day), and non-smokers. All participants were right-handed, as determined by the Flinders handedness survey (FLANDERS) [11]. This study used a within-subject design to reduce error variance in the physiological measures and has sufficient statistical power to answer the research questions. The study protocol was approved by the Ethics Committee of the Graduate School of Engineering, the University of Tokyo. All participants provided written informed consent prior to their participation in this study.

2.2. Stimuli

We used a commercially available vaporizer, caffeinated liquid (caffeine 1%) for test, and non-caffeinated liquid for the sham condition. Both liquids were transparent and indistinguishable by appearance. Moreover, none of the liquids contained nicotine.

2.3. Experimental Task

The letter 3-back working memory tasks [12] were administered as neurobehavioral probes during EEG measurement. The sequences of the uppercase letters were centrally presented with a stimulus duration of 1000 ms and an interstimulus interval of 1000 ms against a black background using Presentation (Neurobehavioral Systems, Inc., Berkeley, CA, USA). Participants were required to press a button with their right finger immediately if the letter currently presented were the same as the previous three times (Figure 1).

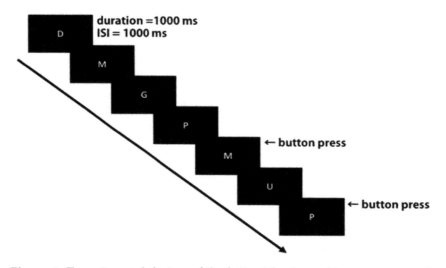

Figure 1. Experimental design of the letter 3-back working memory task.

2.4. Procedures

All participants underwent both caffeine and sham conditions at the same time on two separate days, with an interval of one or more days between the experimental days. The condition order was counterbalanced across participants.

The experiment took place in a shielded room with the participants seated in a comfortable chair, about 90 centimeters from a 29.8" type display MultiSync LCD-PA302W (NEC Corp, Tokyo, Japan; effective display area of 641×401 mm^2). The participants were instructed to relax, prevent excessive body or head movements, and to fix their gaze on the middle of the monitor. After explaining the experiment, it was conducted in the following order while with the participants seated on a chair:

(1) Pre-aspiration task: The participants performed the letter 3-back working memory task for 4 min (120 trials).

(2) The participant performed vaporizer aspiration for 2 min.

(3) Post-aspiration task: The participant performed the letter 3-back working memory task for 4 min (120 trials).

The vaporizer aspiration was performed in eight sets with the following steps constituting a set:

(1) Suck steam for 2 s.

(2) Inhale deeply steam for 3 s.

(3) Exhale from his mouth for 6 s.

(4) Rest for 6 s.

The timings of these steps were indicated on the display. The caffeine content in the aspirated vapor in the caffeine condition was about 0.15 mg. Under either of the conditions (caffeine and sham), the participants were required to rate their subjective evaluation concerning the degree of preference and intensity of aroma on a 4-point scale immediately after vaporizer aspiration.

2.5. EEG Recording and Analysis

EEG signals were continuously recorded using the EEG-1200 (Nihon Kohden Corp., Tokyo, Japan) at a sampling rate of 1000 Hz. Nineteen electrodes were positioned according to the international 10–20 system for electrode placement (at the Fp1, Fp2, Fz, F3, F4, F7, F8, Cz, C3, C4, T3, T4, Pz, P3, P4, T5, T6, O1, and O2 sites; Figure 2) [13], using the average of both earlobes as reference, with a time constant of 10 s.

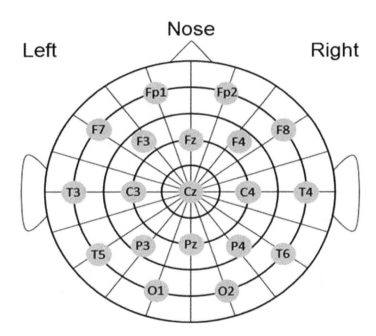

Figure 2. Electroencephalograph electrode positions (Electrode sites of the 10–20 system).

The continuous EEG data were segmented into 4-minute epochs, separately for the pre- and post-aspiration letter 3-back working memory task. The EEG data were exported to EEGLAB14.2b (MATLAB toolbox) [14] for spectral analysis, and were high-pass filtered at 1 Hz using a finite impulse response filter. Electrooculographic artifacts due to blinks or eye movements and electromyographic artifacts were removed using the Automatic Subspace Reconstruction method implemented in the 'clean_rawdata' plugin of EEGLAB [15]. To estimate the average power of the theta band (5–7 Hz), data were processed using the time-frequency algorithm in EEGLAB.

3. Results and Discussion

In order to compare the participants' impressions of the aroma of the vapors in the caffeine and sham conditions, the subjective preference and intensity for aroma were scored (Figures 3 and 4). The paired t-test was performed with the score as the independent variable. There were no significant differences between scores in either of the conditions. We observed that the participants did not feel any difference in the aroma of the vapors under caffeine and sham conditions.

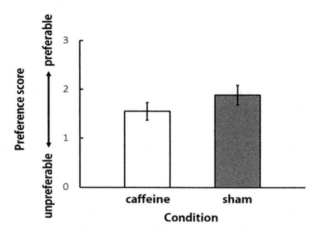

Figure 3. Preference score for the aroma of vapors ($N = 9$).

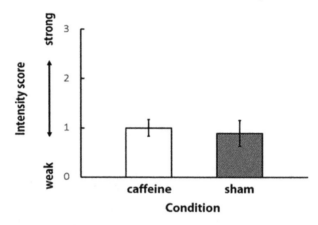

Figure 4. Intensity score for the aroma of vapors ($N = 9$).

In order to compare the behavioral indices in the caffeine and sham conditions, the correct answer rate and the response time in the letter 3-back working memory task were calculated (Figures 5 and 6). In the caffeine condition, the correct answer rate increased post-aspiration, compared to pre-aspiration. Even under the sham condition, the correct answer rate increased post-aspiration; however, this increase was lesser than that under the caffeine condition. There was no difference in the reaction time pre- and post-aspiration under both conditions. In a two-way repeated measures analysis of variance (ANOVA) using treatment (caffeine and sham) and time (pre- and post-aspiration) as the dependent variables, no significant differences were found in the correct answer rate and reaction time.

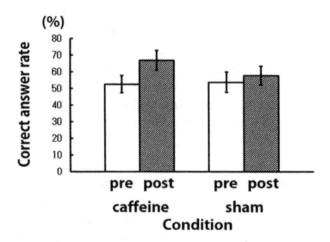

Figure 5. Percentage of correct answer in the letter 3-back working memory task ($N = 9$).

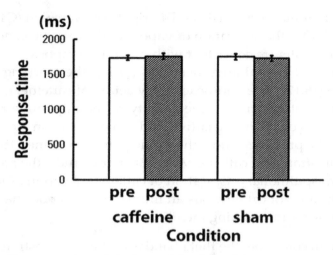

Figure 6. Response time of the letter 3-back working memory task ($N = 9$).

The brain activity in the theta band was calculated for a 4-minute epoch, separately for the pre- and post-aspiration letter 3-back working memory task. A two-way repeated measures ANOVA was performed with treatment (caffeine and sham) and time (pre- and post-aspiration) as the dependent variables, and the log-transformed ($10 \times \log10$ (μV^2)) theta band power (5–7 Hz) as the independent variable. We observed significant interactions for F8, F4, C4, and T4 ($p < 0.05$) (Table 1, Figure 7). Theta-band power differences between post- and pre-aspiration during the letter 3-back working memory task in the caffeine and sham conditions were calculated. The averages of all nine participants in the experiment are presented in Table 1.

Table 1. Theta-band power differences between post- and pre-aspiration during the letter 3-back working memory task in the caffeine and sham conditions ($N = 9$).

| | Treatment Condition | | | |
| | Caffeine ΔPower (Post–Pre) | | Sham ΔPower (Post–Pre) | |
EEG Location	Mean	SE	Mean	SE
F8	0.314	0.225	−0.420	0.231
F4	0.164	0.168	−0.416	0.248
C4	0.173	0.171	−0.335	0.189
T4	0.290	0.199	−0.318	0.239

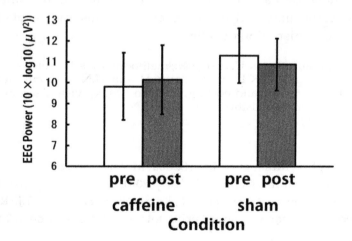

Figure 7. Theta activation at F8 during the letter 3-back working memory task ($N = 9$).

Activity of the right prefrontal cortex (F8 and F4), right central region (C4), and the right temporal region (T4) were enhanced after the aspiration of vapors in the caffeine condition as compared with the sham condition. These results are consistent with previously reported findings, which suggested that the activation of the right frontal area increased during the working memory task after oral administration of caffeine [16,17]. The neuroexcitatory action of caffeine, a non-selective adenosine A1 and A2 receptor antagonist, modulates the activity of the dopamine-rich brain regions of the right hemisphere that are involved in executive and attentional functions required for working memory function [16]. In the previous study, the participants performed the working memory task 20–30 min after oral administration of caffeine, whereas, in this study, the participants performed the task immediately after transpulmonary aspiration of caffeinated vapors. Our findings indicate that transpulmonary administration of caffeine has an immediate effect on the right prefrontal, central, and temporal areas associated with working memory.

With regard to the sham condition, the theta-band activities demonstrated greater deactivation in the post-aspiration task. Previous research has shown the relationship between the sustained effort to focus attention and theta-band activity under working memory load [18]. In the sham condition, it is possible that sustained effort decreased and the theta-band activity decreased with time. On the contrary, the increase in the brain activity for the theta band in the caffeine condition may indicate that caffeine contributes to sustain execution and attention.

In the caffeine condition, the post-aspiration correct answer rate increased more than that of the pre-aspiration. This increase was greater than that observed in the sham condition. However no significant differences were found in the behavioral response. This behavioral effect could be due to the low content of caffeine used in this study rather than the previous study [1–6]. However, as in this study, previous studies of brain function show significant changes in brain activity even without corresponding changes in overt behavior [16,19,20]. The effects of transpulmonary aspiration of caffeine on other brain activity related to resting state, vigilance, attention, and mood are not still clear and need further research.

4. Conclusions

The objective of this study was to investigate the effect of the transpulmonary administration of caffeine on working memory and related brain functions by EEG measurement. The participants performed the letter 3-back working memory tasks before and after vaporizer-assisted aspiration of caffeinated or sham liquid. The transpulmonary administration of caffeine tended to increase the rate of correct answers. Moreover, transpulmonary administration of caffeine was observed to immediately increase the theta-band activity in the right prefrontal, central, and temporal areas during task performance. These results may indicate an efficient and fast means of eliciting the stimulatory effects of transpulmonary administration of caffeine.

Author Contributions: Conceptualization, K.U. and M.N.; methodology, K.U.; software, K.U.; validation, K.U. and M.N.; formal analysis, K.U.; investigation, K.U.; resources, K.U. and M.N.; data curation, K.U.; writing—original draft preparation, K.U.; writing—review and editing, K.U. and M.N.; visualization, K.U.; supervision, M.N.; project administration, M.N.; funding acquisition, K.U. and M.N.

References

1.   Van Dongen, H.P.A.; Price, N.J.; Mullington, J.M.; Szuba, M.P.; Kapoor, S.C.; Dinges, D.F. Caffeine eliminates psychomotor vigilance deficits from sleep inertia. *Sleep* **2001**, *24*, 813–819. [CrossRef] [PubMed]
2.   Ramakrishnan, S.; Laxminarayan, S.; Wesensten, N.J.; Kamimori, G.H.; Balkin, T.J.; Reitman, J. Dose-dependent model of caffeine effects on human vigilance during total sleep deprivation. *J. Theor. Biol.* **2014**, *358*, 11–24. [CrossRef] [PubMed]
3.   Einother, S.J.L.; Giesbrecht, T. Caffeine as an attention enhancer: Reviewing existing assumptions. *Psychopharmacology* **2013**, *225*, 251–274. [CrossRef] [PubMed]

4. Brunyé, T.T.; Mahoney, C.R.; Lieberman, H.R.; Taylor, H.A. Caffeine modulates attention network function. *Brain Cogn.* **2010**, *72*, 181–188. [CrossRef] [PubMed]
5. Nehlig, A. Is caffeine a cognitive enhancer? *J. Alzheimers Dis.* **2010**, *20*, S85–S94. [CrossRef] [PubMed]
6. Haskell, C.F.; Kennedy, D.O.; Wesnes, K.A.; Scholey, A.B. Cognitive and mood improvements of caffeine in habitual consumers and habitual non-consumers of caffeine. *Psychopharmacology* **2005**, *179*, 813–825. [CrossRef] [PubMed]
7. Blanchard, J.; Sawers, S.J.A. The Absolute Bioavailability of Caffeine in Man. *Eur. J. Clin. Pharmacol.* **1983**, *24*, 93–98. [CrossRef] [PubMed]
8. Zandvliet, A.S.; Huitema, A.D.R.; de Jonge, M.E.; den Hoed, R.; Sparidans, R.W.; Hendriks, V.M.; van den Brink, W.; van Ree, J.M.; Beijnen, J.H. Population pharmacokinetics of caffeine and its metabolites theobromine, paraxanthine and theophylline after inhalation in combination with diacetylmorphine. *Basic Clin. Pharmacol.* **2005**, *96*, 71–79. [CrossRef] [PubMed]
9. Arnaud, M.J. Metabolism of caffeine and other components of coffee. In *Caffeine, Coffee, and Health*; Garattini, S., Ed.; Raven Press: New York, NY, USA, 1993; pp. 43–95.
10. Sauseng, P.; Griesmayr, B.; Freunberger, R.; Klimesch, W. Control mechanisms in working memory: A possible function of EEG theta oscillations. *Neurosci. Biobehav. Rev.* **2010**, *34*, 1015–1022. [CrossRef] [PubMed]
11. Okubo, M.; Suzuki, H.; Nicholls, M.E. A Japanese version of the FLANDERS handedness questionnaire. *Shinrigaku Kenkyu* **2014**, *85*, 474–481. [CrossRef] [PubMed]
12. Owen, A.M.; McMillan, K.M.; Laird, A.R.; Bullmore, E.T. N-back working memory paradigm: A meta-analysis of normative functional neuroimaging. *Hum. Brain Mapp.* **2005**, *25*, 46–59. [CrossRef] [PubMed]
13. Klem, G.H.; Luders, H.O.; Jasper, H.H.; Elger, C. The ten-twenty electrode system of the International Federation. The International Federation of Clinical Neurophysiology. *Electroencephalogr. Clin. Neurophysiol. Suppl.* **1999**, *52*, 3–6. [PubMed]
14. Delorme, A.; Makeig, S. EEGLAB: An open source toolbox for analysis of single-trial EEG dynamics including independent component analysis. *J. Neurosci. Methods* **2004**, *134*, 9–21. [CrossRef] [PubMed]
15. Mullen, T.; Kothe, C.; Chi, Y.M.; Ojeda, A.; Kerth, T.; Makeig, S.; Cauwenberghs, G.; Jung, T.P. Real-Time Modeling and 3D Visualization of Source Dynamics and Connectivity Using Wearable EEG. In Proceedings of the 2013 35th Annual International Conference of the IEEE Engineering in Medicine and Biology Society (EMBC), Osaka, Japan, 3–7 July 2013; pp. 2184–2187.
16. Koppelstaetter, F.; Poeppel, T.D.; Siedentopf, C.M.; Ischebeck, A.; Verius, M.; Haala, I.; Mottaghy, F.M.; Rhomberg, P.; Golaszewski, S.; Gotwald, T. Does caffeine modulate verbal working memory processes? An fMRI study. *NeuroImage* **2008**, *39*, 492–499. [CrossRef] [PubMed]
17. Klaassen, E.B.; de Groot, R.H.M.; Evers, E.A.T.; Snel, J.; Veerman, E.C.I.; Ligtenberg, A.J.M.; Jolles, J.; Veltman, D.J. The effect of caffeine on working memory load-related brain activation in middle-aged males. *Neuropharmacology* **2013**, *64*, 160–167. [CrossRef] [PubMed]
18. Gevins, A.; Smith, M.E.; McEvoy, L.; Yu, D. High-resolution EEG mapping of cortical activation related to working memory: Effects of task difficulty, type of processing, and practice. *Cereb. Cortex* **1997**, *7*, 374–385. [CrossRef] [PubMed]
19. Wilkinson, D.; Halligan, P. Opinion—The relevance of behavioural measures for functional-imaging studies of cognition. *Nat. Rev. Neurosci.* **2004**, *5*, 67–73. [CrossRef] [PubMed]
20. Hershey, T.; Black, K.J.; Hartlein, J.; Braver, T.S.; Barch, D.A.; Carl, J.L.; Perlmutter, J.S. Dopaminergic modulation of response inhibition: An fMRI study. *Cogn. Brain Res.* **2004**, *20*, 438–448. [CrossRef] [PubMed]

8

Immunoadsorption for Treatment of Patients with Suspected Alzheimer Dementia and Agonistic Autoantibodies against Alpha1A-Adrenoceptor—Rationale and Design of the IMAD Pilot Study

Sylvia Stracke [1,*,†], Sandra Lange [2,†], Sarah Bornmann [3], Holger Kock [4], Lara Schulze [5], Johanna Klinger-König [5], Susanne Böhm [6], Antje Vogelgesang [3], Felix von Podewils [3], Agnes Föel [3,7], Stefan Gross [8,9], Katrin Wenzel [10], Gerd Wallukat [10], Harald Prüss [11,12], Alexander Dressel [13], Rudolf Kunze [14], Hans J. Grabe [5,7,†], Sönke Langner [2,15,†] and Marcus Dörr [8,9,*,†]

[1] Department for Internal Medicine A, Nephrology, University Medicine Greifswald, Ferdinand-Sauerbruch-Straße, 17475 Greifswald, Germany

[2] Institute of Diagnostic Radiology and Neuroradiology, University Medicine Greifswald, 17475 Greifswald, Germany; sandra.lange@uni-greifswald.de (S.L.); soenke.langner@med.uni-rostock.de (S.L.)

[3] Department of Neurology, University Medicine Greifswald, 17475 Greifswald, Germany; bornmanns@uni-greifswald.de (S.B.); antje.vogelgesang@uni-greifswald.de (A.V.); Felix.vonPodewils@med.uni-greifswald.de (F.v.P.); agnes.floeel@med.uni-greifswald.de (A.F.)

[4] Strategic Research Management, University Medicine Greifswald, 17475 Greifswald, Germany; holger.kock@uni-greifswald.de

[5] Department of Psychiatry and Psychotherapy, University Medicine Greifswald, 17475 Greifswald, Germany; lara.schulze@uni-greifswald.de (L.S.); Johanna.Klinger-Koenig@med.uni-greifswald.de (J.K.-K.); Hans.Grabe@med.uni-greifswald.de (H.J.G.)

[6] Coordinating Centre for Clinical Trials, University Medicine Greifswald, 17475 Greifswald, Germany; Susanne.Boehm@med.uni-greifswald.de

[7] German Center for Neurodegenerative Diseases (DZNE), 17475 Rostock/Greifswald, partner site Greifswald, Germany

[8] Department of Internal Medicine B, University Medicine Greifswald, Ferdinand-Sauerbruch-Straße, 17475 Greifswald, Germany; stefan.gross1@uni-greifswald.de

[9] German Centre for Cardiovascular Research (DZHK), 17475 Greifswald, Germany

[10] Berlin Cures GmbH, 13125 Berlin, Germany; wenzel@berlincures.de (K.W.); wallukat@berlincures.de (G.W.)

[11] German Center for Neurodegenerative Diseases (DZNE) Berlin, 10117 Berlin, Germany; harald.pruess@charite.de

[12] Department of Neurology and Experimental Neurology, Charité—Universitätsmedizin Berlin, 10117 Berlin, Germany

[13] Department of Neurology, Carl-Thiem-Klinikum, 03048 Cottbus, Germany; a.dressel@ctk.de

[14] Science Office, Hessenhagen 2, 17268 Flieth-Stegelitz, Germany; Rudolf.Kunze@gmx.de

[15] Institute of Diagnostic and Interventional Radiology, University Medicine Rostock, 18057 Rostock, Germany

* Correspondence: sylvia.stracke@med.uni-greifswald.de (S.S.); marcus.doerr@uni-greifswald.de (M.D.)

† Denotes equal contribution.

Abstract: Background: agonistic autoantibodies (agAABs) against G protein-coupled receptors (GPCR) have been linked to cardiovascular disease. In dementia patients, GPCR-agAABs against the α1- and ß2-adrenoceptors (α1AR- and ß2AR) were found at a prevalence of 50%. Elimination of agAABs by immunoadsorption (IA) was successfully applied in cardiovascular disease. The IMAD trial (Efficacy of immunoadsorption for treatment of persons with Alzheimer dementia and agonistic autoantibodies against alpha1A-adrenoceptor) investigates whether the removal of α1AR-AABs by a 5-day IA procedure has a positive effect (improvement or non-deterioration) on changes of hemodynamic, cognitive, vascular and metabolic parameters in patients with suspected Alzheimer's clinical syndrome within a one-year follow-up period. Methods: the IMAD trial is designed as an exploratory monocentric interventional trial corresponding to a proof-of-concept phase-IIa study. If cognition capacity of eligible patients scores 19–26 in the Mini Mental State Examination (MMSE), patients are tested for the presence of agAABs by an enzyme-linked immunosorbent assay (ELISA)-based method, followed by a bioassay-based confirmation test, further screening and treatment with IA and intravenous immunoglobulin G (IgG) replacement. We aim to include 15 patients with IA/IgG and to complete follow-up data from at least 12 patients. The primary outcome parameter of the study is uncorrected mean cerebral perfusion measured in mL/min/100 gr of brain tissue determined by magnetic resonance imaging with arterial spin labeling after 12 months. Conclusion: IMAD is an important pilot study that will analyze whether the removal of α1AR-agAABs by immunoadsorption in α1AR-agAAB-positive patients with suspected Alzheimer's clinical syndrome may slow the progression of dementia and/or may improve vascular functional parameters.

Keywords: Alzheimer's clinical syndrome; dementia; immunoadsorption; autoantibodies; α1-Adrenergic receptor

---

1. Introduction

Nearly 50 million people worldwide suffer from Alzheimer's disease (AD) or other forms of dementia, and around 10 million new cases emerge every year, leading to a number of 150 million affected people expected in 2050 [1–3] Dementia has a lifetime prevalence ranging between 5% and 7% for those aged ≥60 years and is a major cause of disability among older adults [4,5] AD is the leading cause of dementia, responsible for two-thirds of all cases [6]. Since no causal treatment for AD is available yet, prevention strategies, psychosocial interventions and symptomatic pharmacological interventions are recommended and are central components of the treatment [7].

Up to now, research of causal therapies is focusing on the knowledge of typical neuropathological features of AD like amyloid plaques and neurofibrillary tangles which are associated with the tau-pathology [8,9]. In particular, the ß-amyloid hypothesis of AD has stimulated the development of therapy concepts directed against the amyloid protein and amyloid deposits in the brain of patients with AD.

One strategy is passive immunization with monoclonal antibodies which bind to ß-amyloid. Although it has been demonstrated that these antibodies may reduce the amyloid burden in the brain of AD patients, positive clinical effects were minimal or absent so far. Many promising compounds like Bapineuzumab, Gantenerumab or Solanezumab have failed in phase III of clinical trials or are still being evaluated (Aducanumab) [10–12].

Other ß-amyloid (Aß)-directed therapies focus on the enzymatic cleavage of the amyloid precursor protein (APP). It is known that ß-secretases contribute essentially to the production of Aß40/42 which is the toxic aggregating form of amyloid. Thus, ß-secretase inhibitors have been identified to be therapeutically beneficial. However, recently, a world-wide clinical trial on the secretase inhibitor Verubecestat was withdrawn because Verubecestat did not improve clinical ratings of dementia among patients with prodromal Alzheimer's disease. Some measures even suggested an impairment of cognition and daily function compared to placebo [13].

The focus on Aß also led to the concept of removing it from plasma by therapeutic plasma exchange (TPE). Aß is bound to serum albumin by >90% which in turn is removed and discarded by TPE [14,15]. TPE-treatment with albumin replacement favored the stabilization of cerebral perfusion in mild to moderate AD patients compared to non-treated controls [15]. The same Spanish group currently conducts a prospective multicenter, randomized, blinded and placebo-controlled, parallel-group, phase IIb/III trial in patients with mild to moderate AD ("Alzheimer's Management by Albumin Replacement (AMBAR)"). This study evaluates TPE with different replacement volumes of therapeutic albumin (5% and 20%), with or without intravenous immunoglobulins and is still ongoing [14]. Another group sought to remove Aß and developed an ex vivo adsorptive filtration system that resulted in an 80–100% reduction of Aßs within 30 min of circulation but has not yet been tested in humans [16].

In view of the numerous negative results, it seems to be necessary to shift attention to new therapeutic targets. In this respect, different pathologies of cognitive decline besides the Aß and the tau-pathologies may be considered. Importantly, clinical, pathological and epidemiological data point to a relevant overlap between cerebrovascular disease (CVD) and Alzheimer's clinical syndrome [17]. Furthermore, cerebral microvascular lesions that are detected as white matter hyperintensities (WMH) on magnetic resonance imaging (MRI) are associated with typical gray matter atrophy patterns of AD in a considerable number of patients [18]. Thus, factors that alter the microenvironment of the endothelium and the smooth muscle cells of blood vessels may compromise the molecular exchange between blood and brain.

Rationale of the Clinical Investigation

Naturally occurring agonistic autoantibodies (agAABs) against G protein-coupled receptors (GPCR) have been linked to cardiovascular disease such as dilated cardiomyopathy, myocarditis, malignant hypertension, vascular renal rejection, diabetes mellitus type 2 or dementia [19]. Agonistic AABs are functional antibodies that can activate the respective receptor. Agonistic AABs differ clearly from non-functional AABs. The latter trigger autoimmune disease in an Fc-receptor mediated manner whereas functional agAABs are able to bind cell receptors and activate intracellular signaling pathways that are normally triggered by endogenous ligands [20]. A pathological example of agAABs is Graves' hyperthyroidism with autoantibodies activating the thyroid-stimulating hormone (TSH)-receptor and with subsequent overproduction of thyroid hormones [21]. Other examples for GPCR-agAABs are AABs directed against adrenoceptors (AR; e.g., ß1AR and ß2AR, α1AR), the angiotensin (2) receptor type 1 (AT-R1) and the endothelin receptor type A (ETA) [19]. The agAABs against AR are directed against the first or second extracellular loop of the receptor. They bind to constant epitopes defined by the amino acid sequence in the respective loop. These AABs belong to the immunoglobulin class G (isotypes 1–3). GPCR-agAABs elicit a long-lasting dimerization of adrenoceptors and continuously activate cellular processes such as phosphorylation of intracellular proteins and modulation of calcium signaling that results e.g., in the case of agAABs against the α1AR in the proliferation of smooth muscle cells and thickening of vessel walls [22]. In response to their natural agonists, the receptor density on the cell membrane is regulated by receptor desensitization. This mechanism is inhibited by agAABs [22]. In an animal model, continuous stimulation triggered by α1AR-AABs leads to cerebrovascular remodeling and obliteration [23].

In a small clinical trial, treatment of Graves' disease with rituximab, a B-cell depleting monoclonal antibody specifically reduced the production of TSH-receptor antibodies [24]. In a case of thyreotoxic crisis, TPE is also used to remove agAABs against TSH-receptor and albumin-bound thyroid hormones [25].

Cerebrovascular remodeling may lead to disturbances in cerebral blood flow and a lack of outflow of Aß. A clearing defect for Aß rather than an Aß-overproduction has been proven experimentally for AD patients [26]. From this view, AABs against the α1AR may interfere with Aß clearance mechanisms and act as a risk factor and a modulating component of dementia in patients with Alzheimer's clinical syndrome.

In line with this, the GPCR-α1AR was also reported to be a target for agAABs in patients with essential and malignant hypertension [27]. In a pilot study in five α1AR-AAB-positive patients with resistant hypertension, removal of these AABs by immunoadsorption lowered the mean arterial blood pressure significantly by approximately 10 mmHg, and the effect was still present after 180 days [28]. In line with this, a recent study in 816 subjects showed that the occurrence of α1AR-AABs predicted arterial stiffness progression even in normotensives over a 5-year period [29].

A disease that has been very well investigated with regard to agAABs is dilated cardiomyopathy (DCM). Among others, agAABs against the GPCR-ß1-adrenoceptor (ß1R) seem to play an important role in DCM. Their elimination from the blood by immunoadsorption (IA) has been transferred to a therapeutic intervention in clinical praxis. Removal of circulating antibodies by IA with subsequent intravenous immunoglobulin G substitution (IA/IgG) has been shown to result in improvement of cardiac function, in better exercise capacity, and in decrease of myocardial inflammation in DCM [30–33]. Removal of functional AABs does not have to be a constant process as in non-functional AAB triggered disease. Already a one-week-course of IA seems to yield a so-called legacy effect that may persist for a long time [34]. In DCM, removal of the agAABs by a one-week-course of IA lasts for up to 12 months and even longer [35,36].

Noticeably, in dementia patients, agAABs against both the α1R- and ß2R-adrenoceptors were also found at a prevalence of approx. 50%. Thus, in a primary care cohort who screened positive for dementia, 40 out of 95 participants were also positive for agAAB (29 subjects with α1AR-AABs and 21 with ß2AR-AABs) [37]. However, agAABs could not discriminate between Alzheimer's Dementia and other forms of dementia. Patients with coronary heart disease were more likely (OR = 4.23) to have α1AR-AABs than those without coronary heart disease. The presence of agAAB against adrenoceptors, especially α1AR-agAABs, in persons suffering from dementia motivated a first pilot trial on the effects of IA on the course of dementia [38]. In this trial, in four out of eight patients an effective depletion of agAAB could be achieved by a 4-day per-protocol IA treatment, while another four patients received a less effective 2–3 day treatment due venous access problems. IA was safe to use in these patients, and the mean change in Mini Mental State Examination (MMSE) score of these patients remained constant over 12 to 18 months.

The IMAD trial (Efficacy of immunoadsorption for treatment of persons with Alzheimer dementia and agonistic autoantibodies against alpha1A-adrenoceptor) aims to ascertain whether the positive effects of IA on slowing down dementia progression can be replicated. Moreover, IMAD will comprehensively examine potential effects of this treatment in patients with Alzheimer's clinical syndrome by a combination of brain and vessel imaging along with cognitive tests and further cardiovascular, cerebrovascular and laboratory examinations.

2. Methods

2.1. Objectives

The IMAD trial is designed as an exploratory monocentric interventional trial corresponding to a proof-of-concept phase-IIa study. The aim of IMAD is to evaluate whether IA with subsequent IgG-substitution (IA/IgG) is related to an improved uncorrected mean brain perfusion after 12 months as a surrogate for potential beneficial effects on disease progression in patients with an Alzheimer's clinical syndrome and mild to moderate cognitive impairment. In addition, potential effects of IA/IgG on cognitive measures as well as cardiovascular, cerebrovascular and laboratory parameters will be investigated.

2.2. Patients

Potential participants for this trial need to have an Alzheimer's clinical syndrome, according to the definition as outlined in Jack et al. [39]. In patients without obvious exclusion criteria, cognitive capacity is again assessed before inclusion using the MMSE. If a mild to moderate impairment (defined by a MMSE score between 19 and 26) is confirmed, patients are tested for the presence of agAABs by an ELISA-based method, followed by a bioassay-based confirmation test (methodological details are given in Section 2.5.8). Patients with a positive test result by the bioassay are eligible for further screening. We aim to include in total 15 patients with IA/IgG and 12 patients with complete follow-up data.

2.3. Inclusion and Exclusion Criteria

Criteria that have to be fulfilled for all participants (inclusion criteria) and reasons that prevent inclusion into the study (exclusion criteria) are summarized in Table 1.

Table 1. Inclusion and exclusion criteria.

	Criteria
Inclusion	- Age 55–85 - Previous or suspected diagnosis of Alzheimer's clinical syndrome - Presence of agAAB against alpha1-adrenoceptor (α1AR) - Mini mental state examination score between 19 and 26 - Written informed consent
Exclusion	- Presence of autoantibodies against the NMDA receptor - Defective blood coagulation at time of inclusion - Severe protein deficiency disorders - Known manifest vitamin/folic acid deficiency (substitution allowed) - Active infectious disease, or sings of ongoing infection with CRP >10 mmol/L - Impaired renal function (serum creatinine >220 μmol/L) - Any disease requiring immunosuppressive drugs or therapeutic antibodies - Non-curative treated malignant disease or another life-threatening disease with poor prognosis (estimated survival less than 2 years), except for basal-cell carcinoma - Unstable angina pectoris, second or third degree atrioventricular block or symptomatic sick sinus syndrome without implanted pacemaker, history of myocardial infarction, bypass or other revascularization procedures, valvular heart defect (≥2. degree) - Severely reduced left ventricular systolic function (LVEF <30%) and/or heart failure symptoms according to NYHA class III/IV - Clinical manifestation of arterial disease, vascular surgery: ACl-Stenosis >60%; PAD > IIb, history of stroke, diffusion disorder or expired territorial stroke in MRI - Endocrine disorder excluding diabetes mellitus - Severe hepatic disorder (Child–Pugh score 5 or more) - Drug therapy against dementia since less than 3 months - Psychopharmacological drug therapy since less than 3 months - Dialysis requirement - MRI contraindications (e.g., pacemaker) - Legal tutelage - Previous treatments with IA or immunoglobulins - ACE-treatment during the IA - Severe mental disorder (bipolar disorder, schizophrenia, depression) requiring treatment - Alcohol or drug abuse - Inability to undergo the study procedure - Participation in any other clinical/interventional study within less than 30 days prior to screening

ACE, angiotensin converting enzyme; ACI, internal carotid artery; agAAB, agonistic autoantibodies; CRP, C reactive protein; IA, immunoadsorption LVEF, left ventricular systolic function; MRI, magnetic resonance imaging; NMDA, N-methyl-D-aspartate; NYHA, New York Heart Association; PAD, peripheral artery disease.

2.4. Study Design

During the screening phase, patients are checked for eligibility according the inclusion and exclusion criteria (Table 1). Patients fulfilling these criteria are comprehensively examined during a baseline visit, followed by IA/IgG treatment. All participants of the IMAD trial are followed up after 1, 6 and 12 months. The complete study flow is illustrated in Figure 1.

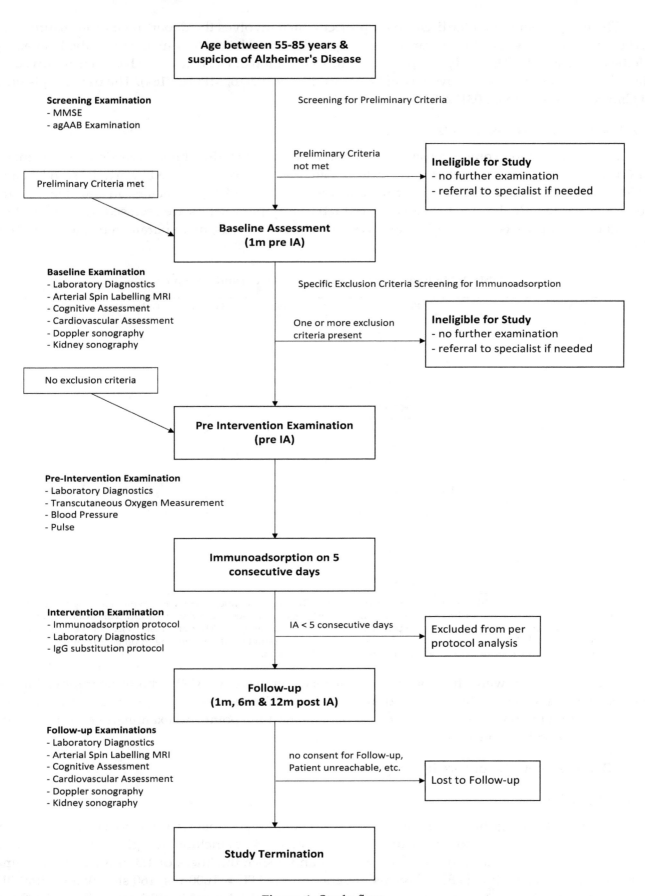

Figure 1. Study flow.

The IMAD trial is an interdisciplinary project which involves the departments and institutes of radiology, neurology, psychiatry, cardiology, nephrology and laboratory medicine of the University Medicine Greifswald. The study complies with the Declaration of Helsinki and it has been approved by the Ethics Committee of the University of Greifswald (MPG 02/16; MPG 02/16a). The trial is registered at ClinicalTrials.gov (NCT03132272).

2.5. Examinations and Assessments

Patients undergo a comprehensive examination program including brain perfusion assessment by MRI (primary outcome parameter: uncorrected mean brain perfusion assessed by arterial spin labeling [ASL]) and assessment of further structural and vascular brain MRI parameters. In addition, several cognitive, cardiovascular, cerebrovascular and laboratory parameters are assessed during baseline and all follow-up visits. Table 2 gives an overview about methods, main parameters and respective time points.

Table 2. Methods, main outcome parameters and time points.

Method	Parameter	Screening	Baseline	Follow-Ups	Comments
Arterial Spin Labelling MRI	Cerebral blood flow		X	X	
MRI Basic protocol	Brain Volume, WMH, CBM; MTA		X	X	
Time-of-flight MR angiography	Vessel anatomy and size		X	X	
Diffusion Tensor Imaging	Fractional anisotropy		X	X	
ADAS-Cog	Cognition		X	X	
MMSE	Cognition	X	X	X	
GDS	Depression		X	X	
VLMT	Cognition		X	X	
Benton Test	Cognition		X	X	
Brachial blood	Brachial blood pressure values	X	X	X	
Pulse wave analysis	Arterial stiffness, central hemodynamics		X	X	
Digital endothelial vascular function and stiffness	Endothelial function and vascular stiffness		X		
Echocardiography	Cardiac function and structure		X		
Transcutaneous oxygen measurement	Oxygenation		X	X	
Kidney sonography	Renal function		X	X	
Doppler Sonography	Carotid Arteria blood flow		X	X	
Liquor analytics	Tau/P-Tau		(X)	(X)	Optional
Liquor analytics	ß-A40/42		(X)	(X)	Optional

IA, immunoadsorption; MRI, magnetic resonance imaging; CBM, cerebral microbleeds; MTA, medial temporal lobe atrophy; DTI, diffusion tensor imaging; ADAS, Alzheimer's Disease Assessment Scale; MMSE, Mini-Mental State Examination; GDS, Geriatric Depression Scale; VLMT, Verbal Learning and Memory Test; LVEF, left ventricular ejection fraction; WMH, white matter hyperintensities; optional parameters are depending upon patient agreement; follow-up visits are conducted 1, 6 and 12 months after IA treatment.

For examinations with a high potential for an observer bias (e.g., MRI, echocardiography), images will be stored and the reading will be done offline in a blinded manner. Specifically, they will be assessed without knowledge of the respective patient and time point. All examinations and methods used are described in more detail in the following sections.

2.5.1. Brain Magnetic Resonance Imaging (MRI)

MR Imaging Protocol

All subjects undergo brain imaging at 1.5T (Magnetom Aera, Semens, Germany) using a 20-channel head coil for image acquisition. Structural MR imaging protocol includes a sagittal 3D T1-weighted sequence with an inplane resolution of 1×1 mm and a slice thickness of 1.3 mm (repetition time [TR] = 1860 ms, echo time [TE] = 3.88 ms, inversion time [TI] = 1000 ms, 160 slices); a sagittal 3D FLAIR dataset with 1×1 mm inplane spatial resolution and 1.1 mm slice thickness (TR = 5000 ms, TE = 214 ms, TI = 1800 ms, field of view [FoV] = 265×265 mm); a diffusion weighted imaging (DWI) sequence with b-values $0/1000$ s/mm^2 (TR = 5600 ms, TE = 113 ms, 1.2×1.2 mm voxel size, 5 mm slice thickness) and a time-of-flight angiography of the circle of Willis with 0.5×0.5 mm spatial resolution with a slice thickness of 0.8 mm (TR = 31 ms, TE = 7.15 ms, FoV = 200 mm).

Cerebral perfusion is assessed using a 2D pseudo-continuous arterial spin-labeling sequence (PICORE Q2T) with 5 mm slice thickness and an in-plane spatial resolution of 4 mm with 64 slices. Other imaging parameters are a post labeling delay of 1.8 s, bolus duration of 700 ms, TR = 2500 ms and TE = 13 ms.

A diffusion tensor imaging (DTI) dataset is acquired in all patients (TR = 4700 ms, TE = 116 ms, b-value $0/1000$ s/mm^2, 12 directions) with a slice thickness of 4 mm and an in-plane spatial resolution of 1.5×1.5 mm.

Total acquisition time is 42 min. All scans are checked by a board certified neuroradiologist for gross abnormalities.

MR Image Analysis

For structural image analysis, all MR datasets are transferred to a dedicated Horos workstation (www.horosproject.org). WMH are evaluated on axial reconstructions of the 3D FLAIR dataset with 3 mm slice thickness according to the Fazekas scale [40]. The Fazekas score are dichotomized into low (Fazekas grade 0–1) and high (Fazekas grade 2–3). Cerebral microbleeds are defined as hypointense lesions smaller than 10 mm on b = 0 diffusion weighted images. Lacunar lesions are defined as small lesions in the deep white and grey matter with a diameter between 3 and 10 mm and cerebrospinal fluid-like signal on all sequences. For quantitative analysis, lacunar lesions and microbleeds are counted by visual inspection and for further statistical analysis dichotomized in present or absent.

Medial temporal lobe atrophy (MTA) score is rated on coronal reformations of the 3D T1w dataset according to previously described criteria [41]. For statistical analysis, the mean MTA score of both sides is dichotomized into high (>1.5) and low (≤1.5) as described elsewhere [42].

Vessel diameter of the internal carotid artery (ICA), the anterior (ACA) and middle cerebral artery (MCA) and the basilar artery (BA) are evaluated by manual measurements. For the ICA, measurements are performed at the level of the cavernous sinus, for the MCA in the median M1 segment, for the ACA immediately distal the anterior communicating artery and for the basilar artery at the level of the origin of the superior cerebellar artery, respectively.

Brain volume estimation are performed using T1w images. Therefore, the measured raw DICOM data are converted into NIFTI (Neuroimaging Informatics Technology Initiative) format using dcm2nii, which is part of the neuroimaging tool MRIcron. Preprocessing using FSL (version 6.0, www.fsl.fmrib.ox.ac.uk/fsl) included correction for gradient nonlinearities, non-brain tissue removal, linear registration to standard space, and tissue segmentation [43]. Evaluation of the pseudo-continuous ASL images is performed as previously described by Binnewijzend et al. [43]. Therefore, ASL images are also corrected for gradient nonlinearities in all three directions and then linearly registered to the brain-extracted T1-weighted images. The brain mask is used to calculate uncorrected mean whole-brain cerebral blood flow (CBF). These volume estimates are then transformed to the ASL data space to correct partial volume-corrected cortical and white matter CBF maps [44]. CBF values are also extracted using regions of interest (ROIs) in the frontal, temporal, occipital and parietal brain areas and the hippocampus based on the MNI152 atlas and the Harvard–Oxford cortical atlas. The primary outcome parameter of the study is uncorrected mean cerebral perfusion measured in mL/min/100 gr of brain tissue determined by ASL.

Preprocessing of DTI data includes also conversion to NIFTI format. Then, the tool eddy correct, part of FSL, is used to correct the diffusion-weighted data with respect to subject motion and deformations introduced by eddy current artifacts of the MRI scanner. Fractional anisotropy (FA) images are created by fitting a tensor model to the raw diffusion data using FSL DTI-FIT. FA analyses was performed on a whole brain basis and using the ROI from CBF-analyses.

2.5.2. Cognitive Assessment

Mini-Mental State Examination (MMSE)

We use MMSE-2 which is a revised version of the original MMSE [45,46] routinely used to measure cognitive decline. The MMSE-2 consists of three versions: the standard version, the brief version and the expanded version of the MMSE. In this study, the standard version is used in order to maximize the benefit of the use of the scale while minimizing the duration of the cognitive assessment. The MMSE-2 shows a sufficient internal consistency (Cronbach's alpha 0.66–0.79) [46].

Alzheimer's Disease Assessment Scale - Cognition (ADAS-Cog)

The Alzheimer's Disease Assessment Scale (ADAS) is commonly used to assess cognitive dysfunction in individuals with Alzheimer's Disease and other types of dementia [47,48]. The ADAS-Cog was developed as a two-part scale: one that measures cognitive impairment and one that measures non-cognitive factors such as mood and behavior. In IMAD, only the cognitive scale of the ADAS-Cog is applied, which consists of 11 parts and measures the cognitive functioning, language, and memory in a 30-min test. Five parallel versions are available to avoid recall bias due to multiple testing. The final score ranges from 0 to 70 points, with higher scores indicating more serious cognitive impairment. The ADAS shows a good internal consistency (Cronbach's alpha 0.61–0.76) [49]. During the baseline visit, a cognitive profile over the 11 dimensions measured by the ADAS-Cog is created. The profile is compared to reference values provided by Graham et al. [48] (Figure 2). According to the reference values, the cognitive profile of patients with mild to moderate AD predominately shows higher impairment in memory, and to a lesser extent, in cognitive functioning. In contrast, language is hardly impaired in this stadium (Figure 2). Thus, patients with a different cognitive profile undergo further examinations to exclude differential diagnoses. For patients included into the IMAD trial, a cognitive change is estimated according to Stern et al. [50] to predict future cognitive decline during the follow-up period. The estimated cognitive change is later compared to the observed cognitive changes over 12 months after IA/IgG.

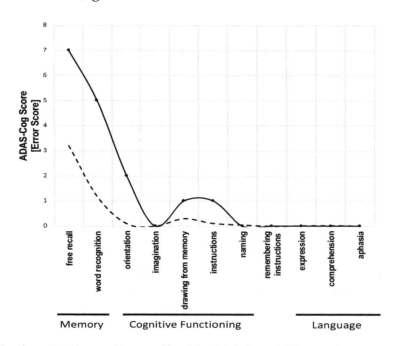

Figure 2. Example of a patient's cognitive profile of the Alzheimer's Disease Assessment Scale–Cognition (ADAS-Cog) with mild to moderate dementia from a patient included in the IMAD trial (own figure). Continuous line, cognitive profile with mild to moderate dementia; dashed line, cognitive profile with no cognitive impairment; grey area, 95% confidence interval for the cognitive profile. Without impairment according to Graham, Emery and Hodges [48].

Verbal Learning and Memory Test (VLMT)

The Verbal Learning and Memory Test (VLMT) allows a short and individual assessment of verbal learning and memory. The VLMT [51] uses 15 semantically independent words to assess verbal memory. In a second step, an interference list with 15 new words is learned and recalled to distract from the first, target list. After 20–30 min a delayed recall of the target list and a recognition test with a new list combining the 30 learned words with 20 semantically and phonemically similar words is done.

Benton Test

The Benton Test (first edition: Benton, 1946) is a visual retention test for clinical use testing the memory of visuo-spatial stimuli. The patient has to reproduce, draw or recognize presented graphic stimuli. In this trial, instruction A (10 figures shown for 10 s) and parallel forms C, D and E are used. The Benton Test has been shown to have a high internal consistency (Cronbach's alpha = 0.94–0.98) and validity [52].

Geriatric Depression Scale (GDS)

The Geriatric Depression Scale (GDS) is used to measure depressive symptoms in older persons. It is a 15-item questionnaire demanding a dichotomous (yes/no) evaluation of depressive symptoms. It was also shown to be applicable for persons with advanced cognitive impairment [53]. The GDS shows a high internal consistency (Cronbach's alpha 0.91).

The standardized questionnaires used in the IMAD trial as well as the respective cut-off values applied are summarized in Table 3.

Table 3. Assessments by standardized questionnaires.

Test	Abbreviation	No Impairment	Severe Impairment	Normal Range
Mini-Mental State Examination	MMSE	30	0	26–30
Alzheimer's Disease Assessment Scale—cognitive Scale	ADAS-Cog	0	70	0–4
Memory		0	22	-
Cognitive Functioning		0	28	-
Language		0	15	-
Verbal Learning and Memory Test	VLMT			
Learning		75	0	48–75
Loss after Interference		0	15	-
Loss after Delay		0	15	0–3
Recognition		0	15	-
Benton Test	Benton Test			
Number Correct Score		10	0	-
Error Score		0	-	-
Geriatric Depression Scale	GDS	0	15	0–5

ADAS-Cog, Alzheimer's Disease Assessment Scale–Cognition; VLMT, GDS, Geriatric Depression Scale; Verbal Learning and Memory Test.

2.5.3. Cardiovascular Examinations

All cardiovascular examinations are conducted according to standardized procedures by certified study nurses and physicians at the cardiovascular examination center of the German Centre for Cardiovascular Disease (DZHK) in Greifswald. The following examinations are part of the IMAD phenotyping:

Brachial Blood Pressure Measurement

Measurements of the brachial blood pressure are taken using an Omron 705 IT (OMRON Healthcare Europe) blood pressure monitor with appropriate cuff size after a resting period of at least 5 min in a sitting position. Accordingly, three measurements are taken on the right arm, with a 3-min break between each measurement [54]. All individual measurements (systolic blood pressure [mmHg], diastolic blood pressure [mmHg], heart rate [/min]) are recorded.

Pulse-Wave Analysis and Central Hemodynamics

To perform cuff-based non-invasive data capturing at the brachial artery, the invasively validated Mobil–O–Graph pulse-wave analysis (PWA) monitor (IEM GmbH, Stolberg, Germany) with inbuilt ARCSolver algorithm is used [55,56]. After conventional blood pressure measurements, the brachial cuff is inflated additionally to the diastolic blood pressure level and held for about 10 s to record pulse waves. Subsequently, central pressure curves are automatically obtained through a transfer function. In total, three measurements are taken, with a 3-min break between each measurement. The following parameters are assessed by this method: pulse-wave velocity (PWV [m/s]), augmentation index (Aix [%]), heart-rate corrected augmentation index (Alx@75 [%]), central systolic blood pressure (cSBP [mmHg]), and central diastolic (cDBP [mmHg]).

Digital Endothelial Vascular Function and Stiffness

Digital pulse amplitude is measured with a pulse amplitude tonometry device placed on the tip of the right index finger (Endo-PAT2000, Itamar Medical, Caesarea, Israel) [57]. This device comprises a pneumatic plethysmograph that applies uniform pressure to the surface of the distal finger, allowing measurement of pulse volume changes. Throughout the study, the inflation pressure of the digital device is electronically set to 10 mm Hg below diastolic blood pressure or 70 mm Hg (whichever is lower). Baseline pulse amplitude is measured for 2 min 20 s. Arterial flow is interrupted for 5 min by a cuff placed on a proximal forearm using an occlusion pressure of 200 mm Hg or 60 mm Hg above systolic blood pressure (whichever is higher). The pulse amplitude is recorded electronically and analyzed by the computerized, automated algorithm of the device that provides the average pulse amplitude for each 30-s interval after forearm cuff deflation up to 4 min [57]. The following parameters which are known markers of endothelial function and vascular stiffness is derived from these measurements: augmentation index (Aix [%]), heart-rate corrected augmentation index (AIx@75% [%]), reactive hyperemia index (RHI) [57].

Transcutaneous Oxygen Pressure (tcPO2)

Transcutaneous oxygen pressure (tcPO2) measurements are performed with the PRÉCISE 8008 device (medicap GmbH, Ulrichstein, Germany). After a resting period of at least 10 min in supine position, four probes are placed at the dorsum of the feet and at the back of both hands. Measurements are taken while patients are breathing ambient air, in a resting supine position at room temperature, between 22 °C and 25 °C. The site on the foot is carefully cleaned before the probes are applied to the skin, using adhesive rings and contact liquid, supplied by the manufacturer. The measurements are performed after calibration and preheating of the transducer to approximate 44 °C [58]. After termination of the procedure tcPO2 [mmHg] values for the four measurement sites are recorded.

Echocardiography

Transthoracic echocardiography as a non-invasive gold standard for the determination cardiac function and morphology is performed by certified physicians (Vingmed Vivid 9, 5S transducer 2.0–5.0 MHz, GE Medical Systems GmbH, Hamburg, Germany). All images and loops are stored digitally and are analyzed offline. The reading of the echocardiograms is performed according to current recommendations [59] includes parameters of left atrial and left ventricular (LV) structure (left atrial diameter in parasternal short axis [mm]; left atrial volume in 4 chamber view [cm^2], enddiastolic/endsystolic thickness of the intraventricular septum and posterial wall [mm], LV mass [g], enddiastolic/endsystolic LV volume [mL]) as well as LV systolic and diastolic function (biplane LV ejection fraction according to Simpsons rule [%], global longitudinal strain [%], peak velocity of the mitral E- and A-wave [cm/s], deceleration time of the mitral E-wave [ms], isovolumetric relaxation time [ms], peak velocity of the excursion of the lateral and septal mitral annulus in the early diastolic phase [cm/s], ratio between the peak velocity of the excursion of the mean lateral/septal mitral annulus in the early diastolic phase and the peak velocity of the mitral E-wave).

2.5.4. Kidney Function and Ultrasound

Kidney function is determined by blood and urinary laboratory tests: estimated glomerular filtration rate by serum creatine and urinary albumin–creatinine ratio.

Renal ultrasound is performed with a HITACHI EUB-7500 machine. Kidney length is determined as the maximum longitudinal dimension. Parenchymal thickness is measured as the shortest distance from the renal sinus fat to the renal capsule at three different points: at the upper and lower pole and at the middle. The parenchymal-pyelon-index is calculated as the sum of ventral and dorsal parenchymal thickness (in a cross-section of the kidney) divided by the width of the central echo complex. The following categories are generally assessed: location, anomalies as agenesis, hypo- or hyperplasia, horseshoe kidney; kidney length; kidney width; parenchymal thickness; surface roughness; echogenicity; parenchymal-pyelon-index; medullary or parenchymal calcification; number and size of cysts, stones, infraction zones and tumors [60].

2.5.5. Ultrasound of the Extracranial Arteries

Ultrasound of the extracranial arteries is performed with a Philips UI 22 machine. Extracranial carotid and vertebral arteries (VA) are examined with linear ultrasound transducers (bandwidth 3–13 MHz). Systolic, diastolic, and mean flow velocities in common carotid artery, internal carotid artery (ICA), and V2 segments of VA are documented after angle correction. We classify ICA stenosis uniformly according to current ultrasound criteria for grading internal carotid artery stenoses of the the German Society of Ultrasound in Medicine (DEGUM) and Transfer to grading system of the North American Symptomatic Carotid Endarterectomy Trial (NASCET) [61]: if peak systolic velocity (PSV) is ≥125 cm/s, ICA stenosis is defined as being equivalent to ≥50% according to North American Symptomatic Carotid Endarterectomy Trial criteria. Occlusion is defined by absence of Doppler and color signal, typical proximal biphasic Doppler spectra, and additional indirect criteria like crossflow. Carotid plaque is defined as any arterial wall irregularity thicker than 1.5 mm or exceeding >50% of the surrounding wall thickness that protruded into the vessel lumen.

VA measurements are taken in the V2 segment and considered abnormal if there is direct evidence of local or indirect evidence of proximal or distal flow abnormalities. Overall, abnormal flow characteristic of the posterior circulation is defined by at least unilateral (1) flow abnormality of the (extracranial) V2 segment of either VA, (2) intracranial VA stenosis or occlusion, or (3) basilar artery (BA) stenosis or occlusion.

2.5.6. Blood and Urine Samples

Blood and urine samples are obtained according to standard operating procedures. In total, 403.7 mL blood and 42.0 mL urine are obtained per participant (250.0 mL for serum analysis, 121.5 mL for plasma analytics, 16 mL EDTA, 16.2 mL Citrate). At the study center, samples are analyzed immediately after blood and urine sampling. Two aliquots of 0.5 mL serum are stored in a freezer (−80 °C) for further analysis.

For sample analyses at independent laboratories (see Section 2.5.8), blood samples (170.0 mL for serum analytics, 49.5 mL for plasma analytics) are collected at the study center. Further sample management is accomplished by biometec GmbH, Greifswald, Germany.

Blood samples are obtained according to standard operating procedures. In total, 29 mL were obtained per participant (8.5 mL for serum analysis, 8 mL for plasma analytics, 10 mL EDTA, 2.5 mL for blood RNA). At the study center they were stored in a freezer at −80 °C). For this analysis, 100 aliquots were available.

2.5.7. Laboratory Parameters

A complete list of the laboratory parameters can be found in the Appendix A (Table A1). Laboratory analytics of blood and urine are carried out in accordance with established standard operating procedures and preanalytical protocols follow the schemes of the GANI_MED (Greifswald Approach to Individualized Medicine) project [62].

2.5.8. Assessment of Autoantibodies

An enzyme-linked immunosorbent assay (ELISA) is used to detect agAAB as described previously [37,63]. Analyses are performed by an independent laboratory (E.R.D.E.-AAK-Diagnostik GmbH, Berlin, Germany) blinded to clinical patient data. In brief, peptides are directed against the ß1-adrenergic receptor loop 1 and ß2- adrenergic receptor loops 1 and 2. Modified peptides are bound to 96-well streptavidin-coated plates. Peptides are coupled to preblocked streptavidin-coated 96-well plates (Perbio Science, Bonn, Germany). Patient serum is added in a 1:100 dilution and incubated for 60 min. As detection antibody a horseradish peroxidase conjugated anti-human IgG antibody is used (Biomol, Hamburg, Germany). Antibody binding is visualized by the 1-Step Ultra TMB ELISA (Perbio Science, Bonn, Germany). The absorbance is measured at 450 nm against 650 nm with an SLT Spectra multiplate reader (TECAN, Crailsheim, Germany).

As confirmation test, a bioassay is used that has been established by Wallukat and Wollenberger for the identification and quantification of GPCR-AABs [64], and that has been modified and standardized as described previously [65,66]. Analyses are performed by an external laboratory (Berlin Cures GmbH, Berlin, Germany) without knowledge about any further patient characteristics or parameters. In this bioassay, the chronotropic response of spontaneously beating cultured neonatal rat cardiomyocytes to patients' IgG-containing GPCR-AABs is recorded [67].

Anti-NMDA (N-methyl-D-aspartate) autoantibodies are determined in the participant's sera by immunohistochemistry according to manufacturer's instruction (Anti-Glutamate-Receptor-IgG (Typ NMDA)–IFFT, EUROIMMUN, Lübeck, Germany).

Additional measurements are performed by biometec GmbH, Greifswald. This includes analyzes of antibodies against oxidized low-density lipoprotein (oxLDL) and β-amyloid, vasculitis marker (aab against myeloperoxidase (anti-MPO), proteinase 3 (anti-PR3), glomerular basement membrane (anti-GBM)), B-cell activity and antibody development (B-cell activating factor (BAFF)) and neurodegeneration (neurogranin).

2.6. Intervention

Immunoadsorption is performed with ADAsorb apheresis devices equipped with Globaffin adsorber columns in the dialysis department of the University Medicine Greifswald.

The Globaffin column is a regenerative twin adsorber system that utilizes peptide ligands (Peptid-GAM®; Fresenius Medical Care, Bad Homburg, Germany) covalently bound to sepharose. These peptide ligands have a strong affinity for Fc fragments of immunoglobulins from any source and selectively remove immunoglobulins and immune complexes from plasma without affecting other plasma proteins. The Globaffin adsorber system has previously been used in antibody mediated disorders, such as dilated cardiomyopathy and acute renal transplant rejection [68].

In contrast to unselective plasma exchange where all plasma components including albumin, clotting factors and immunoglobulins are discarded and replaced with a fluid containing either albumin and colloid or donor plasma, immunoadsorption is a semi-selective device. First, the patient's plasma is separated from blood cells by a membrane. Plasma is then passed over the Globaffin twin adsorber system which selectively remove IgG, IgA, and IgM before the plasma is re-infused to the patient.

Typically, approximately four column volumes (250 mL) are processed before the plasma stream is directed to the second column within the device and the first column undergoes a four-step regeneration, so that the apheresis cycle can be reiterated: (1) replacement of residual plasma by 0.9% NaCl solution; (2) elution of bound immunoglobulin by hydrochloric acid [glycine-HCl] buffer at pH 2.8; (3) neutralization by phosphate buffered saline [PBS] and 4. replacement of PBS by 0.9% NaCl (Figure 3).

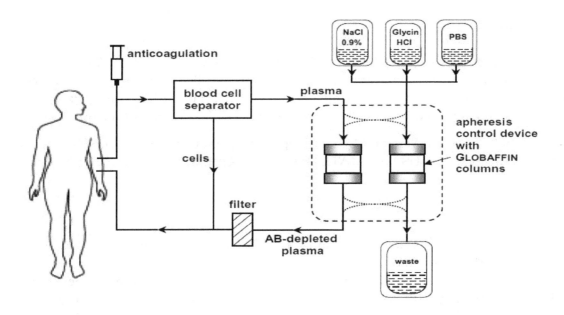

Figure 3. Principle of immunoadsorption. Principle of the immunoadsorption treatment. Reprinted from [68] with permission of John Wiley and Sons.

A separate twin-column pair is assigned to each patient. A total of approximately 2.0-fold of blood plasma volume is processed per day (approximately 4 to 6 h per session) on five consecutive days. After the immunoadsorption series, the patients receive 500 mg per kg body weight intravenous immunoglobulin substitution on day 6 (during approximately 6 h). The dose is determined based on body weight and amounts to 500 mg/kg, depending on the packaging size. The eluates of the regeneration of the columns are collected automatically and are used for detailed immunological analyses. The patients are hospitalized for the immunoadsorption procedures and Ig substitution period in the neurological department of the University Medicine Greifswald.

2.7. Statistical Considerations

The objective of this trial is to assess the effects of IA/IgG in patients with agAABs and dementia in patients with suspected Alzheimer's clinical syndrome. The primary target parameter is uncorrected mean cerebral brain perfusion as assessed by ASL 12 months after treatment.

2.7.1. Statistical Analyses

Analyses will follow an exploratory approach since we plan n = 15 subjects but do not consider a comparison group. Although the main focus of analysis is descriptive, there is an interest in comparing the development of outcomes of 1 month before and 12 months after IA/IgG.

Effect sizes will be estimated using appropriate (generalized) linear mixed regression models. If necessary non-parametric models will be used. To evaluate effect sizes, suggestions according to Cohen (1988) are used [69]. Analyses are performed as intention-to-treat (ITT) and per-protocol (PP).

2.7.2. Missing Data

Missing values are not replaced with substituted values. Due to the small sample size and the exploratory character of the investigation, imputation techniques are not recommended.

2.7.3. Effect Size Consideration

Assuming a prevalence of agAABs of 31.5% and a drop-out rate of 20%, 120 participants have to be checked for eligibility to reach the aim of 15 participants enrolled in the intervention. With a sample size of n = 12, an expected α-error of 5% and a power of 80%, standardized effect sizes of 0.766 can be detected (for one-sided paired t-tests), thus allowing a possible drop out of maximal 3 participants.

For data analyses, Stata (Version 14, StataCorp, College Station, TX, USA), SPSS statistics version 22 (IBM Corp., Armonk, NY, USA) or MATLAB (Version R2015a, Mathworks Inc., Natick, MA, USA) will be used.

3. Discussion

The IMAD study investigates a new pathophysiological and therapeutic aspect of Alzheimer's clinical syndrome, the removal of α1AR-agAABs by immunoadsorption in patients with cognitive impairment and suspected AD. Outcome parameters comprise cerebral blood flow measured by arterial spin labelling MRI (primary), cognition measured by validated cognitive tests and other questionnaires (ADAS-Cog, MMSE, VLMT, Benton Test, GDS) and vascular effects assessed by echocardiography, sonography, blood pressure, pulse wave velocity, plethysmography and transcutaneous oxygen measurement.

Extracorporeal therapies for dementia in Alzheimer's clinical syndrome and CVD are innovative therapeutic options. Recently, three different medical devices have been tested: dialysis, TPE and IA. The Spanish AMBAR study is currently examining whether the peripheral lowering of Aß by TPE and concurrent albumin substitution has an impact on cognitive performance [70]. Kitaguchi and colleagues use dialysis systems [71] and adsorptive double-filtration systems [8] to lower the plasma levels of Aß. Both groups are assuming that the removal of Aß may reduce the cerebral Aß load. By using IA, we contrary aim to target vascular effects of α1AR-agAABs and only secondarily at a probably better clearance of Aß. The IMAD study can profit from the experience of a previously performed open pilot trial [38]. In this earlier study, the applicability of apheresis to dementia patients and safety aspects were examined. The sustainability of the elimination of α1AR-agAABs was proven and the first indications of a stabilization of cognitive performance were observed. The IMAD study now investigates whether the removal of α1AR-AABs by a 5-day IA procedure has a positive effect (improvement or non-deterioration) on impairment-relevant hemodynamic, cognitive, neurological, vascular and metabolic parameters within a one-year follow-up period.

As an exploratory trial, the IMAD study has, owing to feasibility constraints, a small projected sample size in a monocentric, single-arm and unblinded design. Thus, only large effects can reach statistical significance and, even then, the absence of a control group and other trial site(s) will still confine the validity of the results. Nevertheless, this trial may provide important insights whether eliminating or reducing α1AR-agAABs as a contributing factor of dementia-related cerebrovascular impairment opens up a completely new treatment approach for α1AR-agAABs-positive persons along the course of dementia progression in patients with Alzheimer's clinical syndrome. It is of course possible that other agAABs also play a role in the disease course, e.g., ß2AR which has been found in dementia patients in previous studies [37,38].

In this respect, the comprehensive and extensive set of measured endpoints has the potential to indicate possible intervention effects on a broad (patho)physiological spectrum. Indeed, the trial protocol has been devised deliberately to comprise as many measurable physiological and metabolic parameters as possible besides the neurocognitive tests. Therefore, the IMAD trial results will allow to correlate intervention effects with potential physiological or functional mode(s) of action. Such correlations may form the basis of targeted, larger and statistically more robust trials to specifically and precisely uncover the effects of immunoadsorption on affected patients. In the future, the optimal intervention time during the disease progression and the determinants that predict and govern the response profile should be addressed in order to achieve a maximal beneficial effect of IA. In this regard, one challenge will be to pinpoint the actual pathomechanistically active autoantibodies or autoantibodies to delineate less-invasive specific depletion or inactivation schemes.

However, if the IA treatment approach does turn out to have a beneficial capacity for at least a well-defined subgroup of patients at risk of dementia progression in Alzheimer's clinical syndrome, its one-time character (a single week of hospitalization) will certainly be advantageous, discarding or at least attenuating the pharmacotherapeutic need for long-term compliance adherence. For reasons that have not yet been clarified, the GPCR-AABs seldom reoccur after being removed—both in DCM [36,72,73] and in dementia [38].

In the case of a positive outcome of the planned study, functional vascular improvement and cognitive stability or improvement over at least 12 months, knowledge and experience should have been gained to start a well-planned controlled, prospective, multicenter and randomized clinical study. Its data could then be used to prove that IA is suitable for the treatment of mild and moderate dementia with vascular pathological AABs and complements antidementive drug therapies with other targets.

Our study design has potential strengths and limitations that merit further discussion. We see the interdisciplinary approach where knowledge from different disciplines and viewpoints are combined as a unique strength. A further strength resulting directly from this is the comprehensive phenotyping with different end-points to generate a broad spectrum of results that may help design a subsequent multicenter pilot study. As a potential limitation we see the small sample size with low statistical power. For this reason, we are also not able to investigate other potential risk factors (e.g., genetic disposition). As we include patients with cognitive impairment without additional testing of CSF biomarkers we face limitations in the diagnostic classification of their syndromes. Thus, we prefer to label their impairments as suspected or probable AD. On the other hand, we use well-validated neuropsychological testing (MMSE, ADAS-cog, Benton Test, VLMT) and carefully exclude many medical conditions that could lead to secondary and potentially treatable dementia. Moreover, based on the MRI scans we can exclude patients with organic/structural brain damages from the study. In fact, our intention behind this patient selection was the inclusion of patients in their beginning or early phase of probable AD to detect possible changes due to immunoadsorption in physiological and cognitive parameters which might not occur in later states of dementia and to ensure the ability of collaboration and adherence throughout a 12-months follow-up period of the study. Furthermore, we may miss results in the long-term for future associations and detection of causalities due to the relatively short follow up time of 12 months. Additionally, knowledge about the prevalence of agonistic autoantibodies in other forms of dementia and in the general population is limited. Keeping these limitations in mind, our study is designed as an exploratory study and aims at showing proof of principle.

4. Conclusions

IMAD is an important pilot study that will analyze whether the removal of α1AR-agAABs by immunoadsorption in α1AR-agAAB-positive persons slows the progression of dementia in Alzheimer's clinical syndrome and/or improves vascular functional parameters.

Author Contributions: Conceptualization, S.S., S.L. (Sandra Lange), H.K., J.K.-K., S.B., A.V., S.G., A.D., R.K., H.J.G., S.L. (Sönke Langner) and M.D.; Formal analysis, S.G.; Investigation, S.S., S.L. (Sandra Lange), S.B., L.S., J.K.-K., A.V., F.v.P., A.F., K.W., G.W., H.P., H.J.G., S.L. (Sönke Langner) and M.D.; Methodology, M.D.; Project administration, S.L. (Sandra Lange), H.K., S.B. and S.L. (Sönke Langner); Supervision, M.D.; Writing—original draft, S.S., S.L. (Sandra Lange) and M.D.; Writing—review and editing, S.S., S.L. (Sandra Lange), S.B., H.K., L.S., J.K.-K., S.B., A.V., F.v.P., A.F., S.G., K.W., G.W., H.P., A.D., R.K., H.J.G., S.L. (Sönke Langner) and M.D. All authors have read and agreed to the published version of the manuscript.

Acknowledgments: We would like to thank Kristin Werner for assisting the immunoadsorption procedure and study coordination and Bianca Ladwig for supporting the data acquisition and curation.

Conflicts of Interest: AF has received consulting fees from Bayer, Roche, Novartis, and Biogen Idec, and honoraria for oral presentations from Novartis, Böhringer-Ingelheim, Biogen Idec, Paul-Martini-Stiftung, and Daiichi-Sankyo. HP received research support from Diamed and speaker honoraria from Fresenius Medical Care. RK is scientific consultant in therapeutic apheresis for Fresenius Medical Deutschland GmbH, Bad Homburg, Germany. HJG has received travel grants and speakers' honoraria from Fresenius Medical Care, Neuraxpharm, Servier and Janssen Cilag as well as research funding from Fresenius Medical Care. MD has received travel grants and speakers' honoraria from Fresenius Medical Care. All other authors did not report any conflicts of interest related to this manuscript.

Appendix A

Table A1. Laboratory parameters.

Parameter	Screening	Baseline	Immunoadsorption											Follow-Ups
			d1 Pre-IA	d1 Post-IA	d2 Pre-IA	d2 Post-IA	d3 Pre-IA	d3 Post-IA	d4 Pre-IA	d4 Post-IA	d5 Pre-IA	d5 Post-IA	d6 Subst.	
agAB A1AR	X													X
anti oxLDL			X	X	X	X	X	X	X	X	X	X		X
anti MPO			X											X
anti PR3			X											X
anti GBM			X											X
anti NMDA		X												
anti Amyloid ß		X	X	X	X	X	X	X	X	X	X	X		X
Neurogranin			X											
Oxidized low density lipoprotein (oxLDL)			X											
BAFF			X											
Leucocytes		X	X		X		X		X		X		X	X
Erythrocytes		X	X		X		X		X		X		X	X
Hemoglobin		X	X		X		X		X		X		X	X
Hematocrit		X	X		X		X		X		X		X	X
Platelets		X	X		X		X		X		X		X	X
Mean Platelet Volume		X	X		X		X		X		X		X	X
Platelet Distribution Width		X	X		X		X		X		X		X	X
Lymphocytes		X	X		X		X		X		X		X	X
Prothrombin time (Quick)		X	X		X		X		X		X		X	X
International Normalized Ratio (INR)		X	X		X		X		X		X		X	X
Partial Thromboplastine Time (aPTT)		X	X		X		X		X		X		X	X
Mean Cell Volume (MCV)		X	X		X		X		X		X		X	X
Mean Cellular Hemogoblin (MCH)		X	X		X		X		X		X		X	X
Mean Cellular Hemoglobin Concentration (MCHC)		X	X		X		X		X		X		X	X
Red Blood Cell Distribution Curve		X	X		X		X		X		X		X	X
Red Blood Cell Distribution Width (RBCD)		X	X		X		X		X		X		X	X
Sodium		X	X		X		X		X		X		X	X
Potassium		X	X		X		X		X		X		X	X
Calcium		X	X		X		X		X		X		X	X
Phosphate		X	X		X		X		X		X		X	X
Glucose		X	X		X		X		X		X		X	X
Creatinine		X	X		X		X		X		X		X	X
Urea		X	X		X		X		X		X		X	X
Uric Acid		X	X		X		X		X		X		X	X
Total Cholesterol		X	X		X		X		X		X		X	X
High density lipoprotein (HDL)-Cholesterol		X	X		X		X		X		X		X	X
Low density lipoprotein (LDL)-Cholesterol		X	X		X		X		X		X		X	X
Total Triglyzeride		X	X		X		X		X		X		X	X
Alanine Aminotransferase		X	X		X		X		X		X		X	X
Aspartate Aminotransferase		X	X		X		X		X		X		X	X
γ-Glutamyl Transferase		X	X		X		X		X		X		X	X
Total Bilirubin		X	X		X		X		X		X		X	X

Table A1. *Cont.*

Parameter	Screening	Baseline	d1 Pre-IA	d1 Post-IA	d2 Pre-IA	d2 Post-IA	d3 Pre-IA	d3 Post-IA	d4 Pre-IA	d4 Post-IA	d5 Pre-IA	d5 Post-IA	d6 Subst.	Follow-Ups
							Immunoadsorption							
Lipase		X	X		X		X		X		X		X	X
C-reactive Protein (CRP)		X	X		X		X		X		X		X	X
Thyroid (TSH)		X	X		X		X		X		X		X	X
HbA1c		X	X		X		X		X		X		X	X
Albumin		X	X		X		X		X		X		X	X
Protein		X	X		X		X		X		X		X	X
Cystatin C		X	X		X		X		X		X		X	X
Fibrinogen		X	X		X		X		X		X		X	X
Complement C3		X	X		X		X		X		X		X	X
Complement C4		X	X		X		X		X		X		X	X
Factor VIII		X	X		X		X		X		X		X	X
Antithrombin		X	X		X		X		X		X		X	X
Immunoglobulin IgG1		X	X		X		X		X		X		X	X
Immunoglobulin IgG2		X	X		X		X		X		X		X	X
Immunoglobulin IgG3		X	X		X		X		X		X		X	X
Immunoglobulin IgG4		X	X		X		X		X		X		X	X
Immunoglobulin M		X	X		X		X		X		X		X	X
Immunoglobulin A		X	X		X		X		X		X		X	X
Total Immunoglobulin G		X	X	X	X	X	X	X	X	X	X	X	X	X
Total Immunoglobulin		X	X		X		X		X		X		X	X
Vitamin B12		X	X		X		X		X		X		X	X
25-Hydroxy-Vitamin D		X	X		X		X		X		X		X	X
Folic Acid		X	X		X		X		X		X		X	X
Homocysteine		X	X											
Specific gravity (Urine)		X	X		X		X		X		X		X	X
pH (Urine)		X	X		X		X		X		X		X	X
Leucocytes (Urine)		X	X		X		X		X		X		X	X
Nitrite (Urine)		X	X		X		X		X		X		X	X
Protein (Urine)		X	X		X		X		X		X		X	X
Glucose (Urine)		X	X		X		X		X		X		X	X
Ketone (Urine)		X	X		X		X		X		X		X	X
Urobilinogen (Urine)		X	X		X		X		X		X		X	X
Bilirubin (Urine)		X	X		X		X		X		X		X	X
Erythrocytes/Blood (Urine)		X	X		X		X		X		X		X	X
U-Creatine (Urine)		X	X		X		X		X		X		X	X
U-Protein (Urine)		X	X		X		X		X		X		X	X
U-Albumin (Urine)		X	X		X		X		X		X		X	X

References

1. Prince, M. *World Alzheimer Report the Global Impact of Dementia. An Analysis of Prevalence, Incidence, Cost and Trends*; Alzheimer's Disease International: London, UK, 2015.

2. Eggink, E.; van Charante, E.P.M.; van Gool, W.A.; Richard, E. A Population Perspective on Prevention of Dementia. *J. Clin. Med.* **2019**, *8*, 834. [CrossRef] [PubMed]

3. World Health Organization (WHO). Dementia-Key Facts. Available online: https://www.who.int/news-room/fact-sheets/detail/dementia (accessed on 27 May 2020).

4. Vetrano, D.L.; Rizzuto, D.; Calderon-Larranaga, A.; Onder, G.; Welmer, A.K.; Bernabei, R.; Marengoni, A.; Fratiglioni, L. Trajectories of functional decline in older adults with neuropsychiatric and cardiovascular multimorbidity: A Swedish cohort study. *PLoS Med.* **2018**, *15*, e1002503. [CrossRef] [PubMed]

5. Vetrano, D.L.; Rizzuto, D.; Calderon-Larranaga, A.; Onder, G.; Welmer, A.K.; Qiu, C.; Bernabei, R.; Marengoni, A.; Fratiglioni, L. Walking Speed Drives the Prognosis of Older Adults with Cardiovascular and Neuropsychiatric Multimorbidity. *Am. J. Med.* **2019**, *132*, 1207–1215 e6. [CrossRef] [PubMed]

6. Alzheimer's Association. 2020 Alzheimer's Disease Facts and Figures. *Alzheimers Dement.* **2020**, *6*, 391–460.

7. Deutsche Gesellschaft für Psychiatrie, Psychotherapie und Nervenheilkunde (DGPPN); Deutsche Gesellschaft für Neurologie (DGN). S3-Leitlinie "Demenzen". 2016. Available online: https://www.awmf.org/uploads/tx_szleitlinien/038-013l_S3-Demenzen-2016-07.pdf (accessed on 27 May 2020).

8. Brier, M.R.; Gordon, B.; Friedrichsen, K.; McCarthy, J.; Stern, A.; Christensen, J.; Owen, C.; Aldea, P.; Su, Y.; Hassenstab, J.; et al. Tau and Abeta imaging, CSF measures, and cognition in Alzheimer's disease. *Sci. Transl. Med.* **2016**, *8*, 338ra66. [CrossRef] [PubMed]

9. Holtzman, D.M.; Carrillo, M.C.; Hendrix, J.A.; Bain, L.J.; Catafau, A.M.; Gault, L.M.; Goedert, M.; Mandelkow, E.; Mandelkow, E.M.; Miller, D.S.; et al. Tau: From research to clinical development. *Alzheimers Dement.* **2016**, *12*, 1033–1039. [CrossRef]

10. van Dyck, C.H. Anti-Amyloid-beta Monoclonal Antibodies for Alzheimer's Disease: Pitfalls and Promise. *Biol. Psychiatry* **2018**, *83*, 311–319. [CrossRef]

11. Doody, R.S.; Thomas, R.G.; Farlow, M.; Iwatsubo, T.; Vellas, B.; Joffe, S.; Kieburtz, K.; Raman, R.; Sun, X.; Aisen, P.S.; et al. Phase 3 trials of solanezumab for mild-to-moderate Alzheimer's disease. *N. Engl. J. Med.* **2014**, *370*, 311–321. [CrossRef]

12. Salloway, S.; Sperling, R.; Fox, N.C.; Blennow, K.; Klunk, W.; Raskind, M.; Sabbagh, M.; Honig, L.S.; Porsteinsson, A.P.; Ferris, S.; et al. Two phase 3 trials of bapineuzumab in mild-to-moderate Alzheimer's disease. *N. Engl. J. Med.* **2014**, *370*, 322–333. [CrossRef]

13. Egan, M.F.; Kost, J.; Tariot, P.N.; Aisen, P.S.; Cummings, J.L.; Vellas, B.; Sur, C.; Mukai, Y.; Voss, T.; Furtek, C.; et al. Randomized Trial of Verubecestat for Mild-to-Moderate Alzheimer's Disease. *N. Engl. J. Med.* **2018**, *378*, 1691–1703. [CrossRef]

14. Cuberas-Borros, G.; Roca, I.; Boada, M.; Tarraga, L.; Hernandez, I.; Buendia, M.; Rubio, L.; Torres, G.; Bittini, A.; Guzman-de-Villoria, J.A.; et al. Longitudinal Neuroimaging Analysis in Mild-Moderate Alzheimer's Disease Patients Treated with Plasma Exchange with 5% Human Albumin. *J. Alzheimers Dis.* **2018**, *61*, 321–332. [CrossRef] [PubMed]

15. Boada, M.; Lopez, O.; unez, L.N.; Szczepiorkowski, Z.M.; Torres, M.; Grifols, C.; Paez, A. Plasma exchange for Alzheimer's disease Management by Albumin Replacement (AMBAR) trial: Study design and progress. *Alzheimers Dement. (N. Y.)* **2019**, *5*, 61–69. [CrossRef] [PubMed]

16. Kitaguchi, N.; Kawaguchi, K.; Yamazaki, K.; Kawachi, H.; Sakata, M.; Kaneko, M.; Kato, M.; Sakai, K.; Ohashi, N.; Hasegawa, M.; et al. Adsorptive filtration systems for effective removal of blood amyloid beta: A potential therapy for Alzheimer's disease. *J. Artif. Organs.* **2018**, *21*, 220–229. [CrossRef] [PubMed]

17. Attems, J.K.; Jellinger, A. The overlap between vascular disease and Alzheimer's disease–lessons from pathology. *BMC Med.* **2014**, *12*, 206. [CrossRef] [PubMed]

18. Habes, M.; Erus, G.; Toledo, J.B.; Zhang, T.; Bryan, N.; Launer, L.J.; Rosseel, Y.; Janowitz, D.; Doshi, J.; van der Auwera, S.; et al. White matter hyperintensities and imaging patterns of brain ageing in the general population. *Brain* **2016**, *139*, 1164–1179. [CrossRef]

19. Wallukat, G.; Schimke, I. Agonistic autoantibodies directed against G-protein-coupled receptors and their relationship to cardiovascular diseases. *Semin. Immunopathol.* **2014**, *36*, 351–363. [CrossRef]

20. Cabral-Marques, O.; Riemekasten, G. Functional autoantibodies targeting G protein-coupled receptors in rheumatic diseases. *Nat. Rev. Rheumatol.* **2017**, *13*, 648–656. [CrossRef]

21. Nakatake, N.; Sanders, J.; Richards, T.; Burne, P.; Barrett, C.; Pra, C.D.; Presotto, F.; Betterle, C.; Furmaniak, J.; Smith, B.R. Estimation of serum TSH receptor autoantibody concentration and affinity. *Thyroid* **2006**, *16*, 1077–1084. [CrossRef]

22. Wallukat, G.; Fu, M.L.; Magnusson, Y.; Hjalmarson, A.; Hoebeke, J.; Wollenberger, A. Agonistic effects of anti-peptide antibodies and autoantibodies directed against adrenergic and cholinergic receptors: Absence of desensitization. *Blood Press. Suppl.* **1996**, *3*, 31–36.

23. Karczewski, P.; Pohlmann, A.; Wagenhaus, B.; Wisbrun, N.; Hempel, P.; Lemke, B.; Kunze, R.; Niendorf, T.; Bimmler, M. Antibodies to the alpha1-adrenergic receptor cause vascular impairments in rat brain as demonstrated by magnetic resonance angiography. *PLoS ONE* **2012**, *7*, e41602. [CrossRef]

24. El Fassi, D.; Banga, J.P.; Gilbert, J.A.; Padoa, C.; Hegedus, L.; Nielsen, C.H. Treatment of Graves' disease with rituximab specifically reduces the production of thyroid stimulating autoantibodies. *Clin. Immunol.* **2009**, *130*, 252–258. [CrossRef] [PubMed]

25. Beyer, G.; Kuster, I.; Budde, C.; Wilhelm, E.; Hoene, A.; Evert, K.; Stracke, S.; Friesecke, S.; Mayerle, J.; Steveling, A. Hyperthyroid and acute tonsillitis in a 23-year-old woman. *Internist (Berl.)* **2016**, *57*, 717–723. [CrossRef] [PubMed]

26. Mawuenyega, K.G.; Sigurdson, W.; Ovod, V.; Munsell, L.; Kasten, T.; Morris, J.C.; Yarasheski, K.E.; Bateman, R.J. Decreased clearance of CNS beta-amyloid in Alzheimer's disease. *Science* **2010**, *330*, 1774. [CrossRef] [PubMed]

27. Fu, M.L.; Herlitz, H.; Wallukat, G.; Hilme, E.; Hedner, T.; Hoebeke, J.; Hjalmarson, A. Functional autoimmune epitope on alpha 1-adrenergic receptors in patients with malignant hypertension. *Lancet* **1994**, *344*, 1660–1663.

28. Wenzel, K.; Haase, H.; Wallukat, G.; Derer, W.; Bartel, S.; Homuth, V.; Herse, F.; Hubner, N.; Schulz, H.; Janczikowski, M.; et al. Potential relevance of alpha(1)-adrenergic receptor autoantibodies in refractory hypertension. *PLoS ONE* **2008**, *3*, e3742. [CrossRef]

29. Li, G.; Cao, Z.; Wu, X.W.; Wu, H.K.; Ma, Y.; Wu, B.; Wang, W.Q.; Cheng, J.; Zhou, Z.H.; Tu, Y.C. Autoantibodies against AT1 and alpha1-adrenergic receptors predict arterial stiffness progression in normotensive subjects over a 5-year period. *Clin. Sci. (Lond.)* **2017**, *131*, 2947–2957. [CrossRef]

30. Felix, S.B.; Beug, D.; Dörr, M. Immunoadsorption therapy in dilated cardiomyopathy. *Expert. Rev. Cardiovasc. Ther.* **2015**, *13*, 145–152. [CrossRef]

31. Felix, S.B.; Staudt, A.; Dorffel, W.V.; Stangl, V.; Merkel, K.; Pohl, M.; Docke, W.D.; Morgera, S.; Neumayer, H.H.; Wernecke, K.D.; et al. Hemodynamic effects of immunoadsorption and subsequent immunoglobulin substitution in dilated cardiomyopathy: Three-month results from a randomized study. *J. Am. Coll. Cardiol.* **2000**, *35*, 1590–1598. [CrossRef]

32. Herda, L.R.; Trimpert, C.; Nauke, U.; Landsberger, M.; Hummel, A.; Beug, D.; Kieback, A.; Dörr, M.; Empen, K.; Knebel, F.; et al. Effects of immunoadsorption and subsequent immunoglobulin G substitution on cardiopulmonary exercise capacity in patients with dilated cardiomyopathy. *Am. Heart J.* **2010**, *159*, 809–816. [CrossRef]

33. Staudt, A.; Schaper, F.; Stangl, V.; Plagemann, A.; Bohm, M.; Merkel, K.; Wallukat, G.; Wernecke, K.D.; Stangl, K.; Baumann, G.; et al. Immunohistological changes in dilated cardiomyopathy induced by immunoadsorption therapy and subsequent immunoglobulin substitution. *Circulation* **2001**, *103*, 2681–2686. [CrossRef]

34. Staudt, A.; Hummel, A.; Ruppert, J.; Dörr, M.; Trimpert, C.; Birkenmeier, K.; Krieg, T.; Staudt, Y.; Felix, S.B. Immunoadsorption in dilated cardiomyopathy: 6-month results from a randomized study. *Am. Heart J.* **2006**, *152*, 712 e1-6. [CrossRef] [PubMed]

35. Winters, J.L. Apheresis in the treatment of idiopathic dilated cardiomyopathy. *J. Clin. Apher.* **2012**, *27*, 312–319. [CrossRef] [PubMed]

36. Dandel, M.; Wallukat, G.; Englert, A.; Lehmkuhl, H.B.; Knosalla, C.; Hetzer, R. Long-term benefits of immunoadsorption in beta(1)-adrenoceptor autoantibody-positive transplant candidates with dilated cardiomyopathy. *Eur. J. Heart Fail.* **2012**, *14*, 1374–1388. [CrossRef]

37. Thyrian, J.R.; Hertel, J.; Schulze, L.N.; Dörr, M.; Prüss, H.; Hempel, P.; Bimmler, M.; Kunze, R.; Grabe, H.J.; Teipel, S.; et al. Prevalence and Determinants of Agonistic Autoantibodies Against alpha1-Adrenergic

Receptors in Patients Screened Positive for Dementia: Results from the Population-Based DelpHi-Study. *J. Alzheimers Dis.* **2018**, *64*, 1091–1097. [CrossRef] [PubMed]

38. Hempel, P.; Heinig, B.; Jerosch, C.; Decius, I.; Karczewski, P.; Kassner, U.; Kunze, R.; Steinhagen-Thiessen, E.; Bimmler, M. Immunoadsorption of Agonistic Autoantibodies Against alpha1-Adrenergic Receptors in Patients With Mild to Moderate Dementia. *Ther. Apher. Dial.* **2016**, *20*, 523–529. [CrossRef]

39. Jack, C.R.; Bennett, D.A., Jr.; Blennow, K.; Carrillo, M.C.; Dunn, B.; Haeberlein, S.B.; Holtzman, D.M.; Jagust, W.; Jessen, F.; Karlawish, J.; et al. NIA-AA Research Framework: Toward a biological definition of Alzheimer's disease. *Alzheimers Dement.* **2018**, *14*, 535–562. [CrossRef]

40. Fazekas, F.; Chawluk, J.B.; Alavi, A.; Hurtig, H.I.; Zimmerman, R.A. MR signal abnormalities at 1.5 T in Alzheimer's dementia and normal aging. *AJR Am. J. Roentgenol.* **1987**, *149*, 351–356. [CrossRef]

41. Scheltens, P.; Launer, L.J.; Barkhof, F.; Weinstein, H.C.; van Gool, W.A. Visual assessment of medial temporal lobe atrophy on magnetic resonance imaging: Interobserver reliability. *J. Neurol.* **1995**, *242*, 557–560. [CrossRef]

42. Leijenaar, J.F.; Ivan Maurik, S.; Kuijer, J.P.A.; van der Flier, W.M.; Scheltens, P.; Barkhof, F.; Prins, N.D. Lower cerebral blood flow in subjects with Alzheimer's dementia, mild cognitive impairment, and subjective cognitive decline using two-dimensional phase-contrast magnetic resonance imaging. *Alzheimers Dement. (Amst.)* **2017**, *9*, 76–83. [CrossRef]

43. Binnewijzend, M.A.; Kuijer, J.P.; Benedictus, M.R.; van der Flier, W.M.; Wink, A.M.; Wattjes, M.P.; van Berckel, B.N.; Scheltens, P.; Barkhof, F. Cerebral blood flow measured with 3D pseudocontinuous arterial spin-labeling MR imaging in Alzheimer disease and mild cognitive impairment: A marker for disease severity. *Radiology* **2013**, *267*, 221–230. [CrossRef]

44. Asllani, I.; Borogovac, A.; Brown, T.R. Regression algorithm correcting for partial volume effects in arterial spin labeling MRI. *Magn. Reson. Med.* **2008**, *60*, 1362–1371. [CrossRef]

45. Folstein, M.F.; Folstein, S.E.; McHugh, P.R. Mini-mental state. A practical method for grading the cognitive state of patients for the clinician. *J. Psychiatr. Res.* **1975**, *12*, 189–198. [CrossRef]

46. Folstein, M.F.; Folstein, S.E.; White, T.; Messer, M.A. *MMSE-2. Mini-Mental State Examination*, 2nd ed.; PAR Inc.: Lutz, FL, USA, 2010.

47. Rosen, W.G.; Mohs, R.C.; Davis, K.L. A new rating scale for Alzheimer's disease. *Am. J. Psychiatry* **1984**, *141*, 1356–1364.

48. Graham, N.L.; Emery, T.; Hodges, J.R. Distinctive cognitive profiles in Alzheimer's disease and subcortical vascular dementia. *J. Neurol. Neurosurg. Psychiatry* **2004**, *75*, 61–71.

49. Ihl, R.; Mohs, R.; Weyer, G. *Alzheimer's Disease Assessment Scale: ADAS*; Beltz Test: Göttingen, Germany, 1990.

50. Stern, R.G.; Mohs, R.C.; Davidson, M.; Schmeidler, J.; Silverman, J.; Kramer-Ginsberg, E.; Searcey, T.; Bierer, L.; Davis, K.L. A longitudinal study of Alzheimer's disease: Measurement, rate, and predictors of cognitive deterioration. *Am. J. Psychiatry* **1994**, *151*, 390–396.

51. Helmstaedter, C.; Lendt, M.; Lux, S. *VLMT: Verbaler Lern-und Merkfähigkeitstest*; Beltz Test: Göttingen, Germany, 2001.

52. Yesavage, J.A. Geriatric depression scale. *Psychopharmacol. Bull.* **1988**, *24*, 709–711.

53. Yesavage, J.A.; Brink, T.L.; Rose, T.L.; Lum, O.; Huang, V.; Adey, M.; Leirer, V.O. Development and validation of a geriatric depression screening scale: A preliminary report. *J. Psychiatr. Res.* **1982**, *17*, 37–49. [CrossRef]

54. Volzke, H.; Alte, D.; Schmidt, C.O.; Radke, D.; Lorbeer, R.; Friedrich, N.; Aumann, N.; Lau, K.; Piontek, M.; Born, G.; et al. Cohort profile: The study of health in Pomerania. *Int. J. Epidemiol.* **2011**, *40*, 294–307. [CrossRef]

55. Weber, T.; Wassertheurer, S.; Rammer, M.; Maurer, E.; Hametner, B.; Mayer, C.C.; Kropf, J.; Eber, B. Validation of a brachial cuff-based method for estimating central systolic blood pressure. *Hypertension* **2011**, *58*, 825–832. [CrossRef]

56. Wassertheurer, S.; Kropf, J.; Weber, T.; van der Giet, M.; Baulmann, J.; Ammer, M.; Hametner, B.; Mayer, C.C.; Eber, B.; Magometschnigg, D. A new oscillometric method for pulse wave analysis: Comparison with a common tonometric method. *J. Hum. Hypertens* **2010**, *24*, 498–504. [CrossRef]

57. Hamburg, N.M.; Keyes, M.J.; Larson, M.G.; Vasan, R.S.; Schnabel, R.; Pryde, M.M.; Mitchell, G.F.; Sheffy, J.; Vita, J.A.; Benjamin, E.J. Cross-sectional relations of digital vascular function to cardiovascular risk factors in the Framingham Heart Study. *Circulation* **2008**, *117*, 2467–2474. [CrossRef]

58. Deng, W.; Dong, X.; Zhang, Y.; Jiang, Y.; Lu, D.; Wu, Q.; Liang, Z.; Yang, G.; Chen, B. Transcutaneous oxygen pressure (TcPO(2)): A novel diagnostic tool for peripheral neuropathy in type 2 diabetes patients. *Diabetes Res. Clin. Pract.* **2014**, *105*, 336–343. [CrossRef]

59. Recommendations for Cardiac Chamber Quantification by Echocardiography in Adults: An Update from the American Society of Echocardiography and the European Association of, Cardiovascular Imaging. *Eur. Heart J. Cardiovasc. Imaging* **2016**, *17*, 412. [CrossRef]

60. Schmidt, G.G.; Kursbuch, C. *Ultraschall Nach den Richtlinien der DEGUM und der KVR*, 6th ed.; Thieme: New York, NY, USA, 2015.

61. Arning, C.; Widder, B.; von Reutern, G.M.; Stiegler, H.; Gortler, M. Revision of DEGUM ultrasound criteria for grading internal carotid artery stenoses and transfer to NASCET measurement. *Ultraschall Med.* **2010**, *31*, 251–257. [CrossRef]

62. Grabe, H.J.; Assel, H.; Bahls, T.; Dörr, M.; Endlich, K.; Endlich, N.; Erdmann, P.; Ewert, R.; Felix, S.B.; Fiene, B.; et al. Cohort profile: Greifswald approach to individualized medicine (GANI_MED). *J. Transl. Med.* **2014**, *12*, 144. [CrossRef]

63. Karczewski, P.; Hempel, P.; Bimmler, M. Role of alpha1-adrenergic receptor antibodies in Alzheimer's disease. *Front. Biosci. (Landmark Ed.)* **2018**, *23*, 2082–2089.

64. Wallukat, G.A.W. Effects of the serum gamma globulin fraction of patients with allergic asthma and dilated cardiomyopathy on chronotropic beta adrenoceptor function in cultured neonatal rat heart myocytes. *Biomed. Biochim. Acta* **1987**, *46*, S634–S639.

65. Wallukat, G.; Saravia, S.G.M.; Haberland, A.; Bartel, S.; Araujo, R.; Valda, G.; Duchen, D.; Ramirez, I.D.; Borges, A.C.; Schimke, I. Distinct patterns of autoantibodies against G-protein-coupled receptors in Chagas' cardiomyopathy and megacolon. Their potential impact for early risk assessment in asymptomatic Chagas' patients. *J. Am. Coll. Cardiol.* **2010**, *55*, 463–468. [CrossRef]

66. Wallukat, G.; Prüss, H.; Muller, J.; Schimke, I. Functional autoantibodies in patients with different forms of dementia. *PLoS ONE* **2018**, *13*, e0192778.

67. Davideit, H.; Haberland, A.; Bartel, S.; Schulze-Rothe, S.; Muller, J.; Wenzel, K. Determination of Agonistically Acting Autoantibodies to the Adrenergic Beta-1 Receptor by Cellular Bioassay. *Methods Mol. Biol.* **2019**, *1901*, 95–102.

68. Ronspeck, W.; Brinckmann, R.; Egner, R.; Gebauer, F.; Winkler, D.; Jekow, P.; Wallukat, G.; Muller, J.; Kunze, R. Peptide based adsorbers for therapeutic immunoadsorption. *Ther. Apher. Dial.* **2003**, *7*, 91–97. [CrossRef] [PubMed]

69. Cohen, J. *Statistical Power Analysis for the Behavioral Sciences*; Academic Press: New York, NY, USA, 1988.

70. Boada, M.; Anaya, F.; Ortiz, P.; Olazaran, J.; Shua-Haim, J.R.; Obisesan, T.O.; Hernandez, I.; Munoz, J.; Buendia, M.; Alegret, M.; et al. Efficacy and Safety of Plasma Exchange with 5% Albumin to Modify Cerebrospinal Fluid and Plasma Amyloid-beta Concentrations and Cognition Outcomes in Alzheimer's Disease Patients: A Multicenter, Randomized, Controlled Clinical Trial. *J. Alzheimers Dis.* **2017**, *56*, 129–143. [CrossRef] [PubMed]

71. Kitaguchi, N.; Kawaguchi, K.; Nakai, S.; Murakami, K.; Ito, S.; Hoshino, H.; Hori, H.; Ohashi, A.; Shimano, Y.; Suzuki, N.; et al. Reduction of Alzheimer's disease amyloid-beta in plasma by hemodialysis and its relation to cognitive functions. *Blood Purif.* **2011**, *32*, 57–62. [CrossRef] [PubMed]

72. Trimpert, C.; Herda, L.R.; Eckerle, L.G.; Pohle, S.; Muller, C.; Landsberger, M.; Felix, S.B.; Staudt, A. Immunoadsorption in dilated cardiomyopathy: Long-term reduction of cardiodepressant antibodies. *Eur. J. Clin. Investig.* **2010**, *40*, 685–691. [CrossRef]

73. Muller, J.; Wallukat, G.; Dandel, M.; Bieda, H.; Brandes, K.; Spiegelsberger, S.; Nissen, E.; Kunze, R.; Hetzer, R. Immunoglobulin adsorption in patients with idiopathic dilated cardiomyopathy. *Circulation* **2000**, *101*, 385–391. [CrossRef]

9

Comparing Plasma Exchange to Escalated Methyl Prednisolone in Refractory Multiple Sclerosis Relapses

Steffen Pfeuffer [1,*,†], Leoni Rolfes [1,†], Eike Bormann [2], Cristina Sauerland [2], Tobias Ruck [1], Matthias Schilling [1], Nico Melzer [1], Marcus Brand [3], Refik Pul [4], Christoph Kleinschnitz [4], Heinz Wiendl [1] and Sven G. Meuth [1]

1   Neurology Clinic and Institute for Translational Neurology, University of Muenster, 48149 Münster, Germany; leoni.rolfes@ukmuenster.de (L.R.); tobias.ruck@ukmuenster.de (T.R.); matthias.schilling@ukmuenster.de (M.S.); nico.melzer@ukmuenster.de (N.M.); heinz.wiendl@ukmuenster.de (H.W.); sven.meuth@ukmuenster.de (S.G.M.)
2   Institute of Biostatistics and Clinical Research, University of Muenster, 48149 Münster, Germany; eike.bormann@ukmuenster.de (E.B.); cristina.sauerland@ukmuenster.de (C.S.)
3   Department of Internal Medicine D, University of Muenster 48149 Münster, Germany; marcus.brand@ukmuenster.de
4   Department of Neurology, University Duisburg-Essen, 45147 Essen, Germany; refik.pul@uk-essen.de (R.P.); christoph.kleinschnitz@uk-essen.de (C.K.)
*   Correspondence: steffen.pfeuffer@ukmuenster.de
†   Both authors contributed equally.

Abstract: Intravenous methyl prednisolone (IVMPS) represents the standard of care for multiple sclerosis (MS) relapses, but fail to improve symptoms in one quarter of patients. In this regard, apart from extending steroid treatment to a higher dose, therapeutic plasma exchange (TPE) has been recognized as a treatment option. The aim of this retrospective, monocentric study was to investigate the efficacy of TPE versus escalated dosages of IVMPS in refractory MS relapses. An in-depth medical chart review was performed to identify patients from local databases. Relapse recovery was stratified as "good/full", "average" and "worst/no" according to function score development. In total, 145 patients were analyzed. Good/average/worst recovery at discharge was observed in 60.9%/32.6%/6.5% of TPE versus 15.2%/14.1%/70.7% of IVMPS patients, respectively. A total of 53.5% of IVMPS patients received TPE as rescue treatment and 54.8% then responded satisfactorily. The multivariable odds ratio (OR) for worst/no recovery was 39.01 (95%–CI: 10.41–146.18; $p \leq 0.001$), favoring administration of TPE as first escalation treatment. The effects were sustained at three-month follow-ups, as OR for further deterioration was 6.48 (95%–CI: 2.48–16.89; $p \leq 0.001$), favoring TPE. In conclusion, TPE was superior over IVMPS in the amelioration of relapse symptoms at discharge and follow-up. This study provides class IV evidence supporting the administration of TPE as the first escalation treatment to steroid-refractory MS relapses.

Keywords: multiple sclerosis; optic neuritis; plasma exchange; relapse; class IV; steroids

1. Introduction

The treatment of acute multiple sclerosis (MS) relapses has remained unaltered for decades. The use of high-dose short-term intravenous (methyl-) prednisolone (IVMPS; 500–1000 mg per day for three to five days) is the accepted treatment for relapses [1,2]. Of note, adrenocorticotropic hormone (ACTH) gel is an alternative for patients who do not tolerate corticosteroids. Moreover, although it has been suggested that intravenous immunoglobulins (IVIG) may be a therapeutic option if steroids are contraindicated, two well conducted randomized controlled trials showed that IVIG as an add-on treatment with IVMPS did not confer additional benefit [3,4].

Interestingly, around 25% of patients remain with significant disability 14 days after IVMPS treatment initiation [5]. For these patients, one option is IVMPS treatment escalation (up to 2000 mg daily) for a further three to five days, as recommended by the national guidelines [2,6]. An alternative option is therapeutic plasma exchange (TPE), which has been proven effective in one small randomized trial that showed the superiority of TPE over sham treatment [7]. The effectiveness of TPE has been reported for all demyelinating disorders of the CNS, including optic neuritis (ON), clinically-isolated syndrome (CIS) and relapsing-remitting MS (RRMS) [8–10]. Consequently, several guidelines recommend TPE as an adjunctive treatment for increasing the chances of recovery for steroid-refractory relapses [11,12]. However, most studies evaluating TPE lacked an active comparator (such as escalated IVMPS) and comprised heterogeneous treatment regimens. Also, patients with demyelinating diseases other than RRMS were included in the study populations [7–9]. Evidence for IVMPS treatment escalation is to a large part based on a single study that compared MRI endpoints but not clinical endpoints [6]. Furthermore, IVMPS treatment escalation exhibited additional, non-genomic effects in animal models [13]. Robust clinical evidence for the currently recommended treatment sequence (initiation treatment with IVMPS, first escalation treatment with IVMPS, second escalation treatment with TPE) is still lacking [6,11,12].

We here analyzed patients with acute relapses of RRMS, CIS or isolated ON who were treated with escalated IVMPS, TPE, or a combination of both.

2. Experimental Section

2.1. Patients

Between January 2013 and December 2017, all of the in-patients in our department were screened. We identified patients diagnosed with RRMS, CIS, or isolated ON, who received a full course of IVMPS (1000 mg daily for five days without an oral taper) as initial treatment (referred to as "initiation treatment" throughout the manuscript). In a second step, we selected patients who received further relapse treatments (referred to as "escalation treatment" throughout the manuscript) and reviewed their medical chart in detail, using a standardized electronic case report form. All patients included in our analysis were hospitalized in our clinic for both the initiation as well as the escalation treatment.

The inclusion criteria for final analysis were:

(i)   established diagnosis of RRMS or CIS according to 2017 revised McDonald criteria [14] or optic neuritis in absence of any other infectious or inflammatory disease of the CNS (especially neuromyelitis optica spectrum disorders)

(ii)   significant relapse with an increase of the Expanded Disability Status Scale (EDSS) score [15] of at least 1.0 in MS/CIS patients or a decrease of the best-corrected visual acuity (VA) in patients with isolated ON in analogy to a decrease of at least 1 according to the visual function system score (FSS) derived from the EDSS, as inclusion criteria for both initiation and escalation treatment

(iii)   escalation therapy with either 2000 mg methylprednisolone per day for five days, five cycles of therapeutic plasma exchange or a combination thereof following initiation therapy with 1000 mg per day over 5 days

(iv)   completion of escalation treatment within six weeks from relapse onset

Therapeutic plasma exchange was performed with a COM.TEC cell separator (Fresenius Hemo-Care GmbH, Bad Homburg, Germany). All patients received treatment via central venous catheters every other day, for a total of five sessions. Per session, one plasma volume was processed, while human albumin solution (5%) was used for substitution. The blood flow rates were 50–70 mL per min. All patients underwent regional pre-centrifugal anticoagulation with citrate, followed by post-centrifugal calcium application. In four cases, the treatment-free interval was extended by another day due to excessive hypofibrinogenemia.

Patients with the following criteria were excluded:

(i)   pregnancy, as determined by pregnancy test
(ii)   diagnosis of other systemic inflammatory disorders within the observation period
(iii)   onset of relapse symptoms more than one month prior to initiation treatment with IVMPS
(iv)   documentation of a secondary progressive disease course within the observation period

For the patients who received more than one escalation treatment within the observation period, we only evaluated the first relapse to avoid preselection bias.

2.2. Assessment of Effectiveness

To overcome limitations of the EDSS in depicting acute, relapse-associated disability, we decided to classify our patients into different response categories. For statistical analysis we applied FSS-based stratification as proposed by Conway and colleagues, which stratifies treatment responses based on peak- and recovery-FSS distances into "good/full", "partial", or "worst/no" recovery [16]. We show a modified matrix, as previously used, with outcome stratification in Figure S1 [17]. The outcomes were evaluated after treatment completion and at follow-up (3 months after discharge).

Relapses were considered as monosymptomatic when Kurtzke's FSS of the affected system exceeded the other FSS by at least 1 point. Consequently, if this condition was not given, the relapse was regarded as polysymptomatic. In this regard, patients that either showed similar relapse FSSs for pyramidal and cerebellar functions (3 patients) or pyramidal and sensory functions (5 patients), were assigned to their FSS that was EDSS-defining at follow-up. In addition, 4 patients with spinal lesions displayed a similar FSS for bowel and bladder function and pyramidal function. These patients were subjected to the FSS group "pyramidal", as no patients were identified with bowel and bladder dysfunction as monosymptomatic relapse.

2.3. Assessment of Safety

We also screened patients' medical charts for severe adverse events and graded the identified events according to recommendations made in the "Common Terminology Criteria for Adverse Events". The CTCAE classification is as follows: I: asymptomatic testing or mild symptoms without necessity for specific intervention; II: local or noninvasive intervention indicated; III: severe, but not immediately life-threatening event, hospitalization or prolongation of hospitalization necessary; IV: life-threatening event; V: death related to event. The study conduct was ethically approved by the local institutional review board of the University of Muenster, Germany (2017-298-f-S).

2.4. Statistical Analysis

The continuous variables are presented as median and interquartile range and compared between groups using a Kruskal–Wallis test. The categorical variables are presented as absolute and relative frequencies and compared using Fisher's exact test.

To evaluate the influence of multiple variables on the occurrence and outcome of serious adverse events, we applied logistic regression. The results are described with odds ratios (OR), the respective 95% confidence intervals (CI), and Wald-test p-values. Either "worst or no treatment response following first escalation treatment" or "stable course versus further deterioration at follow-up" or "development of severe adverse events" were used as dependent variables.

All analyses are explorative and should be interpreted accordingly. p-values below 0.05 are considered significant; no adjustment for multiple testing was applied. Statistical analysis was conducted with SPSS Version 25 (International Business Machines Corporation (IBM), Armonk, USA).

2.5. Data Availability Statement

Anonymized data will be shared upon request from qualified investigators.

3. Results

3.1. Patients

Between January 2013 and December 2017, a total of 541 patients received initiation treatment for MS relapses. Of those, 193 (35.7%) patients were admitted for escalation treatment and all had a persistent functional deficit as defined above. A total of 127 (65.8%) patients received a second course of IVMPS as a first escalation treatment, while 66 (34.2%) patients were directly subjected to TPE. For our final analysis we could include a total of 145 patients: 99 out of 127 patients who received a second course of IVMPS, and 46 out of 66 patients who were directly subjected to TPE. Of note, 53 out of 99 (53.5%) patients were subjected to TPE as the second escalation treatment. None of the TPE patients were re-exposed to increased doses of IVMPS (for consort plot see Figure 1).

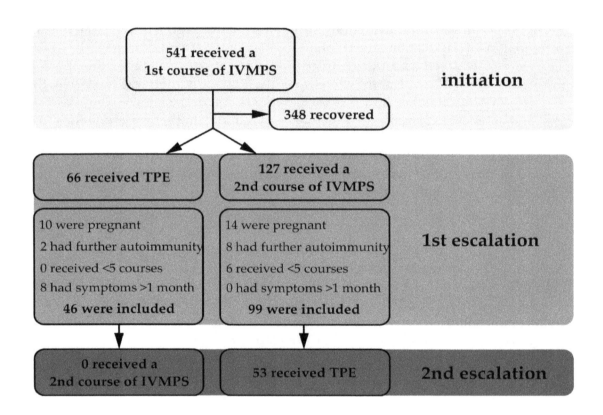

Figure 1. RRMS in-patients who were treated at the study site between January 2013 and December 2017 are described here. The data focus on those patients who received a full course of intravenous methyl prednisolone (5 × 1 g IVMPS) as the first escalation treatment after relapse. Patients who received a lower dosage (e.g., 3 × 1 g IVMPS) were excluded from the primary analysis.

Baseline characteristics of all treatment groups (IVMPS, TPE, and IVMPS + TPE) are shown in Table 1. Patients who did not receive additional TPE presented with lower peak relapse EDSS (median: IVMPS: 2.0; TPE: 3.0; IVMPS+TPE: 3.0; $p = 0.003$). Otherwise, patient characteristics showed no significant differences. The patients were, on average, young and early in their disease course, with only one patient being above 60 years old. The median time from retrospectively identified disease manifestation to current presentation was 1 year, and for 40% of patients it was their first demyelinating event.

Table 1. Rescue therapy patient baseline and follow-up characteristics compared between treatment groups.

	TPE	IVMPS	IVMPS+TPE	p
Patients, No.	46	46	53	-
Age, yr, median (IQR)	33 (29–45)	36 (27–43)	31.5 (27–41)	0.410 *
Male sex, No. (%)	13 (28.3)	14 (30.4)	14 (26.4)	0.922 #
MS duration, yr, median (IQR)				
- since onset	1 (0–3)	1 (0–4)	1 (0–4)	0.574 *
- since diagnosis	0 (0–2)	0 (0–2)	1 (0–3)	0.322 *
Relapses during last two years, median (IQR)	0.5 (0–1)	0 (0–1)	0 (0–1)	0.765 *
first demyelinating event, No. (%)	19 (41.3)	20 (43.48)	18 (33.96)	0.636 #
Baseline EDSS, median (IQR)	0 (0–1)	0 (0–1)	0 (0–2)	0.397 *
Relapse EDSS, median (IQR)	3 (2–3)	2 (2–3)	3 (2–3)	0.003 *
Affected function system, No. (%)				
- visual	25 (54.4)	25 (47.2)	19 (41.3)	
- pyramidal	4 (8.7)	4 (7.6)	8 (17.4)	
- brainstem	8 (17.4)	13 (24.5)	10 (21.8)	0.236#
- cerebellar	3 (6.5)	7 (13.2)	1 (2.2)	
- sensory	6 (13.0)	3 (5.7)	8 (17.4)	
- cerebral	0 (0.0)	1 (1.9)	0 (0.0)	
Time to initiation treatment, d, median (IQR)	3 (1–7)	3 (1–5.25)	3 (1–5)	0.650*
Time to escalation treatment, d, median (IQR)	12.5 (8.75–16)	12 (10–15.25)	11 (8.5–14)	0.087*

Patient baseline characteristics compared between the different treatment groups. No.: Number; yr.: years; IQR: interquartile range. * Significance levels were calculated using a Kruskal–Wallis test. # Significance levels were calculated using Fisher's exact test.

One hundred and thirty-two patients fulfilled the 2017 revised McDonald criteria for the diagnosis of RRMS at relapse onset, whereas eight patients presented with isolated optic neuritis and five patients fulfilled the criteria for CIS. There were no differences in distribution between escalation treatment groups ($p = 0.756$).

Accordingly, the majority of patients did not receive disease modifying treatment (DMT) at relapse onset (62.1%). The treatment approved for mild to moderate courses of RRMS was administered to 22.8% of patients, whereas 15.2% received substances approved for the treatment of active RRMS (for a detailed description of administered DMT, see Table S1). The DMT subset use was evenly distributed between groups ($p = 0.793$). In 137 out of 145 patients the relapse was considered monosymptomatic. The most common relapse presentation was optic neuritis (69 patients; 47.6%). Generally, the frequencies of affected functional systems did not differ significantly between treatment groups ($p = 0.236$). Polysymptomatic relapses occurred in eight patients with infratentorial or spinal lesions and were assigned as outlined in the methods, according to their FSS that was EDSS-defining at follow-up.

3.2. Immediate Effects of Escalation Treatment

According to the previously described FSS-distance related analysis matrix, 28 (60.9%) patients showed good/full recovery following TPE, while 15 (15.2%) patients showed good/full recovery following escalation treatment with IVMPS. Partial recovery was observed in 12 (32.6%) TPE treated patients and in 15 (15.2%) IVMPS treated patients. Finally, no or worst recovery was documented in three (6.5%) TPE treated patients and in 69 (69.7%) IVMPS treated patients ($p < 0.001$, see Figure 2A). Next, 53 (53.5%) patients underwent rescue therapy with TPE following IVMPS, whereas the other patients received no further treatment prior to discharge irrespective of their response. Precise information on why no further treatment was given was not always available; patients' refusal of apheresis treatment was documented as reason in at least eight cases.

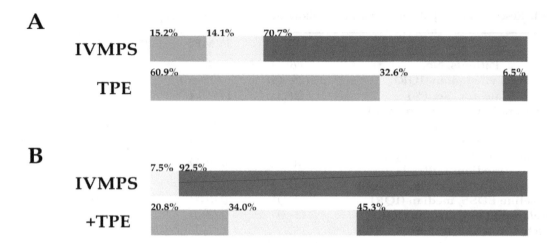

Figure 2. Different response groups following escalation treatment regimens are illustrated (green: good response; yellow: average response; red: worst response). **(A)** Upper bar represents patients who received IVMPS as the first escalation treatment (*n* = 99). Lower bar represents patients who received TPE as the first escalation treatment (*n* = 46). **(B)** Subgroup of patients who received two courses of escalation treatment (*n* = 53). Upper bar shows treatment response after first escalation with IVMPS and lower bar represents results following second escalation with TPE.

After the second escalation treatment with TPE, 25 (47.2%) patients showed a full response and 17 (32.1%) patients remitted partially, while 11 (20.7%) patients were unresponsive to the treatment (see Figure 2B). We performed regression analyses in order to evaluate the possible confounders and to check whether the higher proportion of treatment-resistant patients following IVMPS+TPE versus TPE alone was systematically influenced by different factors/confounders. Logistic regression analysis included "sex", "age", "affected function system (visual vs. other)", "disease duration", "baseline EDSS", and "time to treatment initiation". The adjusted odds ratio for "worst/no" treatment response was 39.01 (95%–CI: 10.42–142.71; *p*<0.001), favoring TPE treatment as the first escalation treatment (for full regression model see Table S2).

3.3. Sustained Effects of Escalation Treatment

Most patients were revisited at our outpatient clinic three months after discharge in order to re-evaluate the outcomes of relapse treatment and to initiate immunomodulatory treatment. A total of 135 (93.1%) patients were evaluated, with no significant differences between groups in terms of attendance (IVMPS: 93.0%; TPE: 90.5%; IVMPS+TPE: 91.8%; *p* = 1.000). The median follow-up duration was 95.5 days (IQR: 86–112), with again no relevant differences between treatment groups (*p* = 0.379). Eight patients reported further relapses with symptoms distinct from previous ones (6 patients/IVMPS group, one patient/TPE group, and one patient/IVMPS+TPE group); and three of these relapses affected the same functional system (optic nerve: two; brainstem: one; onset 53, 64, and 82 days after discharge, respectively). After excluding these patients, we re-evaluated the FSS according to the Conway model. In the IVMPS group, we found a significantly larger proportion of deteriorating patients (41.9%; vs. 12.2% for IVMPS+TPE and 7.1% for TPE; *p* = 0.001). The multivariable odds ratio for further deterioration of relapse symptoms at follow-up was 6.65, favoring the conduction of TPE (95%–CI: 2.52–17.54; *p*<0.001; for full regression model see Table S3).

3.4. Safety

Out of 145 patients, 116 (80.0%) experienced at least one single adverse event (Table 2). IVMPS treatment was frequently associated with hypertension, hyperglycemia, and hypokalemia, making it necessary to regularly substitute potassium (orally). Temporary insulin treatment was necessary in 14 patients (IVMPS: 6; IVMPS+TPE: 8; TPE: 0). Conversely, coagulopathy was associated with apheresis treatment. However, those events were mostly considered °II according to CTCAE. Infections were observed more often in patients who received two courses of IVMPS and among those, four were considered CTCAE °III due to the prolongation of hospitalization. In particular, one case of central venous catheter-associated septicemia required 14 days of vancomycin treatment until full recovery. Hypotension and coagulopathy each resulted in at least one treatment interruption in 28 TPE treated patients, whereas treatment interruption due to hypertension occurred in two IVMPS treated patients (systolic blood pressure>180mmHg each). Notably, we observed thromboembolic events in four out of the 99 patients exposed to escalated IVMPS, including one case of cerebral venous sinus thrombosis.

Table 2. Overview of documented adverse events during hospitalization.

	TPE (n = 46)	IVMPS (n = 46)	IVMPS+TPE (n = 53)
Hypertension (>135 mmHg SBP)	1 (2.2)	11 (19.6)	17 (32.1)
Hyperglycemia (>7.2 mmol/L)	1 (2.2)	20 (43.5)	32 (60.4)
Hypokalemia (<3.5 mmol/L)	4 (8.7)	29 (63.0)	43 (81.1)
Coagulopathy (aPTT>50 s or INR>1.7)	16 (34.8)	2 (4.4)	14 (32.1)
Thrombosis			
- Cerebral venous sinus	-	-	1 (1.9)
- Femoral veins	-	1 (2.2)	1 (1.9)
- Jugular veins/CVC	-	-	1 (1.9)
Infection			
- Thrombophlebitis	1 (2.2)	3 (6.6)	1 (1.9)
- Urinary Tract	4 (8.7)	8 (17.6)	9 (17.0)
- Respiratory Tract	-	2 (4.4)	1 (1.9)
- CVC infection/septicemia	-	-	1 (1.9)
(Temporary) treatment interruption			
- Coagulopathy	4 (8.7)	-	7 (13.2)
- Hypotension	5 (10.9)	-	7 (13.2)
- Hypertension	-	1 (2.2)	1 (1.9)
- Psychosis	-	2 (4.4)	-
- CVC dislocation	1 (2.2)	-	2 (3.8)
Pneumothorax	1 (2.2)	-	-
Patients with at least 1 event	29 (63.0)	38 (82.6)	49 (92.5)

Overview of adverse events documented during hospital stay. Numbers in brackets represent percentages. Numbers in bold indicate CTCAE °III events. TPE: therapeutic plasma exchange, IVMPS: intravenous (methyl-) prednisolone, SBP: systolic blood pressure; aPTT: activated partial thromboplastin time; INR: international normalized ratio; CVC: central venous catheter.

We evaluated whether the amount of previously administered IVMPS (initiation treatment with IVMPS and first escalation treatment with TPE vs. initiation and first escalation treatment with IVMPS and second escalation treatment with TPE) influenced the risk for serious adverse events (defined as CTCAE °III) during TPE treatment. The model resulted in an adjusted odds ratio of 4.63, favoring early treatment with TPE (95%–CI: 1.35–15.91; $p = 0.015$). However, severe adverse events were also more abundant in patients with longer disease duration, higher baseline EDSS, or longer time to treatment initiation (for full regression model see Table S4).

4. Discussion

Several studies have documented the beneficial effects of TPE treatment in acute relapsing MS, but virtually all study designs suffered from significant limitations. Studies were either one-armed, had varying treatment regimens, or consisted of a heterogeneous study population in terms of age, pre-treatment, disability, and disease subgroups (CIS, RRMS, and ON; but also neuromyelitis optica-spectrum disorders and other non-specified entities of CNS-demyelination) [8,9,18,19].

Moreover, a relevant proportion of studies on apheresis treatment solely included ON patients and only a few studies with diverse RRMS patient populations described the affected function systems or acute lesion localization in detail. Consequently, next to escalated IVMPS, the international guidelines recommend TPE as one option for treatment escalation following relapse, while refraining from recommending a specific treatment sequence [11].

Our retrospective cohort is well-defined and representative of more than 500 MS in-patients treated for acute relapses in our hospital within the past 5 years. These MS patients were young and mostly at the beginning of their symptomatic phase and therefore of special interest. Effective therapeutic interventions in this early phase of MS may positively influence long-term outcomes, as both relapse frequency and residual disability can be significantly impacted [20,21].

In our cohort, early apheresis treatment resulted in significantly higher response rates compared to escalation treatment with IVMPS. Interestingly, patients who underwent two courses of IVMPS prior to TPE showed poorer response at discharge compared to patients who only had one course of IVMPS prior to TPE. One explanation could be the longer time to apheresis treatment when conducted as the second instead of as the first escalation treatment. Notably, previous studies recommended the initiation of apheresis no later than six weeks after relapse onset in order to allow for the maximum efficacy of TPE, and all patients in this study were below this threshold [22–24]. We also hypothesize that the restitution of blood–brain barrier function, as induced by excessive doses of corticosteroids, might hamper the drainage of immunoglobulins and further inflammatory factors towards the blood, where they are ultimately cleared by TPE [25]. Ultimately, MS lesion pathology could have differed between patient groups. A so-called "type-2 lesion pattern", which is defined by the presence of immunoglobulins within MS lesions, was identified as a strong predictor for the success of TPE [24]. However, this information is usually not available in clinical routines and markers that have been supposed to be associated therewith, such as the presence of ring-enhancing lesions, could not be evaluated here, as MRI data were not regularly available.

As revealed by follow-up data three months after discharge, patients who underwent apheresis treatment exhibit a lower risk for further deterioration, which is in accordance with a previous report [22]. A likely explanation is the higher capacity of apheresis treatment to stop neuroinflammation and consecutive neuroaxonal degeneration, while IVMPS reverts the conduction block but fails to prevent nerve cell death [26]. This hypothesis is supported by the higher frequency of new relapses in patients who did not receive apheresis treatment, although in the short- and mid-term IVMPS treatment has been associated with a reduction in relapse frequency [27]. However, treatment outcomes after three months were supposed to be representative of long-term residuals, as further recovery was less likely beyond this time point in previous studies [28].

In terms of safety, there are some disadvantages of combining escalated IVMPS and TPE. Patients are exposed to high doses of IVMPS, including all the possible side- effects, without having a demonstrable benefit compared to TPE treatment alone. In line with this; we observed a significant increase of complications for the IVMPS escalation group, including several serious adverse events such as thromboembolism or severe infections.

As is typical for retrospective analyses, potentially unknown confounders that might have guided treatment decisions, such as the personal preferences of the treating consultant as well as the patient, health behaviors, comorbidity and MRI characteristics, challenge our study. In this context, we are not able to retrospectively address the criteria underlying the decision to treat a patient with TPE directly in the first escalation, rather than with escalated doses of IVMPS. Moreover, we have to deal with several limitations, such as bias from the selection and availability of data, recall bias, choice of relevant outcome and the methods of analysis. Furthermore, we have to be aware of limitations concerning the validity of our findings, as it is likely that adverse events are probably underestimated, since it was not known that this information was going to be of interest.

However, a large number of patients in our cohort experienced their first demyelinating event and we analyzed only the first relapse per patient, even though intra-individual differences in steroid-responsiveness over time have recently been described [29]. Furthermore, the previously known poor response to steroids used for relapse treatment was not documented anywhere in our medical charts.

In summary, our study found particular advantages of TPE over escalated IVMPS in escalation treatment of MS relapses. We recommend the rapid admission of steroid-refractory patients to apheresis treatment without escalated IVMPS treatment and identify the need to prospectively evaluate this approach in a contemporary patient cohort.

Author Contributions: S.P.: study concept and design, acquisition of data, analysis and interpretation of data, writing of the manuscript; L.R.: analysis and interpretation of data, writing and critical revision of manuscript for intellectual content; E.B.: analysis and interpretation of data, critical revision of manuscript for intellectual content; C.S.: analysis and interpretation of data, critical revision of manuscript for intellectual content; T.R.: analysis and interpretation of data, critical revision of manuscript for intellectual content; M.S.: acquisition of data, critical revision of manuscript for intellectual content; N.M.: critical revision of manuscript for intellectual content; Marcus Brand: critical revision of manuscript for intellectual content; R.P.: critical revision of manuscript for intellectual content; C.K.: critical revision of manuscript for intellectual content; H.W.: critical revision of manuscript for intellectual content; S.G.M.: study concept and design, critical revision of manuscript for intellectual content. All authors have read and agreed to the published version of the manuscript.

References

1. National Institute for Health and Care Excellence. Multiple Sclerosis: Management of Multiple Sclerosis in Primary and Secondary Care. Available online: www.nice.org.uk/guidance/cg186 (accessed on 3 December 2019).

2. Gold, R.; Chan, A.; Flachenecker, P.; Haghikia, A.; Hellwig, K.; Kappos, L. *DGN/KKNMS Leitlinie zur Diagnose und Therapie der MS*; German Society of Neurology: Berlin, Germany, 2012.

3. Sorensen, P.S.; Haas, J.; Sellebjerg, F.; Olsson, T.; Ravnborg, M.; TARIMS Study Group. IV immunoglobulins as add-on treatment to methylprednisolone for acute relapses in MS. *Neurology* **2004**, *63*, 2028–2033. [CrossRef] [PubMed]

4. Visser, L.H.; Beekman, R.; Tijssen, C.C.; Uitdehaag, B.M.; Lee, M.L.; Movig, K.L.; Lenderink, A.W. A randomized, double-blind, placebo-controlled pilot study of i.v. immunoglobulins in combination with i.v. methylprednisolone in the treatment of relapses in patients with MS. *Mult. Scler.* **2004**, *10*, 89–91. [CrossRef] [PubMed]

5. Stoppe, M.; Busch, M.; Krizek, L.; Then Bergh, F. Outcome of MS relapses in the era of disease-modifying therapy. *BMC Neurol.* **2017**, *17*, 151. [CrossRef]

6. Oliveri, R.L.; Valentino, P.; Russo, C.; Sibilia, G.; Aguglia, U.; Bono, F.; Fera, F.; Gambardella, A.; Zappia, M.; Pardatscher, K.; et al. Randomized trial comparing two different high doses of methylprednisolone in MS: A clinical and MRI study. *Neurology* **1998**, *50*, 1833–1836. [CrossRef] [PubMed]

7. Weinshenker, B.G.; O'Brien, P.C.; Petterson, T.M.; Noseworthy, J.H.; Lucchinetti, C.F.; Dodick, D.W.; Pineda, A.A.; Stevens, L.N.; Rodriguez, M.; et al. A randomized trial of plasma exchange in acute central nervous system inflammatory demyelinating disease. *Ann. Neurol.* **1999**, *46*, 878–886. [CrossRef]

8. Deschamps, R.; Gueguen, A.; Parquet, N.; Saheb, S.; Driss, F.; Mesnil, M.; Vignal, C.; Aboab, J.; Depaz, R.; Gout, O. Plasma exchange response in 34 patients with severe optic neuritis. *J. Neurol.* **2016**, *263*, 883–887. [CrossRef] [PubMed]

9. Ehler, J.; Koball, S.; Sauer, M.; Mitzner, S.; Hickstein, H.; Benecke, R.; Zettl, U.K. Response to Therapeutic Plasma Exchange as a Rescue Treatment in Clinically Isolated Syndromes and Acute Worsening of Multiple Sclerosis: A Retrospective Analysis of 90 Patients. *PLoS ONE* **2015**, *10*, 134583. [CrossRef]

10. Faissner, S.; Nikolayczik, J.; Chan, A.; Hellwig, K.; Gold, R.; Yoon, M.S.; Haghikia, A. Plasmapheresis and immunoadsorption in patients with steroid refractory multiple sclerosis relapses. *J. Neurol.* **2016** *263*, 1092–1098. [CrossRef]

11. Cortese, I.; Chaudhry, V.; So, Y.T.; Cantor, F.; Cornblath, D.R.; Rae-Grant, A. Evidence-based guideline update: Plasmapheresis in neurologic disorders: Report of the Therapeutics and Technology Assessment Subcommittee of the American Academy of Neurology. *Neurology* **2011**, *76*, 294–300. [CrossRef]

12. Sellebjerg, F.; Barnes, D.; Filippini, G.; Midgard, R.; Montalban, X.; Rieckmann, P.; Selmaj, K.; Visser, L.H.;

Sørensen, P.S. EFNS guideline on treatment of multiple sclerosis relapses: Report of an EFNS task force on treatment of multiple sclerosis relapses. *Eur. J. Neurol.* **2005**, *12*, 939–946. [CrossRef]

13. Schmidt, J.; Gold, R.; Schonrock, L.; Zettl, U.K.; Hartung, H.P.; Toyka, K.V. T-cell apoptosis in situ in experimental autoimmune encephalomyelitis following methylprednisolone pulse therapy. *Brain* **2000**, *123*, 1431–1441. [CrossRef] [PubMed]

14. Thompson, A.J.; Banwell, B.L.; Barkhof, F.; Carroll, W.M.; Coetzee, T.; Comi, G.; Correale, J.; Fazekas, F.; Filippi, M.; Freedman, M.S.; et al. Diagnosis of multiple sclerosis: 2017 revisions of the McDonald criteria. *Lancet Neurol.* **2018**, *17*, 162–173. [CrossRef]

15. Kurtzke, J.F. Rating neurologic impairment in multiple sclerosis: An expanded disability status scale (EDSS). *Neurology* **1983**, *33*, 1444–1452. [CrossRef] [PubMed]

16. Conway, B.L.; Zeydan, B.; Uygunoglu, U.; Novotna, M.; Siva, A.; Pittock, S.J.; Atkinson, E.J.; Rodriguez, M.; Kantarci, O.H. Age is a critical determinant in recovery from multiple sclerosis relapses. *Mult. Scler.* **2018**, *25*, 1754–1763. [CrossRef] [PubMed]

17. Rolfes, L.; Pfeuffer, S.; Ruck, T.; Melzer, N.; Pawlitzki, M.; Heming, M.; Brand, M.; Wiendl, H.; Meuth, S.G. Therapeutic Apheresis in Acute Relapsing Multiple Sclerosis: Current Evidence and Unmet Needs—A Systematic Review. *J. Clin. Med.* **2019**, *8*, 1623. [CrossRef] [PubMed]

18. Trebst, C.; Reising, A.; Kielstein, J.T.; Hafer, C.; Stangel, M. Plasma exchange therapy in steroid-unresponsive relapses in patients with multiple sclerosis. *Blood Purif.* **2009**, *28*, 108–115. [CrossRef]

19. Ruprecht, K.; Klinker, E.; Dintelmann, T.; Rieckmann, P.; Gold, R. Plasma exchange for severe optic neuritis: Treatment of 10 patients. *Neurology* **2004**, *63*, 1081–1083. [CrossRef]

20. Scalfari, A.; Neuhaus, A.; Degenhardt, A.; Rice, G.P.; Muraro, P.A.; Daumer, M.; Ebers, G.C. The natural history of multiple sclerosis: A geographically based study 10: Relapses and long-term disability. *Brain* **2010**, *133*, 1914–1929. [CrossRef]

21. Novotna, M.; Paz Soldan, M.M.; Abou Zeid, N.; Kale, N.; Tutuncu, M.; Crusan, D.J.; Atkinson, E.J.; Siva, A.; Keegan, B.M.; Pirko, I.; et al. Poor early relapse recovery affects onset of progressive disease course in multiple sclerosis. *Neurology* **2015**, *85*, 722–729. [CrossRef]

22. Keegan, M.; Pineda, A.A.; McClelland, R.L.; Darby, C.H.; Rodriguez, M.; Weinshenker, B.G. Plasma exchange for severe attacks of CNS demyelination: Predictors of response. *Neurology* **2002**, *58*, 143–146. [CrossRef]

23. Llufriu, S.; Castillo, J.; Blanco, Y.; Ramio-Torrenta, L.; Rio, J.; Valles, M.; Lozano, M.; Castella, M.D.; Calabia, J.; Horga, A.; et al. Plasma exchange for acute attacks of CNS demyelination: Predictors of improvement at 6 months. *Neurology* **2009**, *73*, 949–953. [CrossRef] [PubMed]

24. Keegan, M.; Konig, F.; McClelland, R.; Bruck, W.; Morales, Y.; Bitsch, A.; Panitch, H.; Lassmann, H.; Weinshenker, B.; Rodriguez, M.; et al. Relation between humoral pathological changes in multiple sclerosis and response to therapeutic plasma exchange. *Lancet* **2005**, *366*, 579–582. [CrossRef]

25. Gold, R.; Buttgereit, F.; Toyka, K.V. Mechanism of action of glucocorticosteroid hormones: Possible implications for therapy of neuroimmunological disorders. *J. Neuroimmunol.* **2001**, *117*, 1–8. [CrossRef]

26. Lee, J.M.; Yan, P.; Xiao, Q.; Chen, S.; Lee, K.Y.; Hsu, C.Y.; Xu, J. Methylprednisolone protects oligodendrocytes but not neurons after spinal cord injury. *J. Neurosci.* **2008**, *28*, 3141–3149. [CrossRef] [PubMed]

27. Then Bergh, F.; Kumpfel, T.; Schumann, E.; Held, U.; Schwan, M.; Blazevic, M.; Wismüller, A.; Holsboer, F.; Yassouridis, A.; Uhr, M.; et al. Monthly intravenous methylprednisolone in relapsing-remitting multiple sclerosis - reduction of enhancing lesions, T2 lesion volume and plasma prolactin concentrations. *BMC Neurol.* **2006**, *6*, 19. [CrossRef] [PubMed]

28. Lublin, F.D.; Baier, M.; Cutter, G. Effect of relapses on development of residual deficit in multiple sclerosis. *Neurology* **2003**, *61*, 1528–1532. [CrossRef] [PubMed]

29. Ehler, J.; Blechinger, S.; Rommer, P.S.; Koball, S.; Mitzner, S.; Hartung, H.P.; Leutmezer, F.; Sauer, M.; Zettl, U. Treatment of the First Acute Relapse Following Therapeutic Plasma Exchange in Formerly Glucocorticosteroid-Unresponsive Multiple Sclerosis Patients-A Multicenter Study to Evaluate Glucocorticosteroid Responsiveness. *Int. J. Mol. Sci.* **2017**, *18*, 1749. [CrossRef]

10

Omega-3 Long-Chain Polyunsaturated Fatty Acids Intake in Children with Attention Deficit and Hyperactivity Disorder

Milagros Fuentes-Albero [1]**, María Isabel Martínez-Martínez** [2] **and Omar Cauli** [2,*]

[1] Children's Mental Health Center, Hospital Arnau de Villanova, 46015 Valencia, Spain; milagrosfuentesalbero@yahoo.es

[2] Department of Medicine and Nursing, University of Valencia, 46010 Valencia, Spain; m.isabel.martinez@uv.es

* Correspondence: omar.cauli@uv.es

Abstract: Omega-3 long-chain polyunsaturated fatty acids (LC-PUFA) play a central role in neuronal growth and in the development of the human brain, and a deficiency of these substances has been reported in children with attention deficit hyperactive disorder (ADHD). In this regard, supplementation with omega-3 polyunsaturated fatty acids is used as adjuvant therapy in ADHD. Seafood, particularly fish, and some types of nuts are the main dietary sources of such fatty acids in the Spanish diet. In order to assess the effect of the intake of common foods containing high amounts of omega-3 polyunsaturated fatty acids, a food frequency questionnaire was administered to parents of children with ADHD ($N = 48$) and to parents of normally developing children (control group) ($N = 87$), and the intake of dietary omega-3 LC-PUFA, such as eicosapentaenoic acid (EPA) and docosahexaenoic acid (DHA), was estimated. Children with ADHD consumed fatty fish, lean fish, mollusks, crustaceans, and chicken eggs significantly less often ($p < 0.05$) than children in the control group. The estimated daily omega-3 LC-PUFA intake (EPA + DHA) was significantly below that recommended by the public health agencies in both groups, and was significantly lower in children with ADHD ($p < 0.05$, Cohen's d = 0.45) compared to normally developing children. Dietary intervention to increase the consumption of fish and seafood is strongly advised and it is especially warranted in children with ADHD, since it could contribute to improve the symptoms of ADHD.

Keywords: fish intake; omega-3 fatty acids; nutrients; ADHD; children; diet-deficient

1. Introduction

There is a growing evidence that several mental disorders, although they show an underlying genetic predisposition [1], are probably the product of an interplay between genetic susceptibility and environmental factors [2], of which inadequate nutrition may be a component [3,4]. Among the nutrients that have been consistently shown to be related to mental health and to different psychiatric disorders, mention must be made of omega-3 long-chain polyunsaturated fatty acids (LC-PUFA) [5–7]. A proper physical and mental health and neurodevelopment require a balanced ratio of omega-3 to omega-6 polyunsaturated fatty acids, but the typical diet in many countries provides a much larger intake of food containing omega-6 as compared to omega-3 LC-PUFA, thus often resulting in an imbalance and deficient omega-3 intake [5,8]. The consumption of supplements containing omega-3 LC-PUFA has been shown to be an effective measure in addition to the administration of psychotropic drugs for treating several psychiatric diseases [9–12]. In this regard, it has been demonstrated that omega-3 LC-PUFA such as eicosapentaenoic acid (EPA) and docosahexaenoic acid (DHA) may be helpful in the treatment of attention deficit hyperactive disorder (ADHD) in children [13–17]. Whether the pathophysiology of ADHD may be linked to inadequate bioavailability of omega-3 LC-PUFA, and whether it may be counteracted by dietary supplementation or increased intake of foods containing large amounts of omega-3 LC-PUFA, has gained growing interest in part due to the increasing knowledge of the role of nutrition in psychiatric disorders and in ADHD [18–20]. Dietary guidelines recommend regular fish consumption in all age ranges as the main source of omega-3 LC-PUFA intake [21].

Previous studies refer to the fundamental role afforded by omega-3 LC-PUFA in several essential metabolic functions, given their implication in diverse neuronal processes, as well as in cell growth, the function of cell membrane, hormonal, and immunological cross-talk, and gene expression regulation [8,22,23]. Alteration of some of these functions has been implicated in the physiopathology of ADHD [24]. Several experimental studies suggest that deficiencies of omega-3 LC-PUFA strongly alter brain function, not only during the developmental stages, but also throughout life [25]. There is some evidence to suggest that omega-3 LC-PUFA homeostasis may be impaired in patients with ADHD as a result of deficits and/or imbalances in nutritional intake, genetic alteration, changes in the activity of the enzymes involved in their metabolism, or the influence of some environmental agents [24,25].

Although many studies on omega-3 LC-PUFA supplementation in ADHD have been published in recent years [13,14], most refer to either interventions performed in patients who were given omega-3 LC-PUFA supplements apart from their normal diets. Remarkably, there are few studies on the intake of omega-3 LC-PUFA through diet in patients with ADHD. The present study was therefore designed with the following three main objectives:

1)   Evaluation of the pattern of consumption of the main dietary sources of food containing omega-3 LC-PUFA in children with ADHD and in a control group.
2)   Estimation of the daily intake of omega-3 LC-PUFA (EPA + DHA) in the two groups.
3)   Evaluation of the influence of age, sex, and body mass index (BMI) upon omega-3 LC-PUFA intake.

2. Materials and Methods

2.1. Study Design

An observational case-control study was carried out in Valencia (Spain) in 2016–2017. The study participants were recruited among patients (children and adolescents) with ADHD undergoing child psychiatrist consultation. Neurologically healthy children (control group) were recruited from two public schools in Valencia (Spain). Attention deficit hyperactive disorder was confirmed based on the DSM-IV diagnostic criteria using a standard neurodevelopment examination and interview (Conners scale). The parents of children with ADHD were interviewed during ordinary consultation with the child psychiatrist. Clinical information (diagnosis of ADHD, medication, presence of other comorbidities, anthropometric data) was retrieved by reviewing the medical records in the psychiatrist consultation of children with ADHD. Body mass index was calculated as weight in kilograms divided by the square of height in meters. For children and adolescents, BMI is age- and sex-specific, and is often referred to as BMI-for-age. According to the international guidelines, BMI was grouped into four categories: underweight (BMI less than the 5th percentile), normal or healthy weight (5th percentile to less than the 85th percentile), overweight (85th percentile to less than the 95th percentile), or obese (equal to or greater than the 95th percentile) [26].The children in the control group were sex- and age-matched (proportion 1:2) with the children in the ADHD group. Matching increases the efficiency of the estimates if the matching variables are associated with both the disease and exposure. The study comprised 135 children: 48 with a diagnosis of ADHD (age 5–14 years) and 87 with no ADHD or other psychiatric or neurological disorders (age 4–13 years). Socio-economic variables were measured through three variables: First, occupational social class, widely used in Spain as a measure of socioeconomic position [27]; it was defined using a Spanish adaptation of the British social class classification. In this study, we recoded the social status in three categories: higher, medium and lower. Educational level was recorded as primary or less, secondary, or university. Employment situation was categorized as employed, unemployed, and homemaker.

The study protocol was approved by the local Ethics Committee of the University of Valencia (Valencia, Spain) (protocol number H1397475950160). Parents signed the informed consent in order to participate in the study.

2.2. Diet Assessment

The parents completed the food frequency questionnaire (FFQ) about their children's diet and were also instructed to report all beverage and supplement consumption. The instrument was a semi-quantitative food questionnaire that was comprised of 136 food items, and is validated in Spain [28]. Specifically, the parents were instructed to record estimated portion sizes for each item ingested according to a previously validated [29] visual guide to improve the accuracy of their estimates. Consumptions were assessed by crossing the frequency and the portion size for each food. All food records were analyzed using Nutrition Data Systems-Research free software (DIAL®). Nutrient intake was averaged across the three days and normalized to intake per 1000 kcal, to generate the measures used in subsequent analyses. Energy and nutrient intake was calculated from the Spanish food composition tables [30,31].

2.3. Estimation of Omega-3 LC-PUFA Intake from Fish and Nuts

Parents self-reported fish and nuts consumption in their children. Fish was defined as "any kind of fish, including fish sticks and canned tuna fish, shellfish, crustaceans and mollusks." Participants reported: (a) how often they consumed fish ("did not eat," "once–three times a month," "about once a week," "twice–four times a week," "five–six times a week," "once a day," "twice–three time a day"); and (b) the type of fish they typically consumed.

The items of the three-day semi-quantitative food questionnaire [30] related to fish and seafood consumption and their omega-3 LC-PUFA contents (g/100 g of food item, as the sum of EPA + DHA) were: (a) lean fish: young hake, hake, sea bream, grouper, and sole (0.62); (b) fatty fish: salmon, mackerel, tuna, Atlantic bonito, and sardine (1.87); (c) cod (0.70); (d) smoked and salted fish: salmon and herring (4.44); (e) shellfish: mussel, oyster, and clam (2.20); (f) seafood: shrimp, prawn, and crayfish (0.90), and (g) mollusks: octopus, cuttlefish, and squid (0.71). Omega-3 LC-PUFA intake was calculated as frequency × (EPA + DHA) content for each food item (fish, seafood). We also included common foods in Spanish diets containing high amounts of omega-3 LC-PUFA such as dry fruit nuts: walnuts, hazelnuts, and almonds (6.33) [28,32]. We estimated the intake of EPA + DHA because these fatty acids are administered as nutritional supplements in clinical settings for children/adolescents with ADHD. In addition, we asked the parents about the frequency of consumption of omega-3 LC-PUFA supplements or omega-3 fatty acid-enriched milks. The intake of omega-3 LC-PUFA and fish consumption were adjusted for total energy intake using the residuals method proposed by Willett et al. [33].

2.4. Statistical Analysis

In the univariate analysis, variables were represented as absolute frequencies and percentages for categorical variables, and as the mean ± standard deviation (SD) for continuous (quantitative) variables. In the bivariate analysis, we first checked for normal or non-normal data distribution for quantitative variables using the Shapiro–Wilk ($n < 50$) or Kolmogorov–Smirnoff ($n \geq 50$) tests. As a result of non-normal data distribution, we used nonparametric tests, e.g., the Mann–Whitney U-test (when comparing quantitative variables between two groups) or the Kruskal–Wallis test (when comparing quantitative variables among three or more groups). Correlation analysis between quantitative variables was performed with the nonparametric Spearman test. In order to control the effect of intervening variables, partial correlations were performed. Differences between categorical variables were evaluated with the chi-squared test. In the case of food frequencies, we applied the z-test for differences between proportions to determine which of the five to seven categories differed between the control and ADHD groups. To quantify the effect size for two groups comparison we calculated Cohen's d. Statistical significance was considered to be $p < 0.05$. The SPSS version 24.0 statistical package (SPSS, Inc., Chicago, IL, USA) was used throughout.

3. Results

3.1. Description of the Sample

The characteristics of the study sample are shown in Table 1. Since ADHD shows a clear male predominance over females of about 3:1 to 4:1 in community-based samples of young individuals [1,2,34], we attempted to mimic the difference in sex distribution in our study: females in the ADHD group represented 25.0%, versus 28.7% in the control group. There were no significant differences between the groups regarding sex distribution ($p = 0.64$) or mean age ($p = 0.86$). Regarding the weight distribution of the subjects, 18.5% ($n = 25$) of the sample had low weight (percentile < 5), 36.3% ($n = 49$) showed normal weight (percentile 5–84), 23.7% ($n = 32$) were overweight (percentile 85–94), and 21.5% ($n = 29$) were obese (≥95 percentile). Significant differences in weight distribution were observed between the control and ADHD groups ($p < 0.0001$). In relation to BMI, low weight was significantly more prevalent in the control group compared to the ADHD group ($p < 0.0001$), while obesity was significantly more frequent in the ADHD group compared to the control group ($p < 0.001$) (Table 1).

Table 1. Characteristics of the study sample.

Variable	Control	ADHD	p-Value
Age	10.00 ± 0.27 (range 4–13)	9.54 ± 0.31 (5–14)	$p = 0.86$ (Mann–Whitney test)
Sex	Female $n = 25$ Male $n = 62$	Female $n = 12$ Male $n = 36$	$p = 0.64$ (Chi-squared test)
BMI	18.69 ± 0.39 (range 10.65–30.44)	20.89 ± 0.44 (range 15.50–28.31)	$p = 0.04$ (Mann–Whitney test)
Low weight	26.4%	4.2%	$p < 0.001$ (Chi-squared test)
Normal weight	36.8%	35.4%	
Over weight	25.3%	20.8%	
Obesity	11.5%	39.6%	
Social class	Higher: 26.4% Medium: 55.2% Lower: 18.4	Higher: 31.3% Medium: 52.1% Lower: 16.6%	$p = 0.88$ (Chi-squared test)
Employment situation	Father Employed: 97.7% Unemployed: 2.3% Mother Employed: 50.6% Unemployed: 16.1% Homemaker: 33.3%	Father Employed: 95.8% Unemployed: 4.2% Mother Employed: 58.3% Unemployed: 10.4% Homemaker: 31.3%	$p = 0.95$ (Chi-squared test) $p = 0.78$ (Chi-squared test)
Educational level	Father Primary school: 23.0% Secondary school: 54% University: 23.0% Mother Primary school: 17.2% Secondary school: 56.4% University: 26.4%	Father Primary school: 20.8% Secondary school: 54.2 University: 25.0% Mother Primary school: 12.5% Secondary school: 56.2% University: 31.3%	$p = 0.89$ (Chi-squared test) $p = 0.84$ (Chi-squared test)

No significant differences in the socio-economic variables were observed between parents in the ADHD and control group such as social class, employment situation, and educational level (Table 1).

3.2. Energy Intake and Frequency of Seafood Consumption

The reported average energy intake was approximately 1705 kcal. Of this amount, 51% corresponded to carbohydrates, 34% to fat, and 15% to protein. Fish intake was significantly lower in children/adolescents with ADHD than among the controls for all types of fish and seafood, except codfish. Significant differences were recorded in relation to lean fish (including young hake, hake, blackspot sea bream, goliath grouper, and common sole) ($p < 0.001$) (Figure 1A); the z-scores analysis showed significant differences for the intake categories "once a week" (z-score = 3.05; $p < 0.01$, higher in the control group), "twice–four times a week" (z-score = 2.15; $p < 0.05$, higher in the control group) and "five–six times a week" (z-score = −4.14; $p < 0.001$, higher in the ADHD group). Significant differences were also observed in the case of fatty fish (salmon, mackerel, tuna, bonito, sardine) ($p < 0.001$; chi-squared test) (Figure 1B); the z-scores analysis showed significant differences for the intake categories "did not eat" (z-score = −3.77; $p < 0.001$, higher in the ADHD group), "once–three times a month" (z-score = −3.54; $p < 0.001$, higher in the ADHD group), "once a week" (z-score = 2.55; $p < 0.01$, higher in the control group), and "twice–four times a week" (z-score = 4.39; $p < 0.001$, higher in the control group).

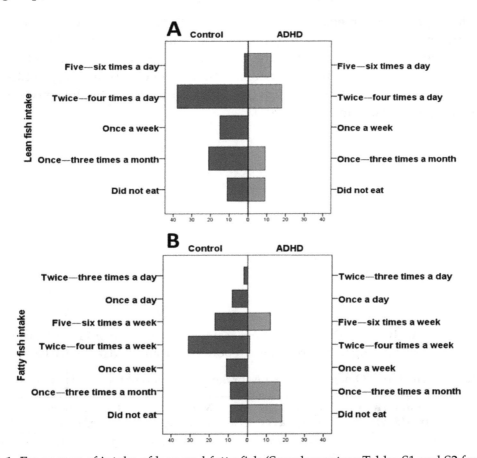

Figure 1. Frequency of intake of lean and fatty fish (Supplementary Tables S1 and S2 for raw).

Significant differences were recorded in the intake of smoked fish (including smoked and salted fish such as salmon and herring) ($p < 0.001$; chi-squared test); the z-scores analysis showed significant differences for the intake category "once a week" (z-score = 2.17; $p < 0.05$, higher in the control group). The same applied to the intake of shellfish (including mussel, oyster, and clam) ($p < 0.05$); the z-scores analysis showed significant differences for the intake category "twice–four times a week" (z-score = 2.02; $p < 0.05$, higher in the control group). Likewise, significant differences were observed in the intake of mollusks (including octopus, common cuttlefish, and squid) ($p < 0.001$); the z-scores analysis showed significant differences for the intake category "once a week" (z-score = 2.82; $p < 0.01$, higher in the control group). Lastly, significant differences were recorded in the intake of crustaceans (including shrimps, prawn, and crayfish) ($p < 0.01$; chi-squared test); the z-scores analysis showed significant differences for the intake categories "once a week" (z-score $= 2.02$; $p < 0.05$, higher in the control group) and "five–six times a week" (z-score $= -2.11$; $p < 0.05$, higher in the ADHD group). In contrast, the intake of codfish was not significantly different between the two groups ($p = 0.23$).

There were no significant differences in relation to the consumption of nuts (referred to those containing higher amounts of omega-3 LC-PUFA, such as walnuts and almonds) ($p = 0.07$), omega-3 LC-PUFA supplements ($p = 0.26$), or omega-3 fatty acid-enriched milk ($p = 0.14$). The intake of omega-3 fatty acids from nuts were not included in the calculation of daily EPA + DHA intake, since these foods contain other omega-3 LC-PUFA different from DHA and EPA, and because no significant differences in the intake of dry fruits were observed between the ADHD and control groups.

Significant differences in food intake were observed between females and males in relation to fatty fish and shellfish (being higher in males compared to females, $p < 0.05$), and eggs (again being higher in males compared to females, $p < 0.01$), but not to other foods ($p > 0.05$).

3.3. Estimation of Omega-3 LC-PUFA (EPA + DHA) Intake

The estimated ingestion of omega-3 LC-PUFA (EPA + DHA) in the diet was 109.87 ± 80.27 mg/day for the control group and 78.42 ± 56.64 mg/day for the children with ADHD ($p < 0.01$, effect size Cohen's d $= 0.45$) (Figure 2). The analysis of the mean intake per day of omega-3 LC-PUFA for each type of fish and seafood is shown in Table 2. There is a significant effects in omega-3 LC-PUFA between the two groups for lean fish ($p < 0.05$), fatty fish ($p < 0.01$), mollusks ($p < 0.05$), and other types of fish and seafood less frequently consumed ($p < 0.05$).

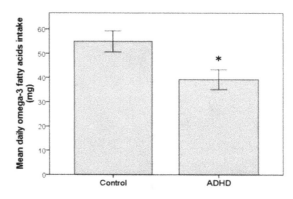

Figure 2. Estimated daily EPA + DHA intake from seafood. Comparison of EPA + DHA intake in the control and ADHD groups. Significant difference reported with an asterisk *, $p < 0.05$.

Table 2. Estimation of Omega-3 LC-PUFA intake form different type of fish and seafood.

Group	Lean Fish (mg/day)	Fatty Fish (mg/day)	Mollusks (mg/day)	Crustaceans (mg/day)	Other Types (mg/day)
Control	45.56 ± 19.81	$40,63 \pm 33.6$	18.28 ± 18.20	3.21 ± 6.22	2.20 ± 5.11
ADHD	38.51 ± 19.22 *	26.42 ± 20.30 **	10.21 ± 15.4 *	3.0 ± 6.43	0.29 ± 2.62 *

*, $p < 0.05$; **, $p < 0.01$ compared to the control group. On considering the daily intake related to weight category, a significant difference was seen to persist between the control and ADHD groups ($p < 0.01$).

There was a significant correlation between the mean daily intake of EPA + DHA and the frequency of intake of fatty fish (rho $= 0.18$, $p < 0.05$) and crustaceans (rho $= 0.17$, $p < 0.05$). No significant differences were observed in the estimated daily amounts of omega-3 LC-PUFA (EPA + DHA) between sexes ($p = 0.17$) or among children in the different weight categories ($p = 0.57$).

In contrast, a significant and direct correlation was observed between the intake of omega-3 LC-PUFA and of the age of the children (rho $= 0.21$, $p < 0.05$; Spearman test). The correlation between mean daily omega-3 LC-PUFA intake and age no longer proved significant ($p > 0.05$, partial correlation) after controlling for the intervening variables, e.g., group, sex, and weight categories, suggesting that these contribute significantly to the association between omega-3 LC-PUFA intake and age.

4. Discussion

Nowadays, several studies showing that food is not only useful for providing energy for bodily functions [35], but it can also prevent or moderate several diseases and a proper diet can improve both physical and mental health [4,5,25,36–38]. Omega-3 LC-PUFA supplementation has been shown to produce beneficial effects in children with ADHD, as summarized by two recent meta-analyses, although some conflicting results have been also reported [12–15]. To our knowledge, no studies have explored whether the intake of the omega-3 LC-PUFA EPA and DHA (expressed as mg/day) through the diet is adequate in children with ADHD. The European Food Safety Authority (EFSA) recommends an average EPA + DHA intake of 250 mg/day in the pediatric population [21]. The Food and Agriculture Organization (FAO)/World Health Organization (WHO) [39] recommends an intake of EPA + DHA about 100–200 mg/day for children aged 2–6 years and 200–250 mg/day from age 6 years onwards. Our study shows worrying results in the form of a low intake of EPA + DHA in both the control group and the ADHD group compared to the amount recommended by the public health organizations (50%–60% reduction with respect to the recommended daily dose) [21,39–41]. Similar findings have also emerged from a recent French population-based study in children (3–10 years) and adolescents (11–17 years) [42]. The mean daily intake of EPA + DHA correlated significantly to age, though on correcting for BMI, which also increases with age, we still observed a low intake of these essential molecules. Interestingly, a lower intake of omega-3 LC-PUFA has also been recently reported in children with autism spectrum disorder [43] suggesting it may be a general nutritional problem affecting the pediatric population rather than a problem conditioned by some specific neuropsychiatric disorder. However, it must be pointed out that the consequences of an omega-3 LC-PUFA (EPA + DHA) deficient diet may have even worse deleterious effects in children with neurodevelopmental disorders, taking into account that omega-3 LC-PUFA supplementation has been shown to afford beneficial effects when added to the pharmacological treatment of ADHD [13–15,38,40]. The analysis and the evolution of ADHD symptoms in children with low versus normal omega-3 LC-PUFA intake deserves future investigations in order to assess its role in ADHD symptomatology. Besides omega-3 LC-PUFA, reduced fish intake could lead to other nutrients deficiencies, such as phospholipids, the neuromodulator amino acid taurine, high-quality source of protein, and beneficial marine carotenoids such as astaxanthin [44], which have been demonstrated to possess anti-oxidant properties and anti-inflammatory effects [44–48], and regular fish intake reduces hyperlipidemia [49], which in turn can improve brain function [50].

Another emerging nutritional concern in our study was the high prevalence of obesity in children with ADHD (40% of the sample compared to 12% of the control group). This finding agrees with those of a recent meta-analysis concluding that the prevalence of obesity in ADHD is 40% higher than in the general population [51,52]. The causes of being overweight and child obesity are multifactorial (diet, sedentary lifestyle, socioeconomic status, disease conditions, neurodevelopmental disorders, etc.), but the core symptoms of children with ADHD might contribute to such increased rates [43,51,52]. Among these factors, ADHD symptoms, such as inattention or impulsivity, can increase the risk of obesity by increasing and dysregulating the food intake pattern in several ways (excessive eating, binge eating, unhealthy food choices, etc.) [51]. Attention deficit disorder may be associated with not remembering whether eating has been done or with a lack of satiation feeling [51,52]. Given the lack of planning and self-regulation skills, the patient can lose control over food and reduce the time spent doing physical exercise [40]. Also, impulsivity may contribute to excessive food intake in ADHD, even in the form of binge eating. This anomalous eating pattern could produce a net increase in adipose tissue, which affects the severity of ADHD and vice versa. Bowling et al. [43] concluded that more ADHD symptoms predict higher fat mass at later ages, which further confirms that more symptoms of impulsivity may contribute to being overweight. Longitudinal studies have explored the direction of the link between ADHD and obesity. Some studies suggested that ADHD precedes, and likely contributes to, subsequent overweightness and obesity [51,52]; however, the reverse pattern has also been demonstrated in preschool children [53]. One of the proposed pathophysiological mechanism by which being overweight may contribute to ADHD relates to sleep-disordered breathing [54], leading to an excessive daytime sleepiness, which in turn may promote inattention via hypoxemia, which in turn contributes to altered prefrontal functioning [52,54]. Finally, a common genetic mechanism between ADHD and obesity has been also proposed [55]. Although the mechanism underlying the association is still unknown, preliminary evidence suggests the role of the dopaminergic reward system [56] or melanocortin system [57]. It is indeed possible that bidirectional pathways are likely involved.

Our study has a number of limitations. First, the cross-sectional observational design involved limits regarding inferences about causality between insufficient intake of omega-3 LC-PUFA and the worsening of ADHD symptoms. Second, there were a number of issues related to the completion of records. Data referred to intake may contain errors due to inaccuracies in recorded quantities and they are based on parents' reports rather than children's. However, we are confident that the self-reported information provided by parents about the nutritional assessment of their children was adequate because they showed interest in the study and they received training and support in filling out the food records. Furthermore, the attrition rate was low. We, therefore, think that the study has a good internal validity. A third limitation is the fact that we did not measure the intake of omega-3 LC-PUFA coming from other sources. Nevertheless, we are confident about the main role of fish and seafood as the principal source of EPA + DHA in the Spanish diet [36,39].

In our sample of children with ADHD and controls (age- and sex-matched with the ADHD subjects), there were considerably more boys than girls (reflecting the characteristic sex ratio observed in ADHD [1,2]), which can rule out a proper analysis for the effects of sex. Both the controls and the ADHD children were recruited not only from the same age group but also from the same geographical region, and had a similar socioeconomic status. Data were collected over the same time period (winter), and this homogeneity reduced potential sources of bias.

Despite these limitations, our study underscores the need for greater attention to the education of parents and children regarding healthy dietary habits in Spain, and as such, education is the most promising and practical complementary management strategy in ADHD. Given that fish consumption is the main source of dietary omega-3 LC-PUFA [58], interventions promoting fish consumption in a balanced diet, as well as other positive eating behaviors, are strongly warranted in the future.

5. Conclusions

The intake of seafood in particular fish, is reduced in children with ADHD compared to typically developing children and this may contribute to reduced intake of some omega-3 LC-PUFA such as EPA and DHA, essential nutrients for a proper brain development and function. Further research is required to clarify associations between ADHD symptomatology, eating patterns and health status.

Author Contributions: Conceptualization, M.F.-A., M.I.M.-M., O.C.; Methodology, M.F.-A., M.I.M.-M.; Formal Analysis, M.F.-A., O.C.; Data Curation M.F.-A., M.I.M.-M.; Writing—Original Draft Preparation, M.F.-A., O.C.; Writing—Review and Editing, M.F.-A., M.I.M.-M., O.C.

Acknowledgments: We express our sincere thanks to all the parents for their time, interest, and goodwill, and all the staff involved in the studies.

References

1. Sciberras, E.; Mulraney, M.; Silva, D.; Coghill, D. Prenatal Risk Factors and the Etiology of ADHD—Review of Existing Evidence. *Curr. Psychiatry Rep.* **2017**, *19*. [CrossRef]
2. Nigg, J.; Nikolas, M.; Burt, S.A. Measured Gene by Environment Interaction in Relation to

Attention-Deficit/Hyperactivity Disorder (ADHD). *J. Am. Acad. Child Adolesc. Psychiatry* **2010**, *49*, 863–873. [CrossRef]

3. Sarris, J.; Logan, A.C.; Akbaraly, T.N.; Amminger, G.P.; Balanzá-Martínez, V.; Freeman, M.P.; Hibbeln, J.; Matsuoka, Y.; Mischoulon, D.; Mizoue, T.; et al. International Society for Nutritional Psychiatry Research. Nutritional medicine as mainstream in psychiatry. *Lancet Psychiatry* **2015**, *2*, 271–274. [CrossRef]

4. Yan, X.; Zhao, X.; Li, J.; He, L.; Xu, M. Effects of early-life malnutrition on neurodevelopment and neuropsychiatric disorders and the potential mechanisms. *Prog. Neuro Psychopharmacol. Boil. Psychiatry* **2018**, *83*, 64–75. [CrossRef]

5. Gow, R.V.; Hibbeln, J.R. Omega-3 Fatty Acid and Nutrient Deficits in Adverse Neurodevelopment and Childhood Behaviors. *Child Adolesc. Psychiatr. Clin. Psychiatry* **2014**, *23*, 555–590. [CrossRef]

6. Grosso, G.; Galvano, F.; Marventano, S.; Malaguarnera, M.; Bucolo, C.; Drago, F.; Caraci, F. Omega-3 Fatty Acids and Depression: Scientific Evidence and Biological Mechanisms. *Oxidative Med. Cell. Longev.* **2014**, *2014*, 1–16. [CrossRef]

7. Parletta, N.; Milte, C.M.; Meyer, B.J. Nutritional modulation of cognitive function and mental health. *J. Nutr. Biochem.* **2013**, *24*, 725–743. [CrossRef]

8. Schuchardt, J.P.; Huss, M.; Stauss-Grabo, M.; Hahn, A. Significance of long-chain polyunsaturated fatty acids (PUFAs) for the development and behaviour of children. *Eur. J. Pediatr.* **2010**, *169*, 149–164. [CrossRef]

9. Cooper, R.E.; Tye, C.; Kuntsi, J.; Vassos, E.; Asherson, P. Omega-3 polyunsaturated fatty acid supplementation and cognition: A systematic review and meta-analysis. *J. Psychopharmacol.* **2015**, *29*, 753–763. [CrossRef]

10. Mischoulon, D.; Freeman, M.P. Omega-3 fatty acids in psychiatry. *Psychiatr. Clin. North Am.* **2013**, *36*, 15–23. [CrossRef]

11. Bloch, M.H.; Hannestad, J. Omega-3 fatty acids for the treatment of depression: Systematic review and meta-analysis. *Mol. Psychiatry* **2012**, *17*, 1272–1282. [CrossRef] [PubMed]

12. Politi, P.; Rocchetti, M.; Emanuele, E.; Rondanelli, M.; Barale, F. Randomized Placebo-Controlled Trials of Omega-3 Polyunsaturated Fatty Acids in Psychiatric Disorders: A Review of the Current Literature. *Drug Discov. Technol.* **2013**, *10*, 245–253. [CrossRef]

13. Bloch, M.H.; Qawasmi, A. Omega-3 Fatty Acid Supplementation for the Treatment of Children with Attention-Deficit/Hyperactivity Disorder Symptomatology: Systematic Review and Meta-Analysis. *J. Am. Acad. Child Adolesc. Psychiatry* **2011**, *50*, 991–1000. [CrossRef] [PubMed]

14. Ramalho, R.; Pereira, A.C.; Vicente, F.; Pereira, P. Docosahexaenoic acid supplementation for children with attention deficit hyperactivity disorder: A comprehensive review of the evidence. *Clin. Nutr. ESPEN* **2018**, *25*, 1–7. [CrossRef]

15. Agostoni, C.; Nobile, M.; Ciappolino, V.; Delvecchio, G.; Tesei, A.; Turolo, S.; Crippa, A.; Mazzocchi, A.; Altamura, C.A.; Brambilla, P. The Role of Omega-3 Fatty Acids in Developmental Psychopathology: A Systematic Review on Early Psychosis, Autism and ADHD. *Int. J. Mol. Sci.* **2017**, *18*, 2608. [CrossRef]

16. Lange, K.W.; Hauser, J.; Makulska-Gertruda, E.; Nakamura, Y.; Reissmann, A.; Sakaue, Y.; Takano, T.; Takeuchi, Y. The Role of Nutritional Supplements in the Treatment of ADHD: What the Evidence Says. *Curr. Psychiatry Rep.* **2017**, *19*, 8. [CrossRef]

17. Königs, A.; Kiliaan, A.J. Critical appraisal of omega-3 fatty acids in attention-deficit/hyperactivity disorder treatment. *Neuropsychiatr. Dis. Treat.* **2016**, *12*, 1869–1882.

18. Arnold, L.E. Fish oil is not snake oil. *J. Am. Acad. Child Adolesc. Psychiatry* **2011**, *50*, 969–971. [CrossRef]

19. Nigg, J.T.; Lewis, K.; Edinger, T.; Falk, M. Meta-analysis of attention-deficit/hyperactivity disorder symptoms, restriction diet and synthetic food color additives. *J. Am. Acad. Child Adolesc. Psychiatry* **2012**, *21*, 86–89. [CrossRef]

20. Stevenson, J.; Buitelaar, J.; Cortese, S.; Ferrin, M.; Konofal, E.; Lecendreux, M.; Simonoff, E.; Wong, I.C.; Sonuga-Barke, E. Research review: The role of diet in the treatment of attention-deficit/hyperactivity disorder—An appraisal of the evidence on efficacy and recommendations on the design of future studies. *J. Child Psychol. Psychiatry* **2014**, *55*, 416–427. [CrossRef]

21. European Food Safety Authority (EFSA). Scientific opinion on dietary reference values for fats, including saturated fatty acids, polyunsaturated fatty acids, monounsaturated fatty acids, trans fatty acids, and cholesterol. *EFSA J.* **2010**, *8*, 1461.

22. Morgane, P.J.; Austin-LaFrance, R.; Bronzino, J.; Tonkiss, J.; Díaz-Cintra, S.; Cintra, L.; Kemper, T.; Galler, J.R.;

Kemper, T. Prenatal malnutrition and development of the brain. *Neurosci. Biobehav. Rev.* **1993**, *17*, 91–128. [CrossRef]

23. Bourre, J.M.; Dumont, O.; Piciotti, M.; Clément, M.; Chaudière, J.; Bonneil, M.; Nalbone, G.; Lafont, H.; Pascal, G.; Durand, G. Essentiality of omega 3 fatty acids for brain structure and function. *World Rev. Nutr. Diet.* **1991**, *66*, 103–117.

24. Burgess, J.R.; Stevens, L.; Zhang, W.; Peck, L. Long-chain polyunsaturated fatty acids in children with attention-deficit hyperactivity disorder. *Am. J. Clin. Nutr.* **2000**, *71*, 327S–330S. [CrossRef] [PubMed]

25. Pusceddu, M.M.; Kelly, P.; Stanton, C.; Cryan, J.F.; Dinan, T.G. N-3 Polyunsaturated Fatty Acids through the Lifespan: Implication for Psychopathology. *Int. J. Neuropsychopharmacol.* **2016**, *19*. [CrossRef] [PubMed]

26. Kuczmarski, R.J.; Ogden, C.L.; Guo, S.S.; Grummer-Strawn, L.M.; Flegal, K.M.; Mei, Z.; Wei, R.; Curtin, L.R.; Roche, A.F.; Johnson, C.L. CDC Growth Charts for the United States: Methods and development. *Vital Health Stat.* **2002**, *246*, 147–148.

27. Domingo-Salvany, A.; Regidor, E.; Alonso, J.; Alvarez-Dardet, C. Proposal for a social class measure. Working Group of the Spanish Society of Epidemiology and the Spanish Society of Family and Community Medicine. *Aten Primaria* **2000**, *25*, 350. [PubMed]

28. Martin-Moreno, J.M.; Boyle, P.; Gorgojo, L.; Maisonneuve, P.; Fernandez-Rodriguez, J.C.; Salvini, S.; Willett, W.C. Development and Validation of a Food Frequency Questionnaire in Spain. *Int. J. Epidemiol.* **1993**, *22*, 512–519. [CrossRef]

29. Le Moullec, N.; Deheeger, M.; Preziosi, P.; Monteiro, P.; Valeix, P.; Rolland-Cachera, M.F.; Potier De Courcy, G.; Christides, J.P.; Cherouvrier, F.; Galan, P.; et al. Validation du manuel-photos utilisé pour l'enquête alimentaire de l'étude SU. VI. MAX. *Cahiers de Nutrition et de Diététique* **1996**, *31*, 158–164.

30. Moreiras, O.; Carbajal, A.; Cabrera, L.; Cuadrado, C. *Tablas de Composición de Alimentos (Food Composition Tables)*; Ediciones Piramide: Madrid, Spain, 2005.

31. Fernandez-Ballart, J.D.; Piñol, J.L.; Zazpe, I.; Corella, D.; Carrasco, P.; Toledo, E.; Perez-Bauer, M.; Martínez-González, M.Á.; Salas-Salvadó, J.; Martín-Moreno, J.M. Relative validity of a semi-quantitative food-frequency questionnaire in an elderly Mediterranean population of Spain. *Br. J. Nutr.* **2010**, *103*, 1808–1816. [CrossRef]

32. Hepburn, F.N.; Exler, J.; Weihrauch, J.L. Provisional tables on the content of omega-3 fatty acids and other fat components of selected foods. *J. Am. Diet. Assoc.* **1986**, *86*, 788–793.

33. Willett, W.C.; Howe, G.R.; Kushi, L.H. Adjustment for total energy intake in epidemiologic studies. *Am. J. Clin. Nutr.* **1997**, *65*, 1220S–1228S. [CrossRef]

34. Willcutt, E.G. The Prevalence of DSM-IV Attention-Deficit/Hyperactivity Disorder: A Meta-Analytic Review. *Neurotherapeutics* **2012**, *9*, 490–499. [CrossRef] [PubMed]

35. Siró, I.; Kápolna, E.; Lugasi, A. Functional food. Product development, marketing and consumer acceptance. A review. *Appetite* **2008**, *51*, 456–467. [CrossRef] [PubMed]

36. SENC, Sociedad Española de Nutrición Comunitaria. Objetivos nutricionales para la población española. *Rev. Esp. Nutr. Comunitaria* **2011**, *4*, 178–199.

37. Kris-Etherton, P.; Taylor, D.S.; Yu-Poth, S.; Huth, P.; Moriarty, K.; Fishell, V.; Hargrove, R.L.; Zhao, G.; Etherton, T.D. Polyunsaturated fatty acids in the food chain in the United States. *Am. J. Clin. Nutr.* **2000**, *71*, 179S–188S. [CrossRef] [PubMed]

38. Wang, L.J.; Yu, Y.H.; Fu, M.L.; Yeh, W.T.; Hsu, J.L.; Yang, Y.H.; Yang, H.T.; Huang, S.Y.; Wei, I.L.; Chen, W.J.; et al. Dietary Profiles, Nutritional Biochemistry Status, and Attention-Deficit/Hyperactivity Disorder: Path Analysis for a Case-Control Study. *J. Clin. Med.* **2019**, *8*, 709. [CrossRef]

39. FAO/FINUT. Grasas y ácidos grasos en Nutrición Humana. Available online: www.fao.org/3/i1953s/i1953s.pdf (accessed on 10 March 2019).

40. Hawkey, E.; Nigg, J.T. Omega-3 fatty acid and ADHD, blood level analysis and meta-analytic extension of suplementation trials. *Clin. Psychol. Rev.* **2014** *34*, 496–505. [CrossRef] [PubMed]

41. Guesnet, P.; Tressou, J.; Buaud, B.; Simon, N.; Pasteau, S. Inadequate daily intakes of *n*-3 polyunsaturated fatty acids (PUFA) in the general French population of children (3–10 years), the INCA2 survey. *Eur. J. Nutr.* **2019**, *58*, 895–903. [CrossRef]

42. Marí-Bauset, S.; Llopis-González, A.; Zazpe-García, I.; Marí-Sanchis, A.; Morales-Suárez-Varela, M. Nutritional status of children with autism spectrum disorders (ASDs), a case control study. *J. Autism. Dev. Disord.* **2015**, *45*, 203–212.

43. Bowling, A.B.; Tiemeier, H.W.; Jaddoe, V.W.V.; Barker, E.D.; Jansen, P.W. ADHD symptoms and body composition changes in childhood: A longitudinal study evaluating directionality of associations. *Pediatr. Obes.* **2018**, *13*, 567–575. [CrossRef]

44. Hosomi, R.; Yoshida, M.; Fukunaga, K. Seafood Consumption and Components for Health. *J. Heal. Sci.* **2012**, *4*, 72–86. [CrossRef]

45. Ouellet, V.; Weisnagel, S.J.; Marois, J.; Bergeron, J.; Julien, P.; Gougeon, R.; Tchernof, A.; Holub, B.J.; Jacques, H. Dietary Cod Protein Reduces Plasma C-Reactive Protein in Insulin-Resistant Men and Women. *J. Nutr.* **2008**, *138*, 2386–2391. [CrossRef]

46. Ouellet, V.; Marois, J.; Weisnagel, S.J.; Jacques, H. Dietary cod protein improves insulin sensitivity in insulin-resistant men and women: A randomized controlled trial. *Diabetes Care* **2007**, *30*, 2816–2821. [CrossRef] [PubMed]

47. Jerlich, A.; Fritz, G.; Kharrazi, H.; Hammel, M.; Tschabuschnig, S.; Glatter, O.; Schaur, R. Comparison of HOCl traps with myeloperoxidase inhibitors in prevention of low density lipoprotein oxidation. *Biochim. Biophys. Acta* **2000**, *1481*, 109–118. [CrossRef]

48. Karppi; Rissanen; Nyyssönen; Kaikkonen; Olsson; Voutilainen; Salonen; Karppi, J.; Rissanen, T.H.; Nyyssönen, K.; et al. Effects of Astaxanthin Supplementation on Lipid Peroxidation. *Int. J. Vitam. Nutr.* **2007**, *77*, 3–11. [CrossRef]

49. Yoshida, H.; Yanai, H.; Ito, K.; Tomono, Y.; Koikeda, T.; Tsukahara, H.; Tada, N. Administration of natural astaxanthin increases serum HDL-cholesterol and adiponectin in subjects with mild hyperlipidemia. *Atherosclerosis* **2010**, *209*, 520–523. [CrossRef]

50. Chung, S.Y.; Moriyama, T.; Uezu, E.; Uezu, K.; Hirata, R.; Yohena, N.; Masuda, Y.; Kokubu, T.; Yamamoto, S. Administration of phosphatidylcholine increases brain acetylcholine concentration and improves memory in mice with dementia. *J. Nutr.* **1995**, *125*, 1484–1489. [PubMed]

51. Cortese, S.; Moreira-Maia, C.R.; Fleur, D.S.; Morcillo-Peñalver, C.; Rohde, L.A.; Faraone, S.V. Association Between ADHD and Obesity: A Systematic Review and Meta-Analysis. *Am. J. Psychiatry* **2016**, *173*, 34–43. [CrossRef]

52. Nigg, J.T.; Johnstone, J.M.; Musser, E.D.; Long, H.G.; Willoughby, M.T.; Shannon, J. Attention-deficit/hyperactivity disorder (ADHD) and being overweight/obesity, new data and meta-analysis. *Clin. Psychol. Rev.* **2016**, *43*, 67–79. [CrossRef] [PubMed]

53. Pérez-Bonaventura, I.; Granero, R.; Ezpeleta, L. The relationship between weight status and emotional and behavioral problems in Spanish preschool children. *J. Pediatr. Psychol.* **2015**, *40*, 455–463. [CrossRef]

54. Bass, J.L.; Corwin, M.; Gozal, D.; Moore, C.; Nishida, H.; Parker, S.; Schonwald, A.; Wilker, R.E.; Stehle, S.; Kinane, T.B. The effect of chronic or intermittent hypoxia on cognition in childhood: A review of the evidence. *Pediatrics* **2004**, *114*, 805–816. [CrossRef] [PubMed]

55. Albayrak, Ö.; Pütter, C.; Volckmar, A.L.; Cichon, S.; Hoffmann, P.; Nöthen, M.M.; Jöckel, K.H.; Schreiber, S.; Wichmann, H.E.; Faraone, S.V.; et al. Common obesity risk alleles in childhood attention-deficit/hyperactivity disorder. *Am. J. Med. Genet. B Neuropsychiatr. Genet.* **2013**, *162*, 295–305. [CrossRef] [PubMed]

56. Liu, L.L.; Li, B.M.; Yang, J.; Wang, Y.W. Does dopaminergic reward system contribute to explaining comorbidity obesity and ADHD? *Med. Hypotheses.* **2008**, *70*, 1118–1120. [CrossRef] [PubMed]

57. Ghanadri, Y.; Eisenberg, I.; Ben Neriah, Z.; Agranat-Meged, A.; Kieselstein-Gross, E.; Mitrani-Rosenbaum, S.; Agranat-Meged, A.; Kieselstein-Gross, E.; Mitrani-Rosenbaum, S. Attention deficit hyperactivity disorder in obese melanocortin-4-receptor (MC4R) deficient subjects: A newly described expression of MC4R deficiency. *Am. J. Med. Genet. B Neuropsychiatr. Genet.* **2008**, *147*, 1547–1553.

58. Meyer, B.J.; Mann, N.J.; Lewis, J.L.; Milligan, G.C.; Sinclair, A.J.; Howe, P.R.C. Dietary intakes and food sources of omega-6 and omega-3 polyunsaturated fatty acids. *Lipids* **2003**, *38*, 391–398. [CrossRef]

11

Gait Asymmetry Post-Stroke: Determining Valid and Reliable Methods Using a Single Accelerometer Located on the Trunk

Christopher Buckley [1], M. Encarna Micó-Amigo [1], Michael Dunne-Willows [2], Alan Godfrey [3], Aodhán Hickey [4], Sue Lord [1,5], Lynn Rochester [1,6], Silvia Del Din [1] and Sarah A. Moore [1,7,8,*]

[1] Institute of Neuroscience/Institute for Ageing, Newcastle University, Newcastle Upon Tyne NE4 5PL, UK; christopher.buckley2@newcastle.ac.uk (C.B.); maria.mico-amigo@newcastle.ac.uk (M.E.M.-A.); sue.lord@aut.ac.nz (S.L.); lynn.rochester@ncl.ac.uk (L.R.); silvia.del-din@newcastle.ac.uk (S.D.D.)

[2] EPSRC Centre for Doctoral Training in Cloud Computing for Big Data, Newcastle University, Newcastle Upon Tyne NE4 5PL, UK; m.dunne-willows@newcastle.ac.uk

[3] Department of Computer and Information Science, Northumbria University, Newcastle upon Tyne NE1 8ST, UK; alan.godfrey@northumbria.ac.uk

[4] Department of Health Intelligence, HSC Public Health Agency, Belfast BT2 7ES, Northern Ireland; Aodhan.Hickey@hscni.net

[5] Auckland University of Technology, 55 Wellesley St E, Auckland 1010, New Zealand

[6] The Newcastle upon Tyne Hospitals NHS Foundation Trust, Newcastle Upon Tyne NE7 7DN, UK

[7] Institute of Neuroscience (Stroke Research Group), Newcastle University, 3-4 Claremont Terrace, Newcastle upon Tyne NE2 4AE, UK

[8] Stroke Northumbria, Northumbria Healthcare NHS Foundation Trust, Rake Lane, North Shields, Tyne and Wear NE29 8NH, UK

* Correspondence: s.a.moore@newcastle.ac.uk

Abstract: Asymmetry is a cardinal symptom of gait post-stroke that is targeted during rehabilitation. Technological developments have allowed accelerometers to be a feasible tool to provide digital gait variables. Many acceleration-derived variables are proposed to measure gait asymmetry. Despite a need for accurate calculation, no consensus exists for what is the most valid and reliable variable. Using an instrumented walkway (GaitRite) as the reference standard, this study compared the validity and reliability of multiple acceleration-derived asymmetry variables. Twenty-five post-stroke participants performed repeated walks over GaitRite whilst wearing a tri-axial accelerometer (Axivity AX3) on their lower back, on two occasions, one week apart. Harmonic ratio, autocorrelation, gait symmetry index, phase plots, acceleration, and jerk root mean square were calculated from the acceleration signals. Test–retest reliability was calculated, and concurrent validity was estimated by comparison with GaitRite. The strongest concurrent validity was obtained from step regularity from the vertical signal, which also recorded excellent test–retest reliability (Spearman's rank correlation coefficients (rho) = 0.87 and Intraclass correlation coefficient (ICC_{21}) = 0.98, respectively). Future research should test the responsiveness of this and other step asymmetry variables to quantify change during recovery and the effect of rehabilitative interventions for consideration as digital biomarkers to quantify gait asymmetry.

Keywords: stroke; asymmetry; accelerometer; gait; trunk; reliability; validity

1. Introduction

Hemiparesis after stroke typically results in reduced walking speed, an asymmetrical gait pattern, and a reduced ability to make gait adjustments that consequentially limit community ambulation and physical activity [1–4]. Reduction in both predisposes an already at risk population to further cardiometabolic disease [5,6]. Therefore, the improvement of gait is a worthwhile and common target for interventions after stroke. Gait asymmetry, if not addressed early in the recovery process, can prolong and increase gait impairment due to compensatory mechanisms, leading to an increasingly asymmetric gait pattern [7]. The latter is inefficient and requires increased energy expenditure. Consequently, falls risk increases, further reducing levels of physical activity [8]. In order to quantify asymmetry and its improvement from targeted rehabilitative interventions, it is essential to have both valid and reliable tools that are able to quantify movement quality/compensatory strategies of the whole body during gait.

Tests such as the 10 m walk [9] and scales such as the Dynamic Gait Index [10] are used to measure gait after stroke. Although useful and practical for application to clinical settings, these tests are susceptible to subjectivity and not specifically designed to capture the cardinal symptoms of gait after stroke, such as asymmetry. Instrumented walkways can objectively measure asymmetry and have shown excellent intra and inter-rater reliability in subacute stroke [11]. Practically, they are costly and need a controlled dedicated environment with a trained specialist to operate; therefore, they are mainly limited to research settings [12]. From a biomechanical perspective, they limit the number of steps collected per trial and solely obtain information of the participant's footfall. They are not designed to measure the movement of the whole body, where synergistic compensatory movement strategy information may be quantified such as compensatory movements of the pelvis [8,13]. Traditionally, gaining this information would rely on three-dimensional motion analysis systems. However, due to the even higher cost, required experience, and time to use relative to instrumented mats, their application is also limited to research settings [12]. Therefore, a need exists for a valid tool that is capable of quantifying whole body asymmetry, while also being feasible for routine clinical adoption.

Wearable accelerometers are a relatively low-cost alternative that are capable of measuring human movement from a variety of contexts while capturing parameters that are difficult to quantify from clinical inspection by the human eye [1,14]. Previous attempts to quantify measures of asymmetry indicative of spatiotemporal information of the feet with accelerometers have shown their feasibility, but also poor concurrent validity with reference standards of Gaitrite [1]. Therefore, the development of algorithms to capture the complex nature of asymmetry post-stroke has been encouraged [1]. Numerous asymmetry variables exist that have been obtained from cyclical acceleration signals during gait such as variables derived from the frequency domain [15,16]. These variables vary according to the complexity of the sensor, the number of sensors used, their location, and the population on which they were tested [17–19]. Relative to the discreet spatiotemporal movement of the feet equivalents, variables quantifying asymmetry from the cyclical signals of the lower back better classified post-stroke gait from controls [16,18,20]. Their advantage stems from considering the acceleration as a complete waveform, not neglecting temporal information outside of the time domain, which may enable a more complete description of the signal and a better characterisation of gait post-stroke [17].

Previously, studies quantifying asymmetry from acceleration signals of the trunk during post-stroke gait typically focus on differences from a control group, adopt a minimal data set of variables, and to our knowledge do not report the concurrent validity or reliability to reference standards. Knowledge of the most robust asymmetry variables that are capable of quantifying similar information to reference standards using clinically feasible tools is important to further the field. This study compares the validity and test–retest reliability of a wide range of novel acceleration-derived variables to quantify asymmetry post-stroke from a single sensor located on the trunk.

2. Materials and Methods

2.1. Study Design and Setting

This cross-sectional study was undertaken in the gait laboratory at the Clinical Ageing Research Unit, Campus for Ageing and Vitality, Newcastle upon Tyne, UK.

2.2. Participants

The study was approved by the Greater Manchester West Research and Ethics Committee (NRES Committee Northwest-Greater Manchester West 15/NW/0731). All subjects gave informed written consent for the study according to the Declaration of Helsinki.

Inclusion criteria: Community-dwelling stroke survivor; at least one month post-stroke onset; mild to moderate gait deficit defined by clinical observation of gait asymmetry including reduced stance time, increased swing time in the affected limb and/or reduced gait speed/balance problems; no changes in gait-related ability over the past month based on self-report and able to walk 10 m with/without a stick.

Exclusion criteria: Medical problems other than stroke impacting on gait e.g., osteoarthritis. Participants were recruited via advertisement or therapist referral. All eligible participants were consecutively invited to participate in the study.

2.3. Demographic and Clinical Measures

The following data were collected at baseline: age, gender, height and weight, date of stroke, stroke type (Oxford Community Stroke Project Classification [21]), stroke impairment (National Institute of Health Stroke Scale [22]), presence of hemiplegia (clinical observation by two independent experienced clinicians), walking stick use, ankle foot orthosis (AFO) use.

2.4. Test Protocol

Participants were asked to walk at their preferred pace in a straight line for 4×10 m intermittent trials (see Figure 1). The trials were repeated on two occasions (Time 1 and Time 2) one week apart (± 2 days). A GaitRite instrumented walkway was positioned in the walk path (dimensions were 7.0 m $\times 0.6$ m, spatial accuracy of 1.27 cm and temporal accuracy of one sample (240 Hz, ~4.17 ms) (GaitRite: Platinum model GaitRite, software version 4.5, CIR systems, NJ, USA)). The participants wore an AX3 wearable sensor located at their fifth lumbar vertebrae (L5). The AX3 is a single tri-axial accelerometer-based wearable (AX3, Axivity, York, UK https://axivity.com/, cost $\approx$ £100, dimensions 23.0 mm $\times 32.5$ mm $\times 7.6$ mm). The AX3 weighs 11 g and has a memory of 512 Mb. AX3 data capture occurs with a sampling frequency of 100 Hz (16-bit resolution) at a range of ± 8 g. Recorded AX3 accelerations were stored locally on the device's internal memory and downloaded upon the completion of each session.

2.5. Asymmetry Variables

Acceleration-derived asymmetry variables were selected based upon their ability to represent levels of asymmetry from signals measured from a single accelerometer located at the trunk. The variables that were selected as representative of asymmetry were the harmonic ratio [16], autocorrelation [20], gait symmetry index [18], and phase plot analysis [23–25] (described in more detail below). Four spatiotemporal variables extracted from GaitRite were selected as measures of asymmetry as defined by Lord et al. [26]. The spatiotemporal asymmetry variables included step time asymmetry, stance time asymmetry, swing time asymmetry, and step length asymmetry, and these were calculated as the absolute difference between consecutive left and right steps.

2.6. Description of Acceleration-Derived Variables

All data analysis relating to the raw acceleration signals was performed using MATLAB (version 9.4.0, R2018a). For a full description for the algorithm and data segmentation techniques applied to the accelerometer data, please see references [27,28]. In brief, the vertical acceleration underwent continuous wavelet transformation to estimate the initial contact and final contact in the gait cycle [28]. To ensure that the steady-state gait was analyzed, the initial and final three steps were removed from the signal. Prior to the calculation of additional variables, the acceleration signals were realigned to the earth's gravitational constant [29,30] and a low-pass Butterworth filter with a cut-off frequency of 20 Hz. A full description of the following variables and the required algorithms is the supplied by the provided references. Additionally, they have been summarised in Appendix A.

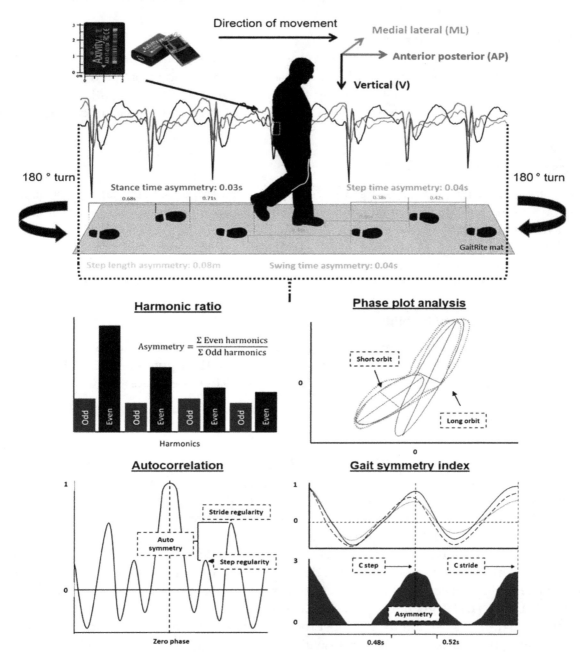

Figure 1. Indication of the instrumentation and the protocol used to collect the acceleration signal and the asymmetry parameters from the GaitRite mat. Also pictured is the acceleration-derived asymmetry variables and the means for the calculation of asymmetry following the processing of the raw acceleration signal.

2.6.1. Harmonic Ratio

The harmonic ratio (HR) describes the step-to-step symmetry within a stride from calculating a ratio of the odd and even harmonics of a signal following fast Fourier transformation [16,31]. This method has been shown previously to reflect increased asymmetry for those post-stroke relative to age and speed-matched controls [16].

2.6.2. Autocorrelation

The unbiased autocorrelation was also calculated due to its ability to reflect the step and stride regularity and the symmetry between the two (autocorrelation symmetry) [20,32,33]. Previously, it has been shown as better capable to characterise hemiplegic gait relative to footfall variables [20,32].

2.6.3. Gait Symmetry Index

The gait symmetry index (GSI) is a more recently proposed variable, which was calculated based upon the concept of the summation of the biased autocorrelation from all three components of movement and a subsequent calculation of step and stride timing asymmetry [18]. It has been shown to be more sensitive than and highly correlated with levels of asymmetry measured with two sensors located at the feet of participants post-stroke [18].

2.6.4. Phase Plot Analysis

Phase plot analysis (aka Poincaré analysis) was performed on vertical components of the acceleration signal [23–25]. This method has had previous applications within electrocardiogram studies. It works by plotting periodic signals as a function of their past values. The resulting ellipses or orbits and the properties thereof can then assess asymmetries in the associated gait. Phase plot analysis also offers the ability to assess intra step correlation i.e., the correlation of signals from immediately successive step cycles, which necessarily corresponds to left-versus-right asymmetry.

2.6.5. Measures Indicative of Stability

Although not indicative of asymmetry, the root mean square of the acceleration signal (Acc RMS) and also its first time derivative (Jerk RMS) were calculated for their potential to highlight synergistic compensatory strategies during gait post-stroke [13,16]. Their test–retest reliability needs to be established in the literature.

2.7. Statistical Analysis

Analysis was completed using SPSS v25 (IBM). The normality of data was tested with a Shapiro–Wilk test. Descriptive statistics (median and interquartile range) were calculated for gait characteristics measured by AX3 and GaitRite. Concurrent validity between the AX3 acceleration-derived variables and those of the GaitRite at Time 1 were tested using Spearman's rank correlation coefficients (RHO). For the AX3 acceleration-derived variables, the test–retest reliability between Time 1 and 2 was established using Spearman's rank correlation coefficients (RHO), intraclass correlation coefficient (ICC_{21}), and limits of agreement (LoA) expressed as a percentage of the mean of the two variables and the 95% LoA. For all analyses, statistical significance was set at $p < 0.05$. Predefined acceptance ratings for ICC_{21} were set at excellent (≥900, 0.0%–4.9%), good (0.750–0.899, 5.0%–9.9%), moderate (0.500–0.749, 10.0%–49.9%), and poor (50.0%) [1,34]. The selection for the most robust variable was based upon the variable with the highest Spearman rank correlation coefficient with the asymmetry variable obtained from the GaitRite while also recording an ICC_{21} greater than 0.8 for test–retest reliability.

3. Results

Twenty-five participants were recruited to the study. Data for two participants who wore a fixed plastic AFO were removed from the analysis, because individual data analysis (including video observations) revealed that the step detection applied were not appropriate for these two participants due to a lack of possible plantar flexion. This was not the case for the remaining participants, as the video analysis confirmed the step detection algorithm was effective to detect both heel strike and toe off [1]. Demographic information for the remaining 23 participants is displayed in Table 1.

Table 1. Participant characteristics.

Demographics (n = 23)	
Gender (male/female)	19/4
Age (years)	63 ± 11
Body mass index	26 ± 4
Stroke characteristics	
Time since stroke (months)	66 ± 48 (range 5–201)
Stroke subtype (OCSP)	
Total anterior circulation	11
Partial anterior circulation	6
Lacunar	3
Posterior circulation	3
Stroke impairment	
NIHSS score (0–40)	4 ± 3 (range 0–11)
NIHSS lower limb score (0–4)	1 ± 0.7 (range 0–3)
Walking speed (m/s)	0. 9 ± 0.4
Marked hemiplegia (Yes/No)	15/8
Walking aid (number (%))	3 (13%)
Push Aequi ankle foot orthosis (number (%))	4 (17%)

Where appropriate mean and standard deviation are displayed, OCSP (Oxford community Stroke Project), NIHSS (National Institute for Health Stroke Scale).

3.1. Concurrent Validity of the Asymmetry Variables

Figure 2 shows the correlation between the asymmetry variables quantified using a GaitRite mat (step time asymmetry, stance time asymmetry, swing time asymmetry, and step length asymmetry) and the acceleration-derived variables proposed to measure asymmetry. Overall, step time asymmetry correlated most with the acceleration-derived variables. Step regularity (vertical acceleration) had the highest concurrent validity with step time asymmetry (−0.87). Six other variables had high levels of agreement (+0.80) (HR V, step regularity (V), step regularity (AP), orbit eccentricity, orbit width deviation, and intra step correlation). Five correlated with step time asymmetry and orbit width deviation correlated with stance time asymmetry. The smallest correlations were achieved by the outputs of the autocorrelation from the medial lateralcomponent of the signal and also a variety of the outputs from the phase plot analysis.

Acceleration-derived variable	GaitRite Asymmetry variables			
	Step time	Stance time	Swing time	Step length
Harmonic ratio (V)	-0.83 **	-0.70 **	-0.73 **	-0.59 **
Harmonic ratio (ML)	-0.47 *	-0.48 *	-0.44 *	-0.26
Harmonic ratio (AP)	-0.76 **	-0.63 **	-0.67 **	-0.44 *
Step regularity (V)	-0.87 **	-0.72 **	-0.72 **	-0.65 **
Step regularity (ML)	-0.23	-0.17	-0.08	-0.29
Step regularity (AP)	-0.83 **	-0.66 **	-0.68 **	-0.52 *
Stride regularity (V)	-0.76 **	-0.65 **	-0.65 **	-0.56 **
Stride regularity (ML)	-0.35	-0.26	-0.17	-0.39
Stride regularity (AP)	-0.45 *	-0.38	-0.37	-0.38
Autocorrelation symmetry (V)	0.54 **	0.38	0.37	0.43 *
Autocorrelation symmetry (ML)	0.23	0.32	0.28	0.17
Autocorrelation symmetry (AP)	-0.57 **	-0.57 **	-0.53 **	-0.49 *
Gait symmetry index	0.62 **	0.48 *	0.50 *	0.36
Orbit eccentricity	-0.81 **	-0.67 **	-0.68 **	-0.38
Relative orbit inclination	0.49 *	0.40	0.35	0.39
Orbit width deviation	0.80 **	0.80 **	0.78 **	0.49 *
Short half orbit eccentricity	0.78 **	0.69 **	0.69 **	0.48 *
Short half orbit segment angle	0.68 **	0.54 **	0.50 *	0.37
Long half orbit eccentricity	0.61 **	0.59 **	0.57 **	0.20
Long half orbit segment angle	0.79 **	0.67 **	0.67 **	0.28
Intra step correlation	-0.83 **	-0.67 **	-0.67 **	-0.45 *

Key: Indication of Spearman's rank correlation coefficient								
-1	-0.75	-0.5	-0.25	0	0.25	0.5	0.75	1

Figure 2. Indication of the correlation between the asymmetry variables quantified using a GaitRite mat and the variables proposed to measure asymmetry from the acceleration signals from the trunk. Black indicates a strong positive or negative correlation. * and ** denotes significance at the 0.05 and 0.01 level, respectively. V = Vertical acceleration, ML = Medial lateral acceleration, and AP = Anterior posterior acceleration.

3.2. Test–Retest Reliability of the Variables

Table 2 demonstrates the test–retest reliability between the wearable variables measured one week apart (Time 1 versus Time 2). The most reliable variables were step regularity (V) and HR (V), both recording an ICC_{21} of 0.98. Taken from the ICC_{21} values, excellent reliability was achieved for 12 out of the 27 variables tested. These came from the majority of autocorrelation outputs except for step regularity (ML), stride regularity (AP), and autocorrelation symmetry (vertical acceleration (V) and medial lateral acceleration (ML)) direction, the GSI, the HR in the V and AP direction, Jerk RMS, and the short half-orbit segment angle form the phase plot analysis. Good reliability was achieved for a further five variables (stride regularity (AP), autocorrelation symmetry (V), relative orbit inclination, short half orbit eccentricity, and long half orbit eccentricity).

Table 2. Test–retest reliability (one week apart) for acceleration-derived variables.

Variables	Median (IQR)			Agreement		
	T1	T2	Median Difference (%)	ICC_{21}	LOA % (95% LoA)	Rho
Harmonic ratio (V)	1.71 (1.37)	1.70 (1.23)	−0.01	0.98 **	1.94 (2.52, 1.36)	0.92 **
Harmonic ratio (ML)	1.38 (0.60)	1.57 (0.72)	0.14	0.71 **	1.56 (2.80, 0.31)	0.71 **
Harmonic ratio (AP)	1.26 (0.97)	1.39 (0.92)	0.10	0.92 **	1.54 (2.34, 0.73)	0.91 **
Step regularity (V)	0.53 (0.47)	0.52 (0.54)	−0.02	0.98 **	0.51 (0.67, 0.34)	0.96 **
Step regularity (ML)	0.42 (0.20)	0.44 (0.18)	0.04	0.73 **	0.44 (0.69, 0.19)	0.61 **
Step regularity (AP)	0.51 (0.43)	0.40 (0.49)	−0.20	0.92 **	0.37 (0.68, 0.07)	0.87 **
Stride regularity (V)	0.70 (0.25)	0.68 (0.27)	−0.03	0.94 **	0.66 (0.85, 0.46)	0.88 **
Stride regularity (ML)	0.59 (0.14)	0.66 (0.20)	0.12	0.93 **	0.57 (0.78, 0.37)	0.73 **
Stride regularity (AP)	0.74 (0.18)	0.75 (0.13)	0.01	0.87 **	0.70 (0.92, 0.48)	0.74 **
Autocorrelation symmetry (V)	0.53 (0.26)	0.52 (0.29)	0.56	0.80 **	0.18 (0.40, −0.03)	0.76 **
Autocorrelation symmetry (ML)	0.10 (0.19)	0.16 (0.25)	0.09	0.59 *	0.19 (0.44, −0.05)	0.49 *
Autocorrelation symmetry (AP)	0.18 (0.15)	0.19 (0.14)	0.61	0.93 **	0.36 (0.62, 0.10)	0.79 **
Gait symmetry index	0.21 (0.37)	0.35 (0.43)	−0.02	0.92 **	0.47 (0.70, 0.23)	0.82 **
Orbit eccentricity	7.79 (6.27)	8.32 (15.13)	0.00	0.72 **	0.97 (1.04, 0.91)	0.70 **
Relative orbit inclination	0.01 (0.01)	0.01 (0.01)	0.07	0.76 **	11.02 (28.02, −5.99)	0.60 **
Orbit width deviation	0.01 (0.02)	0.00 (0.02)	−0.07	0.66 **	0.01 (0.05, −0.02)	0.65 **
Short half orbit eccentricity	5.32 (6.35)	4.12 (5.31)	−0.38	0.73 **	0.02 (0.07, −0.03)	0.87 **
Short half orbit segment angle	0.02 (0.05)	0.01 (0.04)	−0.23	0.95 **	7.74 (15.28, 0.20)	0.57 **
Long half orbit eccentricity	5.20 (10.73)	5.61 (6.55)	−0.16	0.79 **	0.04 (0.13, −0.05)	0.59 **
Long half orbit segment angle	0.89 (0.41)	0.88 (0.20)	0.08	0.45	7.77 (26.32, −10.78)	0.57 **
Intra step correlation	1.05 (0.04)	1.05 (0.04)	−0.01	0.58 *	0.78 (1.29, 0.28)	0.68 **
Acceleration RMS (V)	0.18 (0.09)	0.17 (0.06)	0.00	0.03	1.03 (1.24, 0.83)	0.41
Acceleration RMS (ML)	0.25 (0.15)	0.24 (0.15)	−0.06	0.90 **	0.17 (0.24, 0.10)	0.68 **
Acceleration RMS (AP)	8.53 (8.00)	8.57 (7.47)	−0.04	0.20	0.26 (0.62, −0.10)	0.21
Jerk RMS (V)	6.29 (4.18)	6.36 (4.15)	0.01	0.96 **	9.32 (13.49, 5.14)	0.93 **
Jerk RMS (ML)	6.22 (4.89)	6.42 (6.88)	0.01	0.97 **	7.39 (10.67, 4.11)	0.90 **
Jerk RMS (AP)	1.71 (1.37)	1.70 (1.23)	0.03	0.96 **	7.26 (11.23, 3.28)	0.92 **

* and ** denotes significance at the 0.05 and 0.01 level, respectively. V = Vertical acceleration, ML = Medial lateral acceleration, and AP = Anterior posterior acceleration, RMS = root mean square.

3.3. Selection of the Most Robust Variable

Table 3 highlights the variables that best correlated with spatiotemporal gait variables calculated from GaitRite while also achieving an ICC_{21} greater than 0.8 for test–retest reliability. For the GaitRite variables of asymmetry, step regularity (V) achieved the highest concurrent validity due to its correlation with step time asymmetry (RHO = 0.87 and ICC_{21} = 0.98 **). The second highest concurrent validity was the HR in the vertical direction, which correlated with swing time asymmetry (RHO = 0.73 and ICC_{21} = 0.98 **).

Table 3. Indication of what wearable sensor variable recorded the highest Spearman's rank correlation coefficient with each variable obtained by the GaitRite mat. The Spearman's rank correlation coefficient between the two devices and the intraclass correlation coefficient is displayed for each variable.

	GaitRite Variable	Acceleration Derived Variable	Spearman's Rank Correlation Coefficient (RHO)	ICC_{21} (Test–Retest)
Asymmetry	Step time (s)	Step regularity (V)	0.87	0.98 **
	Swing time (s)	Harmonic ratio (V)	0.73	0.98 **
	Stance time (s)	Step regularity (V)	0.72	0.98 **
	Step length (m)	Step regularity (V)	0.65	0.98 **

** denotes significance at the 0.01 level. V = Vertical acceleration.

4. Discussion

This study examined the concurrent validity and reliability of a comprehensive range of asymmetry variables derived from a single accelerometer located on the trunk and identified step regularity as the most robust outcome. Step regularity showed strong concurrent validity and excellent test–retest reliability when compared with GaitRite outcomes reflecting asymmetry. This contrasts with previous work based on the AX3 sensor, which achieved poor to moderate criterion validity (Spearman's rank correlation coefficient of RHO = 0.01 to 0.601) for variables engineered to replicate spatiotemporal asymmetry variables calculated from GaitRite [1]. Although clinically more challenging to interpret than traditional spatiotemporal variables, our results support the adoption of novel variables to quantify asymmetry as robust digital variables for measuring asymmetrical gait post stroke.

With one exception (HR correlation with swing time asymmetry), variables calculated from performing an autocorrelation procedure on the original acceleration signal were more strongly correlated with GaitRite asymmetry. Hodt–Billington and colleagues [20] found that autocorrelation variables taken from the trunk were better at discriminating gait post-stroke from controls relative to GaitRite variables of asymmetry. The strength of the autocorrelation procedure may stem from analysing continuous successive steps. Complex measures such as gait asymmetry are not simply portrayed within a single discreet gait cycle; this concept has been highlighted before, whereby continuous measures have been described to highlight different asymmetry causes, symptoms, and gait strategies such as particular compensatory techniques [17]. Data from our study indicate that participants with high asymmetry produced poor forward propulsion from the affected limb, instead of relying on the more dominant limb to achieve progression at the end of each stride. This can be observed by the lack of step regularity and its diminution relative to stride regularity in the AP, ML, and V directions, replicating the gait strategy described by Balasubramanian et al. [35]. The autocorrelation method is well designed to reflect this synergistic gait strategy, which might explain the high correlation found from this sample of participants. However, this strategy will likely vary among a broader range of participants and throughout recovery. Other methods may better reflect true levels of asymmetry at different stages of recovery from acute, early subacute, late subacute, and chronic stroke, meaning that they should still be considered as potential variables [17,20].

Previously, Iosa et al. [16] assessed symmetry together with upright gait stability post-stroke and showed that relative to speed-matched controls, higher instabilities (Acceleration RMS) and reduced symmetry of trunk movements (as measured using the HR) were recorded. In this study, HR in the vertical direction was the only HR variable that performed favourably to autocorrelation variables due to its correlation with swing time asymmetry (RHO = −0.73) while also recording excellent reliability (ICC_{21} = 0.98). Since we did not assess control subjects, we could not determine the best measure to characterise gait post-stroke and highlight the compensatory mechanisms adopted relative to healthy controls. This is a broader aim for ongoing work. However, it has been previously highlighted that compensation strategies may be beneficial to increase gait ability, but this occurs at the compromise of stability. Thus, variables such as Acceleration and Jerk RMS should always be considered in addition to variables directly linked to asymmetry, aiming to provide a more holistic description of gait patterns [13,16]. Future research should explore this relationship so that a holistic, multivariate wearable approach can better assess gait strategies during recovery post-stroke. This potentially would quantify what movements are beneficial to gait, while also highlighting the impact of compensation strategies, consequently quantifying separate movements that can be targeted for rehabilitation.

Although previously suggested as a variable representative of asymmetry in stroke [18], the GSI performed relatively poorer to the previously discussed variables, despite also being based on the autocorrelation (biased) of accelerometry. This was unexpected, as GSI theoretically is designed to detect the asymmetry within temporal footfall parameters. Equally, the autocorrelation symmetry variables did not perform better than step regularity alone, despite being designed to the capture the difference between step and stride regularity and therefore the symmetry between them. Potentially, the GSI and the autocorrelation symmetry did not quantify the synergistic movement strategy that the step regularity variable was suited to highlight and the reason for its favourable concurrent validity. The GSI and the autocorrelation symmetry variables may be better suited to highlight different compensatory synergies at different stages of recovery such as during acute, early subacute, late subacute, and chronic stages, and therefore should not be neglected in future research.

Select phase plot variables achieved RHO values greater than 0.8 when compared to GaitRite asymmetry values and also demonstrated good to excellent reliability, therefore highlighting their ability to quantify symmetry post-stroke. Adaption to the algorithms to the other directional components other than vertical and comparison with controls would better test their application as a biomarker. Similar to the other variables capable of quantifying movements in the AP and ML direction, there is the possibility that they can highlight a new domain of asymmetry separate from the asymmetry footfall asymmetry variables captured by GaitRite. Future research should explore this upper and lower body relationship post-stroke to examine the similarities and differences during gait and determine if added value is obtained [36,37].

All data were collected in a controlled environment; however, wearable technology is not limited by the testing environment and for improved ecological validity; obtaining data from the participant's community is desired [38]. To this goal, future research should utilise the variables tested in the laboratory in the participant's free-living environment. For free-living gait, the majority of walking bouts for people with Parkinson's disease and older adults have been found to be below 10 s, and it has been inferred that these bouts are when the participants are indoors [39]. One limitation with autocorrelation is that it relies on successive steps in a straight line. For free-living data, variables such as the HR may be more useful during these short walking bouts due to their ability to be calculated from a single stride in addition to successive steps [31,40]. Future research should assess the ability of these variables to accurately and reliably quantify asymmetry during short walking bouts or if tested refined spaces, as for this population, the median (and interquartile range) bout length was 16.3 (6.2) seconds for data collected over seven days [1].

4.1. Limitations

The relatively small sample size and limited heterogeneity with respect to time post-stroke did not allow us to determine what variables are the best at quantifying asymmetry for a more general sample or recovery stage-specific populations [41]. Future work is required on a larger sample size that ranges in time since stroke to discover what variables are the most capable to perform as objective biomarkers over all stages of recovery as one variable may not be appropriate for all, and compensatory strategies may change between the different stages of stroke recovery. Equally, future research should confirm that these results are replicable with different accelerometers with differing sampling frequencies, ranges, and resolutions. Further limitations stem from the reliance of the step detection algorithm. Data from two participants was not analysed due to their use of a fixed AFO that impacted on heel strike and the performance of the algorithm, which was based on the detection of initial and final contact within the gait cycle. Future research should integrate/develop step detection algorithms for participants requiring fixed AFOs to broaden application. Alternatively, the variables should be developed so that the cyclical nature of a signal may divide gait cycles (similar to the method used for phase plots) as opposed to methods that rely on detecting the initial and final contact of the foot.

4.2. Applications

These results provide evidence that asymmetry can accurately and reliably be calculated using a single accelerometer. Although much work is needed for accelerometers to be routinely adopted [42,43], these results give evidence that asymmetry can be objectively quantified using a tool applicable for many purposes. Consequently, the variables tested here may then act as a digital biomarker to quantify the impact of targeted interventions proposed to improve gait timing mechanisms and gait asymmetry (e.g., auditory rhythmical cueing) [44]. Accelerometers provide a potentially low burden method for clinicians to collect data from a variety of environments, increasing the ability to objectively quantify asymmetry during stroke rehabilitation. Alongside application within the clinic, accelerometer data can be collected on gait asymmetry in naturalistic environments, thus removing the Hawthorn effect/observer bias associated with clinical testing. With increased development, these variables may provide continuous asymmetry focussed feedback for self-progress specific to each participant during rehabilitation.

5. Conclusions

Gait asymmetry after stroke can be measured robustly using a single wearable sensor on the trunk. Step regularity is the most valid and reliable asymmetry outcome, which is quantified by performing autocorrelation on the vertical component of the signal. The variables tested performed favourably to previous studies that also used GaitRite as the reference. Consequently, their adoption, in addition to other wearable-derived spatiotemporal variables of gait, are encouraged as they provide a more holistic description of gait that appears to indicate compensatory movement post-stroke. Future research is encouraged on larger populations where asymmetry is expected, during recovery/interventions to identify which wearable variables are biomarkers for gait asymmetry and compensatory mechanisms during gait. This will allow for increased accuracy in determining effective interventions.

Author Contributions: Conceptualisation, C.B., S.D.D., L.R. and S.A.M.; methodology, C.B., M.E.M.-A., M.D.-W., A.G., A.H., S.L., L.R., S.D.D., and S.A.M.; software, C.B., S.D.D., M.E.M.-A., M.D.-W., A.G., and A.H.; validation, C.B., A.H., A.G., and S.D.D.; formal analysis, C.B., S.D.D., and S.A.M.; investigation, C.B., A.G., A.H., L.R., S.D.D., and S.A.M.; resources, S.A.M., and L.R.; data curation, C.B., M.E.M.-A., M.D.-W., A.G., A.H., S.D.D.; writing—original draft preparation, C.B.; writing—review and editing, C.B., M.E.M.-A., M.D., A.G., A.H., S.L., L.R., S.D.D., and S.A.M.; visualisation, C.B., S.D.D.; supervision, S.A.M., S.D.D., L.R., and S.L.; project administration, S.A.M.; funding acquisition, S.A.M. and L.R. All authors have read and agreed to the published version of the manuscript.

Acknowledgments: We would like to thank the following for their contribution: Patients who took part in the study; Staff from local NHS trusts who assisted with recruitment to the study and lastly, Lisa Alcock for her assistance during in data collection.

Appendix A

Appendix A.1. Acceleration-Derived Variable Definitions

Table A1. Indication for the variables used from the signal-derived variables and their respective definitions.

Variable	Definition
Harmonic ratio (V, ML, AP)	The step-to-step symmetry within a stride from calculating a ratio of the odd and even harmonics of a signal following fast Fourier transformation.
Step regularity (V, ML, AP)	Estimated as the normalized unbiased autocovariance for a lag of one step time. Thus, this feature reflects the similarity between subsequent steps of the acceleration pattern over a step. Values of this feature close to 1.0 (maximum possible value) reflect repeatable patterns between subsequent steps.
Stride regularity (V, ML, AP)	Estimated as the normalized unbiased autocovariance for a lag of one stride time. Thus, this feature reflects the similarity between subsequent strides of the acceleration pattern over a stride cycle.
Autocorrelation symmetry (V, ML, AP)	Difference between step and stride regularity designed to quantify the level of symmetry between them and indicative of symmetry during a straight walk.
Gait symmetry index	Calculated based upon the concept of the summation of the biased autocorrelation from all three components of movement and a subsequent calculation of step and stride timing asymmetry.
Orbit eccentricity (V)	Average eccentricity of all fully fitted ellipses.
Relative orbit inclination (V)	Average angle subtended by alternating fitted ellipses within a bout of gait.
Orbit width deviation (V)	Standard deviation of minor axes lengths of all fully fitted ellipses. Analogous to Principle Component Analysis (second component).
Short half orbit eccentricity (V)	Difference in eccentricity of two ellipses fitted to each half-cycle of a full orbit in the phase plot. Averaged over all orbits in a bout's phase plot.
Short half orbit segment angle (V)	Difference in inclination of two ellipses fitted to each half-cycle of a full orbit in the phase plot. Averaged over all orbits in a bout's phase plot.
Long half orbit eccentricity (V)	Difference in eccentricity of two ellipses fitted to each half-cycle of a full orbit in the phase plot. Averaged over all orbits in a bout's phase plot.
Long half orbit segment angle (V)	Difference in inclination of two ellipses fitted to each half-cycle of a full orbit in the phase plot. Averaged over all orbits in a bout's phase plot.
Intra step correlation (V)	Average correlation of acceleration signal corresponding to step i with that of step i-1. I.e., a lag-1 autocorrelation where a single lag is one step cycle's duration.
Acceleration RMS (V, ML, AP)	The calculation of the root mean square of the acceleration signal.
Jerk RMS (V, ML, AP)	The calculation of the root mean square of the first time derivative of the acceleration signal (jerk).

Appendix A.2. Explanation and Equation for Each Acceleration Derived Variable for Asymmetry

Appendix A.2.1. Harmonic Ratio

The harmonic ratio is a measure based upon the premise that a stride contains two steps and therefore, during continuous walking, accelerations should repeat in multiples of two. The variable quantifies how well these accelerations are repeated in each stride compared to when accelerations do not repeat and are therefore out of phase. Therefore, the ratio of in and out-of-phase accelerations is a measure of how symmetric the participant is walking. To calculate the harmonic ratio, it is required to evaluate the harmonic content of the acceleration signal using the stride frequency from the analysis of frequency components. Following a fast Fourier transform (using the FFT function in MATLAB), a ratio be can created from the first 20 harmonics extracted from the Fourier series. Due to the AP and V components of the signals being biphasic, the ratio for these components is determined by the sum of the even harmonics (in phase movement) divided by the sum of the odd harmonics (out-of-phase movement).

$$HR_{AP, V} = \frac{\Sigma \text{ Amplitudes of even harmonics}}{\Sigma \text{ Amplitudes of odd harmonics}}$$

For the ML component of the signal due to only showing only one dominant acceleration peak within a stride cycle (whereby the odd harmonics are in-phase and even harmonic out-of-phase), the opposite is performed.

$$HR_{ML} = \frac{\Sigma \text{ Amplitudes of odd harmonics}}{\Sigma \text{ Amplitudes of even harmonics}}$$

As a gait measure, a higher harmonic ratio indicates a better symmetry between steps within a single stride For the AP and V components.

Appendix A.2.2. Autocorrelation

Autocorrelation is calculated taking the complete signal of the time when the participant was in contact with the GaitRite mat. Plots of an autocorrelation estimate are used to inspect the structure of a cyclic component within a time series. To do this, the generic unbiased autocorrelation function of the sample sequence x(i) was computed using the below equation:

$$Ad(m) = \frac{1}{N - |m|} \sum_{i=1}^{N-|m|} x(i) \cdot x(i+m)$$

where N is the number of samples and m is the time lag expressed as number of samples.

Since phase shifts can be performed with identical results in both positive and negative directions relative to the original time series, an autocorrelation plot is conventionally organized symmetrically with the zeroth shift located centrally. This central value was used to normalize the signal so that its maxima was one. For a time series of trunk accelerations during walking, autocorrelation coefficients can be produced to quantify the peak values at the first and second dominant period, representing phase shifts equal to one step and one stride, respectively (see Figure 1 as an example). A tailored MATLAB code was used to detect these peaks, particularly using the signals power density to determine the windows in which the peaks would occur. For the symmetry between the step and stride regularity, the absolute difference was calculated as a measure of asymmetry instead of the ratio, which is more conventionally used. This was because the between-step and between-stride autocorrelations may approach zero if the regularity between neighboring steps or neighboring strides is low.

Appendix A.2.3. Gait Symmetry Index (GSI)

Differently from the aforementioned autocorrelation measures, the gait symmetry index (GSI) uses a second-order Butterworth low-pass filter with the cut-off frequency of 10 Hz to filter the complete time series and then uses the biased version of the autocorrelation function as displayed below:

$$Ad(m) = \frac{1}{N} \sum_{i=1}^{N-|m|} x(i) \cdot x(i+m).$$

The maximum time lag was 4 s (400 samples), which approximates 2.5 times a single stride duration in post hemiplegic stroke patients. This window length was chosen to capture the repetition of stride cycles in very slow walking. A coefficient of stride cycle repetition (Cstride) was the sum of the positive autocorrelation coefficients of the three axes as a function of the equation displayed below:

$$\text{Cstride(t)} = \text{ADv(t)} + \text{ADml(t)} + \text{ADap(t)}; \quad \text{if AD(t)} < 0, \text{AD(t)} = 0.$$

The coefficient of step repetition (Cstep) was the norm of autocorrelation coefficients as a function of the equation displayed below:

$$\text{Cstep(t)} = \sqrt{\text{ADv(t)} + \text{ADml(t)} + \text{ADap(t)}}; \text{if AD(t)} < 0, \text{AD(t)} = 0.$$

One stride time (Tstride) equals t when the Cstride had the maximum value. The hypothesis was that in a perfect symmetric gait pattern, two consecutive steps have the same step duration of $0.5 \times$ Tstride. Thus, the maximum value of Cstep was set at $\sqrt{3}$ when the autocorrelation coefficient of each acceleration axis was 1 at zero-lag (t = 0). The gait symmetry index (GSI) was Cstep ($0.5 \times$ Tstride) normalized to its value at zero-lag, as indicated in the below equation:

$$\text{Cstep(t)} = \text{Cstep}(0.5 * \text{Tstride}) / \sqrt{3}.$$

Appendix A.2.4. Phase Plot Analysis

To create an ellipse to apply the following models, the vertical acceleration signal was first transformed to a horizontal–vertical coordinate system and filtered with a low-pass fourth order Butterworth filter at 20 Hz. Following piecewise integration, the full vertical excursion signal must be restored via concatenation of the resultant integrals. Here, the phase shift is introduced. We restore two such vertical excursion signals, one of which is exactly one step cycle lagged behind the other i.e.,:

$$PP1(tt) = PP0(tt - nn)$$

where n is the number of data points comprising a step interval in the vertical excursion signal and $PP1$ and $PP0$ are the lagged and original vertical excursion signal, respectively.

The following conic model is fitted to the two-dimensional phase plot data. This fitting is performed on each orbit in turn.

$$ax^2 + by^2 + cxy + dx + ey + f = 0$$

In the case of ellipse fitting to phase plot data, x and y are taken to be $PP1$ and $PP0$.
The above model defines an ellipse subject to the following constraint.

$$c^2 - 4ab < 0$$

This constraint is used to ensure that an elliptical conic is fitted to the data as opposed to a hyperbola or parabola. The model defined by the conic equation can be fitted using ordinary least squares to find an estimate of $\hat{A} = \left(\hat{a}, \hat{b}, \hat{c}, \hat{d}, \hat{e} \right)$. f is set equal to 1 to avoid a trivial solution.

The above form of an ellipse does not lend itself well to geometric interpretation, so the following parameterisation is implemented:

$$\frac{(x - g)^2}{r_1^2} + \frac{(y - k)^2}{r_2^2} = 1.$$

However, this form does not account for inclined ellipses. To account for the significant inclination of ellipses, the following rotated coordinate system is introduced:

$$x' = (x - g)\cos(\theta) + (y - k)\sin(\theta)$$

$$y' = (y - k)y\cos(\theta) + (x - g)\sin(\theta).$$

This form of ellipse and rotated coordinate system ensure more straightforward interpretation of the ellipses and more intuitive feature extraction.

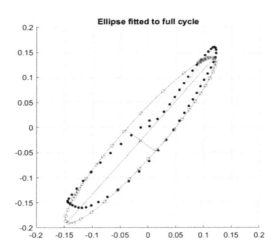

Figure A1. A single orbit with a fitted conic (ellipse).

This Figure A1 shows one such ellipse fitted to a single orbit of a phase plot. From this ellipse, we can extract features relating to the eccentricity and inclination. In general, phase plots consist of many orbits and their respective fitted ellipses (Figure A2). Further features can be extracted by assessing the relative inclination of ellipses from alternating orbits. In general, these inclinations oscillate about the value $\theta = \frac{\pi}{4}$.

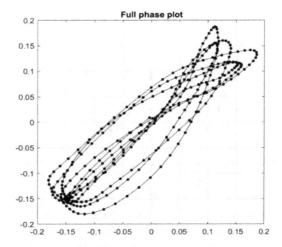

Figure A2. Complete phase plot comprising 7 continuous gait cycles.

Features extracted from ellipses fitted to entire orbits are considered primary features. Ellipses can be fitted to partial orbits; for example, two separate ellipses can be fitted to both halves of an orbit where the orbit in question is halved according to its major/minor axes. This leads to four additional ellipses fitted to each orbit of a phase plot (Figure A3). As an example, take the two ellipses fitted to either half of the shown orbit following halving via the minor axis (Figure A3, lower two figures). Features are extracted from these ellipses by extracting their relative characteristics e.g., their inclination relative to the other, the ratio of their areas, etc. Features extracted from ellipses fitted to partial orbits in this way are considered secondary phase plot features.

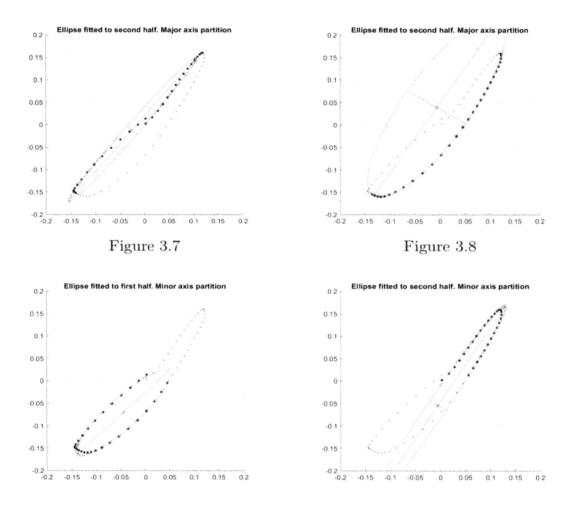

Figure 3.7   Figure 3.8

Figure A3. Indication of the different conic (ellipses) fitted to the major/minor axis and the first/second halves.

References

1. Moore, S.A.; Hickey, A.; Lord, S.; Del Din, S.; Godfrey, A.; Rochester, L. Comprehensive measurement of stroke gait characteristics with a single accelerometer in the laboratory and community: A feasibility, validity and reliability study. *J. Neuroeng. Rehabil.* **2017**, *14*, 130. [CrossRef] [PubMed]

2. Gallanagh, S.; Quinn, T.J.; Alexander, J.; Walters, M.R. Physical Activity in the Prevention and Treatment of Stroke. *ISRN Neurol.* **2011**, *2011*, 1–10. [CrossRef] [PubMed]

3. Patterson, K.K.; Gage, W.H.; Brooks, D.; Black, S.E.; McIlroy, W.E. Evaluation of gait symmetry after stroke: A comparison of current methods and recommendations for standardization. *Gait Posture* **2010**, *31*, 241–246. [CrossRef] [PubMed]

4. Fini, N.A.; Holland, A.E.; Keating, J.; Simek, J.; Bernhardt, J. How physically active are people following stroke? Systematic review and quantitative synthesis. *Phys. Ther.* **2017**, *97*, 707–717. [CrossRef]

5. Bull, F.; Goenka, S.; Lambert, V.; Pratt, M. *Physical Activity for the Prevention of Cardiometabolic Disease*; The International Bank for Reconstruction and Development/The World Bank: Washington, DC, USA, 2017; ISBN 9781464805189.

6. Lee, I.M.; Shiroma, E.J.; Lobelo, F.; Puska, P.; Blair, S.N.; Katzmarzyk, P.T.; Alkandari, J.R.; Andersen, L.B.; Bauman, A.E.; Brownson, R.C.; et al. Effect of physical inactivity on major non-communicable diseases worldwide: An analysis of burden of disease and life expectancy. *Lancet* **2012**, *380*, 219–229. [CrossRef]

7. Patterson, K.K.; Parafianowicz, I.; Danells, C.J.; Closson, V.; Verrier, M.C.; Staines, W.R.; Black, S.E.; McIlroy, W.E. Gait Asymmetry in Community-Ambulating Stroke Survivors. *Arch. Phys. Med. Rehabil.* **2008**, *89*, 304–310. [CrossRef]

8. Balaban, B.; Tok, F. Gait Disturbances in Patients with Stroke. *PM R* **2014**, *6*, 635–642. [CrossRef]

9. Wade, D.T. Measurement in neurological rehabilitation. *Curr. Opin. Neurol. Neurosurg.* **1992**, *5*, 682–686.

10. Lin, J.-H.; Hsu, M.-J.; Hsu, H.-W.; Wu, H.-C.; Hsieh, C.-L. Psychometric Comparisons of 3 Functional Ambulation Measures for Patients with Stroke. *Stroke* **2010**, *41*, 2021–2025. [CrossRef]

11. Wong, J.S.; Jasani, H.; Poon, V.; Inness, E.L.; McIlroy, W.E.; Mansfield, A. Inter- and intra-rater reliability of the GAITRite system among individuals with sub-acute stroke. *Gait Posture* **2014**, *40*, 259–261. [CrossRef]

12. Buckley, C.; Alcock, L.; McArdle, R.; Ur Rehman, R.Z.; Del Din, S.; Mazzà, C.; Yarnall, A.J.; Rochester, L. The role of movement analysis in diagnosing and monitoring neurodegenerative conditions: Insights from gait and postural control. *Brain Sci.* **2019**, *9*, 34. [CrossRef] [PubMed]

13. Iosa, M.; Fusco, A.; Giovanni, M.; Paolicci, S. Development and decline of upright gait stability. *Front. Aging Neurosci.* **2014**, *6*, 14. [CrossRef] [PubMed]

14. Wright, R.L.; Brownless, S.B.; Pratt, D.; Sackley, C.M.; Wing, A.M. stepping to the Beat: Feasibility and Potential efficacy of a home-Based auditory-cued step Training Program in chronic stroke. *Front. Neurol.* **2017**, *8*, 412. [CrossRef] [PubMed]

15. Buckley, C.; Galna, B.; Rochester, L.; Mazzà, C. Upper body accelerations as a biomarker of gait impairment in the early stages of Parkinson's disease. *Gait Posture* **2018**, *71*, 289–295. [CrossRef] [PubMed]

16. Iosa, M.; Bini, F.; Marinozzi, F.; Fusco, A.; Morone, G.; Koch, G.; Martino Cinnera, A.; Bonnì, S.; Paolucci, S. Stability and Harmony of Gait in Patients with Subacute Stroke. *J. Med. Biol. Eng.* **2016**, *36*, 635–643. [CrossRef] [PubMed]

17. Viteckova, S.; Kutilek, P.; Svoboda, Z.; Krupicka, R.; Kauler, J.; Szabo, Z. Gait symmetry measures: A review of current and prospective methods. Biomed. Signal Process. *Control* **2018**, *42*, 89–100.

18. Zhang, W.; Smuck, M.; Legault, C.; Ith, M.A.; Muaremi, A.; Aminian, K. Gait Symmetry Assessment with a Low Back 3D Accelerometer in Post-Stroke Patients. *Sensors* **2018**, *18*, 3322. [CrossRef]

19. Huang, X.; Mahoney, J.M.; Lewis, M.M.; Guangwei, D.; Piazza, S.J.; Cusumano, J.P. Both coordination and symmetry of arm swing are reduced in Parkinson's disease. *Gait Posture* **2012**, *35*, 373–377. [CrossRef]

20. Hodt-Billington, C.; Helbostad, J.L.; Moe-Nilssen, R. Should trunk movement or footfall parameters quantify gait asymmetry in chronic stroke patients? *Gait Posture* **2008**, *27*, 552–558. [CrossRef]

21. Bamford, J.; Sandercock, P.; Dennis, M.; Burn, J.; Warlow, C. Classification and natural history of clinically identifiable subtypes of cerebral infarction. *Lancet* **1991**, *337*, 1521–1526. [CrossRef]

22. Brott, T.; Adams, H.P.; Olinger, C.P.; Marler, J.R.; Barsan, W.G.; Biller, J.; Spilker, J.; Holleran, R.; Eberle, R.; Hertzberg, V.; et al. Measurements of acute cerebral infarction: A clinical examination scale. *Stroke* **1989**, *20*, 864–870. [CrossRef] [PubMed]

23. Esser, P.; Dawes, H.; Collett, J.; Howells, K. Insights into gait disorders: Walking variability using phase plot analysis, Parkinson's disease. *Gait Posture* **2013**, *38*, 648–652. [CrossRef] [PubMed]

24. Dunne-Willows, M.; Watson, P.; Shi, J.; Rochester, L.; Del Din, S. A Novel Parameterisation of Phase Plots for Monitoring of Parkinson's Disease. In Proceedings of the 2019 41st Annual International Conference of the IEEE Engineering in Medicine and Biology Society, Berlin, Germany, 23–27 July 2019; IEEE Explore: Berlin, Germany, 2019.

25. Brennan, M.; Palaniswami, M.; Kamen, P. Do existing measures of Poincare plot geometry reflect nonlinear features of heart rate variability? *IEEE Trans. Biomed. Eng.* **2001**, *48*, 1342–1347. [CrossRef] [PubMed]

26. Lord, S.; Galna, B.; Rochester, L. Moving forward on gait measurement: Toward a more refined approach. *Mov. Disord.* **2013**, *28*, 1534–1543. [CrossRef] [PubMed]

27. Del Din, S.; Godfrey, A.; Rochester, L. Validation of an Accelerometer to Quantify a Comprehensive Battery of Gait Characteristics in Healthy Older Adults and Parkinson's Disease: Toward Clinical and at Home Use. *IEEE J. Biomed. Health Inform.* **2016**, *20*, 838–847. [CrossRef] [PubMed]

28. McCamley, J.; Donati, M.; Grimpampi, E.; Mazzà, C. An enhanced estimate of initial contact and final contact instants of time using lower trunk inertial sensor data. *Gait Posture* **2012**, *36*, 316–318. [CrossRef]

29. Buckley, C.; Galna, B.; Rochester, L.; Mazzà, C. Quantification of upper body movements during gait in older adults and in those with Parkinson's disease: Impact of acceleration realignment methodologies. *Gait Posture* **2017**, *52*, 265–271. [CrossRef]

30. Moe-Nilssen, R. A new method for evaluating motor control in gait under real-life environmental conditions. Part 1: The instrument. *Clin. Biomech.* **1998**, *13*, 328–335. [CrossRef]

31. Bellanca, J.L.; Lowry, K.A.; Vanswearingen, J.M.; Brach, J.S.; Redfern, M.S. Harmonic ratios: A quantification of step to step symmetry. *J. Biomech.* **2013**, *46*, 828–831. [CrossRef]

32. Moe-Nilssen, R.; Helbostad, J. Interstride trunk acceleration variability but not step width variability can differentiate between fit and frail older adults. *Gait Posture* **2005**, *21*, 164–170. [CrossRef]

33. Tura, A.; Raggi, M.; Rocchi, L.; Cutti, A.G.; Chiari, L. Gait symmetry and regularity in transfemoral amputees assessed by trunk accelerations. *J. Neuroeng. Rehabil.* **2010**, *7*, 4. [CrossRef] [PubMed]

34. Fleiss, J.L. *The Design and Analysis of Clinical Experiments*; John Wiley & Sons, Inc.: Hoboken, NJ, USA, 1999; ISBN 0471820474.

35. Balasubramanian, C.K.; Bowden, M.G.; Neptune, R.R.; Kautz, S.A. Relationship between step length asymmetry and walking performance in subjects with chronic hemiparesis. *Arch. Phys. Med. Rehabil.* **2007**, *88*, 43–49. [CrossRef] [PubMed]

36. Boström, K.J.; Dirksen, T.; Zentgraf, K.; Wagner, H. The Contribution of Upper Body Movements to Dynamic Balance Regulation during Challenged Locomotion. *Front. Hum. Neurosci.* **2018**, *12*, 8. [CrossRef] [PubMed]

37. Mahaki, M.; Bruijn, S.M.; van Dieën, J.H. The effect of external lateral stabilization on the use of foot placement to control mediolateral stability in walking and running. *PeerJ* **2019**, *7*, e7939. [CrossRef] [PubMed]

38. Van de Port, I.; Punt, M.; Meijer, J.W. Walking activity and its determinants in free-living ambulatory people in a chronic phase after stroke: A cross-sectional study. *Disabil. Rehabil.* **2018**, *16*, 1–6. [CrossRef] [PubMed]

39. Del Din, S.; Godfrey, A.; Galna, B.; Lord, S.; Rochester, L.; Del-Din, S.; Godfrey, A.; Galna, B.; Lord, S.; Rochester, L. Free-living gait characteristics in ageing and Parkinson's disease: Impact of environment and ambulatory bout length. *J. Neuroeng. Rehabil.* **2016**, *13*, 1–12. [CrossRef]

40. Tamburini, A.P.; Storm, F.; Buckley, C.; Bisi, C.; Stagni, R.; Mazzà, C.; Tamburini, P.; Storm, F.; Buckley, C.; Bisi, M.C.; et al. Moving from laboratory to real life conditions: Influence on the assessment of variability and stability of gait. *Gait Posture* **2018**, *59*, 248–252. [CrossRef]

41. Bernhardt, J.; Hayward, K.S.; Kwakkel, G.; Ward, N.S.; Wolf, S.L.; Borschmann, K.; Krakauer, J.W.; Boyd, L.A.; Carmichael, S.T.; Corbett, D.; et al. Agreed Definitions and a Shared Vision for New Standards in Stroke Recovery Research: The Stroke Recovery and Rehabilitation Roundtable Taskforce. *Neurorehabil. Neural Repair* **2017**, *31*, 793–799. [CrossRef]

42. Espay, A.J.; Bonato, P.; Nahab, F.B.; Maetzler, W.; Dean, J.M.; Klucken, J.; Eskofier, B.M.; Merola, A.; Horak, F.; Lang, A.E.; et al. Technology in Parkinson's disease: Challenges and opportunities. *Mov. Disord.* **2016**, *31*, 1272–1282. [CrossRef]

43. Patterson, M.R.; Whelan, D.; Reginatto, B.; Caprani, N.; Walsh, L.; Smeaton, A.F.; Inomata, A.; Caulfield, B. Does external walking environment affect gait patterns? In Proceedings of the 2014 36th Annual International Conference of the IEEE Engineering in Medicine and Biology Society, Chicago, IL, USA, 26–30 August 2014; Volume 2014, pp. 2981–2984.

44. Yoo, G.E.; Kim, S.J. Rhythmic Auditory Cueing in Motor Rehabilitation for Stroke Patients: Systematic Review and Meta-Analysis. *J. Music Ther.* **2016**, *53*, 149–177. [CrossRef]

32

Safety and Tolerability of Plasma Exchange and Immunoadsorption in Neuroinflammatory Diseases

Johannes Dorst [1,*], Frank Fillies [1], Jens Dreyhaupt [2], Makbule Senel [1] and Hayrettin Tumani [1]

[1]   Department of Neurology, University of Ulm, 89081 Ulm, Germany; frank.fillies@uni-ulm.de (F.F.); makbule.senel@uni-ulm.de (M.S.); hayrettin.tumani@uni-ulm.de (H.T.)

[2]   Institute for Epidemiology and Medical Biometry, University of Ulm, 89081 Ulm, Germany; jens.dreyhaupt@uni-ulm.de

*   Correspondence: Johannes.dorst@uni-ulm.de

Abstract: Plasma exchange (PE) and immunoadsorption (IA) are frequently used for treatment of various autoimmune-mediated neurological diseases, including multiple sclerosis (MS), chronic inflammatory demyelinating polyneuropathy (CIDP), and Guillain–Barré syndrome (GBS). Although both methods are generally regarded as well-tolerated treatment options, evidence for safety and tolerability is low for most indications and largely relies on small case series. In this study, we retrospectively analysed adverse events (AEs) and laboratory changes in 284 patients with various neurological indications who received either PE ($n = 65$, 113 cycles) or IA ($n = 219$, 435 cycles) between 2013 and 2020 in our Neurology department. One standard treatment cycle for PE as well as IA consisted of five treatments on five consecutive days. During every treatment, the 2.0–2.5-fold individual plasma volume (PV) was treated in IA, while in PE, the 0.7-fold individual PV was replaced by human albumin solution. Overall, both methods showed an excellent safety profile; no deaths of life-threatening adverse events were recorded. Severe AEs (corresponding to grade 3 on the Common Terminology Criteria for Adverse Events grading scale v5.0) including three patients with sepsis, one pneumonia, and one pneumothorax were present in 5/435 IA cycles (1.1%); in the PE group, no severe AEs were recorded. Furthermore, although advantageous tolerability is generally considered the main advantage of IA over PE, we found that overall frequency of AEs (including grades 1 and 2) was higher in IA (67.1% of all cycles) compared to PE (35.4%; $p < 0.001$). The low incidence of AEs in PE might be caused by the lower PV exchanged during each treatment (0.7-fold) compared to previous studies which predominantly exchanged the 1.0–1.5-fold PV. In order to verify this hypothesis as well as confirming the efficacy of this lower-dosed scheme, prospective studies comparing different treatment regimens are needed.

Keywords: therapeutic plasma exchange; immunoadsorption; neurological diseases; multiple sclerosis; chronic inflammatory demyelinating polyneuropathy

1. Introduction

Plasma exchange (PE) and immunoadsorption (IA) are used in various autoimmune-mediated neurological diseases in order to remove autoimmune antibodies and other pathological constituents from the patients' blood. Currently, indications include multiple sclerosis (MS), myasthenia gravis, autoimmune encephalitis, chronic inflammatory demyelinating polyneuropathy (CIDP), Guillain–Barré syndrome (GBS), and many others. Although PE constitutes the standard technique for most diseases, IA is increasingly recognized as a more specific alternative and generally appreciated for its potentially advantageous safety profile. However, safety and tolerability of both methods have rarely been directly compared under standardized, monocentric conditions.

Originally, both treatment options primarily aimed at removing auto-antibodies from the blood, although various additional immune-modulating mechanisms like up- and downregulation of anti- and pro-inflammatory interleukins have been discussed [1]. Substantial methodological differences have to be considered which may affect efficacy as well as safety. Since in PE the plasma is removed and substituted by a volume replacement solution (human albumin or fresh frozen plasma (FFP)), all circulating proteins are removed, including coagulation factors. In contrast, IA relies on adsorbers which selectively bind human immunoglobulins (Ig) while largely sparing other plasma proteins; the processed plasma is led back to the patient, and no replacement solution is needed. Theoretically speaking, these factors should favor IA in terms of adverse events (AEs), while on the other hand the preservation of pro-inflammatory cytokines and other pathogenetically important proteins may weaken its efficacy dependent on the specific immunology of the respective disease, which is however, not fully understood in many cases. Furthermore, it has been shown that even in IA other plasma proteins are also affected which might explain its efficacy in diseases which are not regarded to be primarily antibody-mediated [2].

Apart from the method itself, specific techniques and treatment regimens have to be taken into account when assessing efficacy and safety of PE and IA. Various regenerable (protein A, recombinant proteins) and non-regenerable (tryptophan, phenylalanine) IA adsorbers are routinely used in clinical practice which feature different binding characteristics with regard to immunoglobulin classes, subclasses, and other plasma proteins [3,4]. For example, protein A adsorbers have a stronger binding affinity to IgG compared to IgA and IgM [3]. Furthermore, various treatment regimens can be applied for PE and IA with regard to number and frequency of treatments as well as the plasma volume (PV) treated during each session. Usually, 5–7 treatments are performed in both PE and IA, while treatment frequencies vary between daily and 2-day applications depending on fibrinogen levels. In IA, processing of the 2.0–2.5-fold individual PV constitutes the standard [5], which allows a daily treatment regimen for regenerable protein A and recombinant protein adsorbers, while a two-day treatment regimen with fixed PV (usually 2 or 2.5 L) is usually applied for non-regenerable tryptophan and phenylalanine adsorbers (due to loss of fibrinogen) [6–8]. In PE, various regimens with different PVs have been used. For example, the original randomized controlled trial (RCT) which built the foundation for the use of PE in MS applied 7 treatments within 14 days, exchanging the 1.1-fold PV during each session [9], while a more recent RCT showed that a daily treatment regime with 5 sessions and replacement of the 0.7-fold PV during each session was also effective [5]. Importantly, across all neurological indications there are no RCTs which directly compare different treatment regimens, and only few regimens have been tried; therefore, it seems very likely that the optimal regimen with regard to efficacy and safety has not yet been found.

Furthermore, specific peri- and intra-procedural measures vary between centers. In order to prevent blood in the extracorporeal circuit from clotting, heparin and/or citrate are most commonly used which carry various potential complications like heparin-induced thrombopenia and hypocalcemia. Some centers replace immunoglobulins after each treatment in order to account for the immunodeficiency induced by the therapy, while others rely on the periprocedural prophylactic administration of antibiotics. For all these measures, no reliable evidence exists.

Previous studies comparing PE and IA with regard to safety and tolerability in neurological diseases predominantly reported either no differences [6,8,10], or advantages for IA [11,12]. Since PE is unspecific, various complications due to loss of coagulation factors and other plasma constituents have been reported such as thrombosis, bleeding, hypotension (due to volume-shift), and sepsis [13,14]. Furthermore, the need of a volume replacement solution carries the risk of severe allergic reactions [13]. Life-threatening complications have been reported in 0.12% of patients [14], and a higher risk of adverse events in patients with neurological diseases compared to non-neurological diseases has been described [13]. On the other hand, IA has repeatedly been described as a safe and well-tolerated procedure [3,4,15]. Two studies in myasthenia gravis found that side effects were reduced in IA compared to PE [11,12]. In MS, the majority of studies did however not report any differences between

IA and PE with regard to safety [5,6,8] which was confirmed by a recent meta-analysis [10]. The only prospective study comparing IA and PE in CIDP [16] reported a good safety profile for both methods and comparable incidences of AEs. One retrospective study reported that both PE and IA were safely applied in 19 patients with GBS [17]. In summary, safety data for PE and IA in neurological diseases largely rely on studies with rather low numbers of subjects, which might explain the large range of reported incidences of AEs as well as the diverging assessments of safety profiles for both methods.

Considering the lack of RCTs regarding the use of PE and IA in neurological diseases, the extensive differences with regard to treatment regimens and peri-procedural measures, and the absence of reliable therapeutic standards for specific disease entities, it is of crucial importance to collect systematic clinical data. In this study, we retrospectively analyzed tolerability and safety data (including adverse events and laboratory abnormalities) in 284 patients (548 treatment cycles, 2470 treatments) with various neurological indications who were treated with either PE ($n = 65$) or IA ($n = 219$) between 2013 and 2020 in our center. We primarily aimed at (1) verifying the advantageous safety and tolerability profile of IA as proposed by previous studies and (2) evaluating our specific PE-regimen which features a comparatively low PV treated per session (0.7-fold) compared to previous publications, allowing daily treatments.

2. Methods

2.1. Patients

All patients who were treated with either PE or IA between 2013 and 2020 in the Department of Neurology, University of Ulm, were analysed. All clinical information including medical history, neurological status, adverse events, laboratory data, and clinical scales were collected by reviewing the complete medical records of each patient, including discharge letters, diagnostic findings, and monitoring documents. We included patients with all neurological diagnoses who received at least one treatment of PE or IA. Overall, 284 patients (65 PE, 219 IA) were identified. Because some patients received more than one cycle, 548 cycles (113 PE, 435 IA) were performed and analysed. Reasons for multiple cycles per patient included chronic diseases like CIDP which necessitate the application of multiple cycles in regular time intervals, or insufficient treatment response. One cycle consisted of 5 treatments, resulting in a total of 2740 treatments (565 PE, 2175 IA) which were separately documented and analysed.

All patients with MS fulfilled the 2017 MacDonald diagnostic criteria for MS [18] or CIS at the time of treatment. Patients with CIDP fulfilled the European Fedaration of Neurological Societies (EFNS) criteria for possible, probable, or definite CIDP. Patients with GBS showed the typical clinical picture including rapidly progressive bilateral limb weakness and sensory deficits, hypo-/areflexia, electrophysiological signs of demyelination, and increased protein levels in cerebrospinal fluid. Patients with other diseases were likewise diagnosed based on the respective internationally accepted guidelines.

2.2. Indication for PE/IA

All patients were treated in the Neurological Department of Ulm University, Neurological Center of Apheresis and Therapies (Neurologisches Apherese- und Therapiezentrum, NATZ). The decision to perform PE or IA was based on individual evaluation, taking into account diagnosis, clinical and diagnostic findings, and response to previous treatments. In patients with MS or clinically isolated syndrome (CIS), prerequisite for apheresis was the unsuccessful application of at least one cycle of high-dose intravenous methyl-prednisolone (MP). In cases of incomplete improvement, a second cycle of high-dose intravenous MP was performed in some patients. In CIDP, apheresis was only applied in therapy-refractory cases, i.e., patients who deteriorated despite MP and/or IVIg therapy (usually both). In case of a positive treatment effect, apheresis was applied in regular time intervals, based on the individual course of disease, i.e., PE/IA was performed when symptoms began to worsen again after the initial improvement. In GBS, apheresis was used as a first-line therapy as an alternative to

IVIg. In some cases, PE/IA was performed after an initial unsuccessful application of IVIg. In all other indications, apheresis was usually performed as an escalation therapy after unsatisfying response to the first-line/standard therapies. The decision for the specific method (PE or IA) was individually made based on current evidence, personal preference/experience, pathophysiological considerations, and comorbidities/contraindications in a process of shared decision-making after in-depth information of each individual patient about all therapeutic options. In 21 patients (8 MS, 2 CIDP, 3 GBS, and 8 other) PE was switched to IA, and in 22 patients (4 MS, 4 CIDP, 3 GBS, and 11 other) IA was switched to PE after one initial unsuccessful cycle.

2.3. Procedures

PE and IA were both applied on 5 consecutive days. The majority of patients received a Shaldon catheter in the right jugular vein. In patients who received several cycles over a prolonged period of time (mainly CIDP), a cubital arteriovenous shunt was used in a few cases. Heparin and citrate were used as anticoagulants, and no prophylactic antibiotics or post-procedural IVIg were given. Before each treatment, a systemic infection was ruled out by blood and urine analysis, and ACE inhibitors were paused at least 3 days before IA. Patients were extensively informed about risks as well as alternative treatment options and gave their written informed consent. During each treatment, a continuous monitoring was performed including blood pressure, heart rate, and oxygen saturation. Laboratory testing including blood count, CRP, electrolytes, liver, and kidney parameters were routinely done on a daily basis during PE/IA.

During PE, a fixed PV of 2 L (corresponding to a mean individual 0.7-fold PV) was exchanged until 07/2018; afterwards, we instead exchanged the 0.7-fold individual PV. Since comparative studies regarding different treatment regimens for PE/IA are completely lacking, these parameters are mainly based on local experience and expertise. A COM.TEC cell separator (Fresenius Kabi Deutschland GmbH, Bad Homburg, Germany) was used during PE.

During IA, the 2.0-fold individual plasma volume was processed on the first day, and the 2.5-fold individual plasma volume was processed on days 2–5. The individual plasma volume was calculated according to the formula published by Sprenger et al. [19]. Three different regenerable double-column adsorbers were used: protein A (Immunosorba, Fresenius Medical Care, Bad Homburg, Germany), Peptid-GAM (Globaffin, Fresenius Medical Care, Bad Homburg, Germany), and recombinant proteins (Miltenyi Biotec, Bergisch Gladbach, Germany). All three adsorbers selectively bind human immunoglobulins while largely sparing other plasma proteins. The choice of adsorber was mainly based on availability. ADAsorb (medicap clinic GmbH, Ulrichstein, Germany) and Life 21 (Miltenyi Biotec, Bergisch Gladbach, Germany) were used as immunoadsorption devices; COM.TEC (Fresenius Kabi Deutschland GmbH, Bad Homburg, Germany) and ART Universal (Fresenius Medical Care, Bad Homburg, Germany) were used for cell separation.

2.4. Outcome Parameters

Adverse events were retrospectively collected by reviewing the medical reports and monitoring curves of each patient and treatment. Laboratory changes were assessed based on daily laboratory reports. Adverse events were classified as Grade 1–5 according to the Common Terminology Criteria for Adverse Events grading scale v5.0.

Efficacy parameters before and after treatment were collected as documented in the medical reports. In patients with MS, these include the Expanded Disability Status Scale (EDSS) and the Multiple Sclerosis Functional Composite (MSFC) as the best validated and frequently used standardized clinical scales. In patients with CIDP, we routinely performed the CIDP score [20], which incorporates the Inflammatory Neuropathy Cause and Treatment (INCAT) score [21], the Oxford muscle strength grading score, and vibration sensitivity testing with a 256-Hz Ryder-Seiffel tuning fork. Since no generally accepted and adequately validated standardized scale exists for GBS, evaluation of efficacy in these patients was based on neurological examination before and after PE/IA and classified as large, partial, equivocal, or no improvement. For other indications, no systematic evaluation of efficacy was done due to low numbers of patients. Efficacy data refer to subgroups of patients with sufficient clinical data and have been published previously [5,20,22].

2.5. Statistical Analysis

Adverse events and laboratory changes were evaluated per cycle. Adverse events were additionally analysed on a per-patient basis in order to exclude bias based on the per-cycle approach (i.e., one patient may present one specific AE during multiple cycles, causing an overestimation of this AE). Statistical analysis was based on absolute/relative frequencies (categorial variables) and median/interquartile range (continuous variables). For evaluation of laboratory changes, we calculated the change between baseline and second day of PE/IA (not shown) as well as fifth day of PE/IA (before last treatment); we also recorded the share of cycles/patients with pathological values for each laboratory parameter.

Changes of patient related continuous data were investigated with the Wilcoxon signed rank test. Group comparisons for patient related continuous data were performed using the Mann–Whitney-U-test. Group comparisons for patient related categorical data were carried out with the chi-square test or Fisher's exact test as appropriate. Group comparisons for cycle related continuous data were investigated using linear mixed effects regression models in order to account for patients receiving multiple cycles. Group comparisons for cycle related binary data were investigated using mixed effects regression models for binary outcomes.

The level of significance was set as $p \leq 0.05$ (two-sided). To estimate treatment effects, we calculated median differences including a two-sided 95% confidence interval. Statistical analyses were done using SAS, version 9.4, and GraphPad Prism, version 7.05. Because of the explorative nature of this study, all results from statistical tests have to be interpreted as hypothesis-generating rather than proof of efficacy. No adjustment for multiple testing was done.

3. Results

3.1. Demographics and Clinical Characteristics

Demographic and clinical characteristics are depicted in Table 1. PE and IA patients were not different with regard to age, sex distribution, and body mass index (BMI). For more detailed clinical information for patients with the most common diagnoses (MS, CIDP, and GBS) see Tables S1–S3. Prognostic factors in patients with MS, CIDP, and GBS were evenly distributed between PE and IA.

Table 1. Baseline Characteristics.

	IA	PE	Total	p
Patients (cycles)	219 (435)	65 (113)	284 (548)	
Treatments per cycle	5	5		
Processed PV per treatment	2.0–2.5-fold	0.7-fold		
Age (years)	51.0 (36.0 to 62.0)	45.5 (34.5 to 63.0)	50.0 (36.0 to 62.0)	0.68
Sex				0.89
male	94 (42.9%)	27 (41.5%)	121 (42.6%)	
female	125 (57.1%)	38 (58.5%)	163 (57.4%)	
BMI (kg/m^2)	24.3 (21.8 to 27.8)	25.2 (21.6 to 27.5)	24.6 (21.8 to 27.8)	0.67
Diagnosis				
MS	72 (32.9%)	21 (32.3%)	93 (32.7%)	
CIS	28 (12.8%)	10 (15.4%)	38 (13.4%)	
NMOSD	3 (1.4%)	2 (3.1%)	5 (1.8%)	
AE	15 (6.8%)	2 (3.1%)	17 (6.0%)	
CIDP	30 (13.7%)	4 (6.2%)	34 (12.0%)	

Table 1. *Cont.*

	IA	PE	Total	*p*
GBS	17 (7.8%)	10 (15.4%)	27 (9.5%)	
MG	4 (1.8%)	0	4 (1.4%)	
SPS	3 (1.4%)	1 (1.5%)	4 (1.4%)	
SLE	1 (0.5%)	2 (3.1%)	3 (1.1%)	
Other	46 (21.0%)	12 (18.4%)	58 (20.4%)	

IA—immunoadsorption; PE—plasma exchange; PV—individual plasma volume; BMI—body mass index; MS—multiple sclerosis; CIS—clinically isolated syndrome; NMOSD—neuromyelitis optica spectrum disorder; AE—autoimmune encephalitis; CIDP—chronic inflammatory demyelinating polyneuropathy; GBS—Guillain–Barré syndrome; MG—myasthenia gravis; SPS—stiff person syndrome; SLE—systemic lupus erythematodes.

3.2. Adverse Events

Overall, both methods showed an excellent safety profile; no treatment-associated deaths or life-threatening adverse events were recorded. Severe AEs (corresponding to grade 3 on the Common Terminology Criteria for Adverse Events grading scale) in the IA group included three patients with sepsis, one severe pneumonia, and one pneumothorax, corresponding to 5/435 affected IA cycles (1.1%). In the PE group, no severe AEs were recorded.

Importantly, all three patients with sepsis were diagnosed with CIDP, two-thirds were older than 80 years and multimorbid. One patient had type 2 diabetes mellitus and recurrent urinary infections in medical history. Primary focus was the Shaldon catheter in all three cases. All patients recovered with antibiotic treatment. One severe pneumonia occurred in a 49 year old female with severe myasthenic crisis who was monitored on intensive care unit and dependent on non-invasive ventilation when IA was initiated; she eventually recovered. The pneumothorax (IA group) was a complication of Shaldon catheter placement and necessitated a Bülau drainage as well as a short stay on intensive care unit. The patient recovered completely and received several IA cycles afterwards without any further complications.

Surprisingly, we found that mild and moderate adverse events per cycle (grade 1 and 2; Table 2) were more frequent in the IA group (67.1%) compared to PE (35.4%; $p < 0.001$). With the exception of fatigue, all adverse events were more frequent in the IA group. Most common were intermittent hypotonia (24.0% of all patients), hematoma caused by Shaldon placement (16.4%), and mild infections (6.9%). All adverse events were uncomplicated and did not necessitate any specific therapy. Thrombotic events included deep venous thromboses, most commonly of the Shaldon-affected jugular vein, which were treated with oral anticoagulants and healed without permanent consequences in all cases. Thrombotic events were most frequently seen in patients with GBS.

Table 2. Adverse Events per Cycle.

Adverse Event	MS PE (n = 27)	MS IA (n = 100)	CIDP PE (n = 18)	CIDP IA (n = 80)	GBS PE (n = 15)	GBS IA (n = 22)	Overall PE (n = 113)	Overall IA (n = 435)	Total (n = 550)
Hypotonia	7.4	23.0	5.6	16.3	0.0	31.8	8.8	28.0	24.0
Hematoma (Shaldon)	3.7	18.0	16.7	6.3	13.3	9.1	11.5	17.7	16.4
Mild Infections	0.0	4.0	5.6	7.5	20.0	13.6	5.3	7.4	6.9
Technical Complications	0.0	6.0	0.0	7.5	0.0	13.6	0.8	5.7	4.7
Nausea	3.7	3.0	0.0	1.3	0.0	9.1	3.5	4.8	4.5
Tachycardia	0.0	3.0	0.0	7.5	13.3	4.5	1.8	4.6	4.0
Edema	0.0	3.0	0.0	3.8	0.0	4.5	0.0	4.8	3.8
Allergic Skin Reaction	0.0	10.0	5.6	2.5	0.0	4.5	0.8	4.6	3.8
Thrombosis	3.7	0.0	0.0	3.8	6.7	13.6	2.7	3.4	3.3
Thoracic Pain	0.0	3.0	0.0	1.3	0.0	13.6	0.8	3.9	3.3
Fatigue	0.0	0.0	5.6	1.3	6.7	0.0	3.5	1.1	1.6
Thrombosis	3.7	0.0	0.0	3.8	6.7	13.6	2.7	3.4	3.3

Data are %. Table presents all adverse events that occurred in >3% of patients in at least one of the treatment groups. IA—immunoadsorption; PE—plasma exchange; MS—Multiple Sclerosis; CIDP—Chronic Inflammatory Demyelinating Polyneuropathy; GBS—Guillain–Barré syndrome.

Per-patient analysis yielded similar results as per-cycle analysis (not shown). Albeit CIDP patients were older and had more co-morbidities compared to MS, we did not detect any meaningful disease-specific characteristics with regard to AEs.

3.3. Laboratory Changes

Median laboratory changes between the day of last treatment (before last treatment) compared to baseline of each cycle in both groups are displayed in Table 3. While loss of thrombocytes was more pronounced in IA, loss of erythrocytes was more pronounced in PE. IA patients showed larger decreases of potassium and calcium; sodium was rather stable in PE as well as IA. The substitution of proteins masks the assumedly larger loss of plasma proteins in PE compared to IA. Importantly, fibrinogen levels were similar in PE and IA. As described previously, we found that in the IA group IgG was removed more effectively than IgA and IgM; consistently, IgG reduction was more pronounced in IA, while IgA and IgM reduction were more pronounced in PE. Supplementing the absolute changes, Table 4 displays the share of patients above/below the pathological threshold for each laboratory parameter per group which yielded congruent results.

Table 3. Laboratory Changes.

Parameter	PE (n = 113)		IA (n = 435)		P
Leukocytes (G/L)	−0.3	(−1.6 to 0.9)	0.1	(−1.4 to 1.3)	0.98
Erythrocytes (T/L)	−0.55	(−0.72 to −0.21)	−0.35	(−0.59 to −0.14)	**<0.001**
Hemoglobin (g/L)	−15	(−23 to −8)	−10	(−17 to −4)	**<0.001**
Hematocrit (%)	−4	(−2 to −6)	−3	(−1 to −5)	**<0.001**
Thrombocytes (G/L)	−53	(−90 to −26)	−91	(−128 to −55)	**<0.001**
MPV(fL)	0.1	(−0.3 to 0.4)	0.4	(0.1 to 0.8)	**<0.001**
Quick (%)	−24	(−37 to −12)	−10	(−39 to 2)	0.18
INR	0.13	(0.07 to 0.44)	0.06	(−0.01 to 0.37)	0.66
pTT (s)	11.6	(4.6 to 32.3)	6.5	(3.1 to 26.0)	0.52
Fibrinogen (g/L)	−1.7	(−1.9 to −0.1)	−1.6	(−3.4 to −0.8)	0.96
Sodium (mmol/L)	1	(−1 to 3)	2	(1 to 4)	**0.003**
Potassium (mmol/L)	−0.23	(−0.60 to 0.08)	−0.47	(−0.77 to −0.17)	**<0.001**
Calcium (mmol/L)	0.02	(−0.08 to 0.10)	−0.17	(−0.25 to −0.06)	**<0.001**
Urea (mmol/L)	−0.12	(−0.98 to 0.76)	−0.94	(−2.14 to 0.05)	**0.019**
Creatinine (µmol/L)	−1.5	(−8.5 to 1.8)	2	(−5.5 to 8)	**0.002**
GFR (ml/min)	2.0	(−3.5 to 10.5)	−2.5	(−13 to 7.3)	**0.002**
AST (U/L)	9.0	(−6.25 to 13.8)	1.0	(−4.0 to 10.0)	0.98
ALT (U/L)	−6.0	(−13.0 to 7.0)	−3.5	(−9.3 to 9.0)	0.85
GGT (U/L)	−17.0	(−27.5 to −12.0)	−9.0	(−22.0 to −4.0)	0.92
AP (U/L)	−39.0	(−43.0 to −26.0)	−19.0	(−30.3 to −12.0)	**0.03**
Bilirubin (µmol/L)	3.5	(0.5 to 5.3)	0.1	(−2.4 to 11.4)	0.09
Protein (g/L)	−5.9 *	(−9.4 to −1.8)	−19.9	(−23.9 to −15.8)	**<0.001**
CRP (mg/L)	0.08	(−1.02 to 1.40)	0.81	(−0.28 to 3.81)	0.23
IgA (mg/L)[#]	−866	(−572 to −1100)	−1362	(−1197 to −1536)	**<0.001**
IgG (mg/L)[#]	−6639	(−5428 to −7367)	−5770	(−5562 to −6582)	**<0.001**
IgM (mg/L)[#]	−711	(−316 to −924)	−713	(−324 to −1066)	**0.008**

Median laboratory changes (IQR) between the day of last treatment compared to baseline of each cycle in both groups. IA—immunoadsorption; PE—plasma exchange; MPV—mean platelet volume; INR—international normalized ratio; pTT—partial thromboplastin time; GFR—glomerular filtration rate; AST—aspartate aminotransferase; ALT—alanine aminotransferase; GGT—gamma glutamyl transferase; AP—alkaline phosphatase; CRP—C-reactive protein; * after substitution with human albumin solution; [#] Immunoglobulins A, G, and M were measured in a subset of 61 MS patients who participated in a randomized controlled study [5]. Bold p-values mark significant values.

Table 4. Pathological Laboratory Parameters at Last Day of Apheresis (Before Last Treatment).

Parameter	PE (n = 113)	IA (n = 435)	p
Leukocytes (G/L)	18.3%	19.0%	0.64
Erythrocytes (T/L)	53.9%	38.5%	**0.05**
Hemoglobin (g/L)	58.7%	46.0%	0.08
Hematocrit (%)	54.8%	45.8%	0.09
Thrombocytes (G/L)	12.6%	41.5%	**<0.001**
MPV(fL)	4.9%	6.1%	0.46
Quick (%)	44.8%	37.5%	0.15
INR	90.0%	91.0%	0.82
pTT (s)	78.6%	79.9%	0.85
Fibrinogen (g/L)	80.0%	66.7%	0.82
Sodium (mmol/L)	5.8%	0.3%	0.13
Potassium (mmol/L)	9.7%	27.0%	**0.001**
Calcium (mmol/L)	5.2%	17.8%	0.11
Urea (mmol/L)	8.3%	7.1%	0.90
Creatinine (µmol/L)	23.4%	28.1%	0.80
GFR (ml/min)	85.3%	82.6%	0.42
AST (U/L)	33.3%	23.8%	0.07
ALT (U/L)	18.2%	20.6%	0.49
GGT (U/L)	0.0%	15.7%	0.15
AP (U/L)	100.0%	88.5%	0.64
Bilirubin (µmol/L)	16.7%	11.4%	0.52
Protein (g/L)	92.0%*	99.1%	**0.004**
CRP (mg/L)	24.5%	40.3%	0.23

Share of patients with values below or above the pathological threshold for each parameter at last day of apheresis in each group. IA—immunoadsorption; PE—plasma exchange; MPV—mean platelet volume; INR—international normalized ratio; pTT—partial thromboplastin time; GFR—glomerular filtration rate; AST—aspartate aminotransferase; ALT—alanine aminotransferase; GGT—gamma glutamyl transferase; AP—alkaline phosphatase; CRP—C-reactive protein; * after substitution with human albumin solution. Bold p-values mark significant values.

3.4. Efficacy

Efficacy data for patients with sufficient standardized data have previously been published. These data refer to subsets of the study population investigated in the current study and were treated with the same IA and PE protocols.

In steroid-refractory MS, we conducted a randomized controlled trial in 61 patients (31 IA vs. 30 PE, 5 treatments on 5 consecutive days as outlined above) [5]. We found a significant improvement of symptoms after four weeks compared to pre-treatment in both groups as measured by MSFC and EDSS. In the PE group, median MSFC improved from 0.22 (−0.27 to 0.55) to 0.57 (0.15 to 0.82; $p < 0.001$), and median EDSS improved from 3.0 (2.0 to 3.5) to 2.0 (1.0 to 3.5; $p < 0.001$). In the IA group, median MSFC improved from 0.09 (−0.19 to 0.39) to 0.63 (0.21 to 0.90; $p < 0.001$), and median EDSS improved from 3.0 (2.0 to 4.0) to 2.0 (1.0 to 3.1; $p < 0.001$). Although improvement started earlier in the PE group, MSFC improvement (0.385 vs. 0.265; $p = 0.03$) and response rates (86.7% vs. 76.7%) after four weeks were larger in the IA group.

In CIDP, we performed a prospective observational study in 17 patients with therapy-refractory courses (insufficient response to steroids and/or IVIg) who underwent IA [20]. Overall, median CIDP scores improved from 308.0 (266.0 to 374.5) pre-treatment to 330.0 (290.0 to 393.5; $p = 0.02$) after two weeks. Furthermore, we were able to stabilize disease progression in 6/7 patients who received long-term IA treatments in regular intervals. Before IA, these patients lost 6.7 (3.0 to 13.1) points of CIDP score per month, while during IA, they lost 0.1 (0.0 to 0.8) points. Due to the insufficient number of patients treated with PE, we cannot provide any comparative results.

A retrospective analysis of 20 patients with GBS [22] yielded response rates of 61.5% for IA and 71.4% for PE after the last treatment based on the documented neurological examinations.

4. Discussion

This study aimed at evaluating safety and tolerability of PE and IA as main options of apheresis in autoimmune-mediated neurological diseases. Pre-existing evidence suggested that IA may be superior to PE in this regard, although comparative studies with high numbers of patients are missing. For this purpose, we analysed data from 284 patients (548 cycles, 2740 treatments) who were treated with either PE or IA between 2013 and 2020 in our center under standardized conditions. Importantly, we used an adjusted protocol for PE, aiming for a comparatively small volume of exchanged plasma volume per day (0.7-fold individual PV per day) compared to other commonly used regimens which imply higher volumes (1.0–1.5-fold individual PV per day). This protocol is based on our own clinical experience, including a randomized controlled trial in MS [5] which suggested an excellent safety and good efficacy profile for this specific regimen. The retrospective nature of this study has to be mentioned as a limitation, since we cannot exclude that AEs occurred or diagnoses changed after discharge. We regard the high number of treatments under standardized, monocentric conditions and the continuous, systematic recording of safety data as strengths of this study.

Overall, we found that both methods were very safe across all neurological indications, since we did not record any life-threatening complications or deaths, and grade 3 AEs were recorded in only 1.1% of IA cycles while in PE, we did not record any grade 3 AEs. Therefore, the incidence of serious AEs was even rarer in PE compared to IA. Surprisingly, we found that the share of mild and moderate AEs, including thrombosis, hypotonia, allergic reactions, nausea, and vegetative symptoms were also lower in PE which contradicts the common conception of IA as a better tolerated method of apheresis. However, a closer look at current literature reveals that this question has not been conclusively answered as highlighted by several studies in MS [6,8] as well as a recent meta-analysis [10] which found similar incidences of adverse events. The generally favourable safety profile of both PE and IA should also be considered when weighing against alternative treatment options, for example whether a second high-dose MP cycle should be performed in steroid-refractory MS relapse before apheresis. As highlighted by a recent publication [23], sparing a second MP cycle and applying apheresis directly may be superior in terms of efficacy and safety.

Data about complication rates of PE are heterogenous, varying between 4.2% and 25.6% [13,24–26], most likely due to heterogenous treatment regimens with regard to PV treated per session, type and dosage of applied anticoagulants, type of venous access (peripheral or central), and type of volume substitution (human albumin or FFP). Basic-Jukic et al. found moderate allergic reactions in 1.6% of 509 patients treated with PE as well as severe anaphylactic reactions in five cases; accordingly, Schneider-Gold et al. found a higher incidence of allergic reactions in patients with myasthenia gravis treated with PE compared to IA [11]. However, the incidence of allergic reactions in PE may presumably be lowered by using human albumin solution instead of FFP, since allergic reactions are commonly associated with FFP [27], but very rarely with human albumin solution [28]. Accordingly, the incidence of allergic reactions was extremely low in our PE study population (0.8%), and lower compared to IA (4.6%). Since no volume substitution is needed in IA, the higher incidence of allergic reactions in IA may be associated with the higher amounts of anticoagulants needed for IA, especially heparin. Furthermore, it cannot be ruled out completely that adsorber substances may be reinfused.

Importantly, in order to utilize the advantageous safety profile of human albumin solution compared to FFP in PE, it is essential to limit fibrinogen loss by either reducing the frequency of treatments (i.e., performing treatments on a two-day instead of a daily basis) or reducing the PV processed during each treatment. Based on our data, it was possible to perform daily PE treatments with 0.7-fold PV without any treatment interruptions while maintaining acceptable fibrinogen plasma levels, i.e., fibrinogen levels remained above 0.8 g/L before each treatment. Applying this scheme, we found comparable fibrinogen levels in PE and IA, suggesting that (1) fibrinogen loss in PE can be sufficiently controlled by attenuating PV per treatment, and (2) significant loss of fibrinogen is also present in IA. In line with our finding of similar and acceptable fibrinogen levels in both PE and IA, we did not record any bleeding complications with both measures, while the incidence of thrombotic events was similar (2.7% in PE, 3.4% in IA). Therefore, we can conclude that maintaining higher fibrinogen levels during PE may contribute to improve safety, since bleeding complications have previously been described to occur more frequently in PE (3.1% of treatments) compared to IA (1.3%) [15].

In addition to allergic reactions and bleeding complications, infections induced by the immune-modulating effects of PE/IA are a major concern. Based on our data, both measures were very safe in this regard. We found severe infections with consecutive sepsis in three patients who were all diagnosed with CIDP; two of them were >80 years old. Therefore, we conclude that these clinical characteristics constitute risk factors which have to be considered. Mild infections occurred in only 5.3% (PE) and 7.4% (IA), respectively. These data corroborate the conception that peri-procedural prophylactic application of antibiotics or immunoglobulins is not needed. We could not confirm the finding of Schneider-Gold et al. who found a higher frequency of respiratory infections in PE compared to IA [11]. Again, different treatment regimens (0.7-fold vs. up to 1.5-fold PV treated in PE patients) do most likely account for this discrepancy, since treating lower PVs per session implies a higher preservation of antibodies and other anti-infective plasma proteins. Accordingly, we found that overall reduction rates of immunoglobulins were about similar in PE and IA; regarding subclasses, we found that reduction rates of IgA and IgM were higher in PE, while reduction rate of IgG was higher in IA. This was expected since the applied IA adsorbers feature a higher IgG affinity [29].

Regarding mild adverse events such as hypotonia, nausea, and palpitations, we generally found higher incidences in the IA group. This finding is not necessarily caused by technical differences of PE and IA, but may simply be explained by the significantly prolonged treatment times in IA. Applying the treatment regimens outlined above and dependent on the patient's individual PV, one IA treatment requires about the double amount of time compared to PE due to the excessive amount of blood treated during each session. Apart from the higher incidence of adverse events which are associated with longer treatment times, this also implies a larger burden for the patient.

Subclinical laboratory changes were unproblematic in all cases and did not necessitate specific treatment, with the exception of potassium and protein substitution which are routinely done in PE as well as IA. Interestingly, we found a higher incidence of anemia in PE, but a higher incidence of thrombopenia in IA, confirming previous findings [5]. The latter may possibly be explained by the higher demand for heparin during IA, since the external blood circuit has to be maintained for a longer timeframe and heparin may cause heparin-induced thrombopenia (HIT). While cell count abnormalities can be contributed to the procedures themselves, changes of plasma constituents like liver transaminases or urea do not necessarily imply organic disturbances, but rather signify that these substances are removed by the procedures. Regarding electrolytes, hypokalemia and hypocalcemia (due to citrate binding) are both known phenomena in PE and IA. In our study electrolyte disturbances were more frequent in the IA group.

Despite the lower incidence of AEs and laboratory abnormalities found for the low-PV PE treatment regimen compared to IA, this finding has to be interpreted carefully because of the following limitations of this study: First, the safety profile was compared with IA, which is quite a novel therapeutic approach itself, especially with regard to neurological diseases. A superiority of our PE regimen compared to other commonly applied regimens can however only be proven by conducting a direct comparative prospective study. Secondly, lowering the PV treated each day may compromise the efficacy of the procedure, which cannot be adequately analysed by means of a retrospective study design. We investigated the efficacy of this approach in a randomized controlled study in patients with steroid-refractory MS relapse versus IA [5]. Indeed, we found that after four weeks, IA patients showed a significantly larger improvement of the MSFC; however, the difference between PE and IA was rather small.

In summary, we conclude that:

1. PE and IA constitute safe and generally well-tolerated therapeutic options in autoimmune-mediated neurological diseases.

2. Contrary to previous publications, we found a lower incidence of adverse events in the PE group—possibly due to the low-volume per treatment regimen (0.7-fold PV per day), which allows to use human albumin solution while maintaining sufficient fibrinogen levels.

3. Safety and efficacy of this specific PE treatment regimen have to be further evaluated by means of a directly comparative, prospective study.

4. This study highlights the importance to consider specific treatment regimens with regard to safety and efficacy in general when assessing apheresis studies.

Author Contributions: Conceptualization, J.D. (Johannes Dorst); data curation, J.D. (Johannes Dorst) and F.F.; formal analysis, J.D. (Johannes Dorst), F.F., and J.D. (Jens Dreyhaupt); investigation, J.D. (Johannes Dorst) and F.F.; methodology, J.D. (Johannes Dorst), F.F., and J.D. (Jens Dreyhaupt); project administration, J.D. (Johannes Dorst); resources, J.D. (Johannes Dorst), M.S., and H.T.; supervision, J.D. (Johannes Dorst); validation, J.D. (Johannes Dorst), F.F., J.D. (Jens Dreyhaupt), M.S., and H.T.; visualization, J.D. (Johannes Dorst); writing—original draft, J.D. (Johannes Dorst); writing—review and editing, J.D. (Johannes Dorst), F.F., J.D. (Jens Dreyhaupt), M.S., and H.T.; and funding acquisition, N/A. All authors have read and agreed to the published version of the manuscript.

Acknowledgments: The authors would like to thank Helmut Lehner and his team for their excellent care for the patients in our Neurological Center of Apheresis and Therapies (NATZ).

References

1. Baggi, F.; Ubiali, F.; Nava, S.; Nessi, V.; Andreetta, F.; Rigamonti, A.; Maggi, L.; Mantegazza, R.; Antozzi, C. Effect of IgG immunoadsorption on serum cytokines in MG and LEMS patients. *J. Neuroimmunol.* **2008**, *201–202*, 104–110. [CrossRef] [PubMed]

2. Trebst, C.; Bronzlik, P.; Kielstein, J.T.; Schmidt, B.M.; Stangel, M. Immunoadsorption therapy for steroid-unresponsive relapses in patients with multiple sclerosis. *Blood Purificat.* **2012**, *33*, 1–6. [CrossRef] [PubMed]

3. Belak, M.; Borberg, H.; Jimenez, C.; Oette, K. Technical and clinical experience with protein A immunoadsorption columns. *Transfus. Sci.* **1994**, *15*, 419–422. [CrossRef]

4. Hohenstein, B.; Passauer, J.; Ziemssen, T.; Julius, U. Immunoadsorption with regenerating systems in neurological disorders –A single center experience. *Atheroscler. Suppl.* **2015**, *18*, 119–123. [CrossRef] [PubMed]

5. Dorst, J.; Fangerau, T.; Taranu, D.; Eichele, P.; Dreyhaupt, J.; Michels, S.; Schuster, J.; Ludolph, A.C.; Senel, M.; Tumani, H. Safety and efficacy of immunoadsorption versus plasma exchange in steroid-refractory relapse of multiple sclerosis and clinically isolated syndrome: A randomised, parallel-group, controlled trial. *EClinicalMedicine* **2019**, *16*, 98–106. [CrossRef]

6. Muhlhausen, J.; Kitze, B.; Huppke, P.; Muller, G.A.; Koziolek, M.J. Apheresis in treatment of acute inflammatory demyelinating disorders. *Atheroscler. Suppl.* **2015**, *18*, 251–256. [CrossRef]

7. Schimrigk, S.; Faiss, J.; Köhler, W.; Günther, A.; Harms, L.; Kraft, A.; Ehrlich, S.; Eberl, A.; Fassbender, C.; Klingel, R.; et al. Escalation therapy of steroid refractory multiple sclerosis relapse with tryptophan immunoadsorption - Observational multicenter study with 147 patients. *Eur. Neurol.* **2016**, *75*, 300–306. [CrossRef]

8. Lipphardt, M.; Muhlhausen, J.; Kitze, B.; Heigl, F.; Mauch, E.; Helms, H.-J.; Müller, G.A.; Koziolek, M.J. Immunoadsorption or plasma exchange in steroid-refractory multiple sclerosis and neuromyelitis optica. *J. Clin. Apher.* **2019**, *30*, 381–391. [CrossRef]

9. Weinshenker, B.G.; O'Brien, P.C.; Petterson, T.M.; Noseworthy, J.H.; Lucchinetti, C.F.; Dodick, D.W.; Pineda, A.A.; Stevens, L.N.; Rodriguez, M. A randomized trial of plasma exchange in acute central nervous system inflammatory demyelinating disease. *Ann. Neurol.* **1999**, *46*, 878–886. [CrossRef]

10. Lipphardt, M.; Wallbach, M.; Koziolek, M.J. Plasma exchange or immunoadsorption in demyelinating diseases: A meta-analysis. *J. Clin. Med.* **2020**, *9*, 1597. [CrossRef]

11. Schneider-Gold, C.; Krenzer, M.; Klinker, E.; Mansouri-Thalegani, B.; Müllges, W.; Toyka, K.V.; Gold, R. Immunoadsorption versus plasma exchange versus combination for treatment of myasthenic deterioration. *Ther. Adv. Neurol. Disord.* **2016**, *9*, 297–303. [CrossRef] [PubMed]

12. Kohler, W.; Bucka, C.; Klingel, R. A randomized and controlled study comparing immunoadsorption and plasma exchange in myasthenic crisis. *J. Clin. Apher.* **2011**, *26*, 347–355. [CrossRef] [PubMed]

13.   Bramlage, C.P.; Schröder, K.; Bramlage, P.; Ahrens, K.; Zapf, A.; Müller, G.A.; Koziolek, M.J. Predictors of complications in therapeutic plasma exchange. *J. Clin. Apher.* **2009**, *24*, 225–231. [CrossRef] [PubMed]

14.   Basic-Jukic, N.; Kes, P.; Glavas-Boras, S.; Brunetta, B.; Bubic-Filipi, L.; Puretic, Z. Complications of therapeutic plasma exchange: Experience with 4857 treatments. *Ther. Apher. Dial.* **2005**, *9*, 391–395. [CrossRef]

15.   Zöllner, S.; Pablik, E.; Druml, W.; Derfler, K.; Rees, A.; Biesenbach, P. Fibrinogen reduction and bleeding complications in plasma exchange, immunoadsorption and a combination of the two. *Blood Purif.* **2014**, *38*, 160–166. [CrossRef]

16.   Lieker, I.; Slowinski, T.; Harms, L.; Hahn, K.; Klehmet, J. A prospective study comparing tryptophan immunoadsorption with therapeutic plasma exchange for the treatment of chronic inflammatory demyelinating polyneuropathy. *J. Clin. Apher.* **2017**, *32*, 486–493. [CrossRef]

17.   Marn Pernat, A.; Buturovic-Ponikvar, J.; Svigelj, V.; Ponikvar, R. Guillain-Barre syndrome treated by membrane plasma exchange and/or immunoadsorption. *Ther. Apher. Dial.* **2009**, *13*, 310–313. [CrossRef]

18.   Thompson, A.J.; Banwell, B.L.; Barkhof, F.; Carroll, W.M.; Coetzee, T.; Comi, G.; Correale, J.; Fazekas, F.; Filippi, M.; Freedman, M.S.; et al. Diagnosis of multiple sclerosis: 2017 revisions of the McDonald criteria. *Lancet Neurol.* **2018**, *17*, 162–173. [CrossRef]

19.   Sprenger, K.B.; Huber, K.; Kratz, W.; Henze, E. Nomograms for the prediction of patient's plasma volume in plasma exchange therapy from height, weight, and hematocrit. *J. Clin. Apher.* **1987**, *3*, 185–190. [CrossRef]

20.   Dorst, J.; Ludolph, A.C.; Senel, M.; Tumani, H. Short-term and long-term effects of immunoadsorption in refractory chronic inflammatory demyelinating polyneuropathy: A prospective study in 17 patients. *J. Neurol.* **2018**, *265*, 2906–2915. [CrossRef]

21.   Merkies, I.S.; Schmitz, P.I.; van der Meche, F.G.; Samijn, J.P.; van Doorn, P.A. Clinimetric evaluation of a new overall disability scale in immune mediated polyneuropathies. *J. Neurol. Neurosurg. Psychiatry* **2002**, *72*, 596–601. [CrossRef] [PubMed]

22.   Davies, A.J.; Fehmi, J.; Senel, M.; Tumani, H.; Dorst, J.; Rinaldi, S. Immunoadsorption and plasma exchange in seropositive and seronegative immune-mediated neuropathies. *J. Clin. Med.* **2020**, *9*, 2025. [CrossRef] [PubMed]

23.   Pfeuffer, S.; Rolfes, L.; Bormann, E.; Sauerland, C.; Ruck, T.; Schilling, M.; Melzer, N.; Brand, M.; Pul, R.; Kleinschnitz, C.; et al. Comparing plasma exchange to escalated methyl prednisolone in refractory multiple sclerosis relapses. *J. Clin. Med.* **2020**, *9*, 35. [CrossRef] [PubMed]

24.   Mokrzycki, M.H.; Kaplan, A.A. Therapeutic plasma exchange: Complications and management. *Am. J. Kidney Dis.* **1994**, *23*, 817–827. [CrossRef]

25.   Samtleben, W.; Blumenstein, M.; Liebl, L.; Gurland, H.J. Membrane plasma separation for treatment of immunologically mediated diseases. *Trans. Am. Soc. Artif. Intern. Organs* **1980**, *26*, 12–16.

26.   Sprenger, K.B.; Rasche, H.; Franz, H.E. Membrane plasma separation: Complications and monitoring. *Artif. Organs* **1984**, *8*, 360–363.

27.   Pandey, S.; Vyas, G.N. Adverse effects of plasma transfusion. *Transfusion* **2012**, *52* (Suppl. 1), 65S–79S. [CrossRef]

28.   Vincent, J.L.; Wilkes, M.M.; Navickis, R.J. Safety of human albumin—serious adverse events reported worldwide in 1998-2000. *Br. J. Anaesth.* **2003**, *91*, 625–630. [CrossRef]

29.   Gjörstrup, P.; Watt, R.M. Therapeutic protein A immunoadsorption. A review. *Transfus. sci.* **1990**, *11*, 281–302. [CrossRef]

13

Wearable Electronics Assess the Effectiveness of Transcranial Direct Current Stimulation on Balance and Gait in Parkinson's Disease Patients

Mariachiara Ricci [1], Giulia Di Lazzaro [2], Antonio Pisani [2], Simona Scalise [2], Mohammad Alwardat [2], Chiara Salimei [2], Franco Giannini [1] and Giovanni Saggio [1,*]

[1]   Department of Electronic Engineering, University of Rome "Tor Vergata", 00133 Rome, Italy; rccmch01@uniroma2.it (M.R.); giannini@ing.uniroma2.it (F.G.)
[2]   Department of Systems Medicine, University of Rome "Tor Vergata", 00133 Rome, Italy; giulia.dilazzaro@students.uniroma2.eu (G.D.L.); pisani@uniroma2.it (A.P.); simona.scalise@alumni.uniroma2.eu (S.S.); mohammadsamimohammad.alwardat.alwardatmohammad01@alumni.uniroma2.eu (M.A.); chiara.salimei@alumni.uniroma2.eu (C.S.)
*   Correspondence: saggio@uniroma2.it

Abstract: Currently, clinical evaluation represents the primary outcome measure in Parkinson's disease (PD). However, clinical evaluation may underscore some subtle motor impairments, hidden from the visual inspection of examiners. Technology-based objective measures are more frequently utilized to assess motor performance and objectively measure motor dysfunction. Gait and balance impairments, frequent complications in later disease stages, are poorly responsive to classic dopamine-replacement therapy. Although recent findings suggest that transcranial direct current stimulation (tDCS) can have a role in improving motor skills, there is scarce evidence for this, especially considering the difficulty to objectively assess motor function. Therefore, we used wearable electronics to measure motor abilities, and further evaluated the gait and balance features of 10 PD patients, before and (three days and one month) after the tDCS. To assess patients' abilities, we adopted six motor tasks, obtaining 72 meaningful motor features. According to the obtained results, wearable electronics demonstrated to be a valuable tool to measure the treatment response. Meanwhile the improvements from tDCS on gait and balance abilities of PD patients demonstrated to be generally partial and selective.

Keywords: balance; gait; Parkinson's disease; transcranial direct current stimulation; wearable electronics; IMUs

1. Introduction

Wearable electronics are gaining increasing attention and importance as a valid tool for healthcare practitioners in medical treatment [1–3] and patient monitoring [4–6]. In particular, wearable sensors have been applied for assessing the motor performance of patients with neurodegenerative disorders, as it is for Parkinson's disease, in both home and clinical environments [7–12].

Parkinson's disease (PD) can be characterized by motor deficiencies, such as bradykinesia and a combination of rest tremor, rigidity, as well as gait and balance impairment [13]. In routine clinical care, the evaluation of those deficiencies is mainly based on severity-rating standardized scales, such as the Movement Disorder Society Unified Parkinson's disease rating scale (MDS-UPDRS) [14], based on patients' reports and clinicians' vision-based evaluations, and clinical investigators determine the effectiveness of a therapy of a drug by using the MDS-UPDRS score [15]. Inconveniently, patient reports can be affected by mood and unfamiliarity with forms, and clinicians' evaluations can be biased by personal beliefs, experiences, and a priori expectations, resulting in inter- and intra-rater score variability [15,16]. Furthermore, the MDS-UPDRS is quantified according to a discrete scale (0–4, unity step) only, and the human eyes of clinicians hardly detect subtle motor changes during the monitoring of patients. These limitations compel investigators to employ more rigorous, and thus costly, clinical trial designs, with a random assignment of patients, thus blinding investigators to treatment assignment.

The aforementioned limitations can be in some way reduced or overcome through the use of wearable inertial sensors (hereafter wearables), which provide measures of human postures and kinematics, paving the way for objective assessment in clinical trials [17]. In fact, wearables can gather motion parameters in a continuous (analog) or high-step density (digital) scale, and avoid intra- and inter-rater variability, thereby reducing the sample size and simplifying the assessment of the patients, objectively quantifying a possible beneficial effect of a therapeutic intervention. For this reason, even if wearables are still poorly used (only 2.7% of ongoing clinical trials [15]), there is growing attention given to this technological tool, and some pharmaceutical companies are working to develop their own devices [18–20].

Our work approaches the utilization of wearables in the particular case of objectively demonstrating the therapeutic beneficial effects, if any, of transcranial direct current stimulation (tDCS) treatment on the motor impairments of patients affected by Parkinson's disease.

The proven appeal of tDCS is evident as it is a non-invasive, inexpensive, painless brain stimulation technique with many clinical and research applications, ranging from the treatment of depression to neurorehabilitation [21,22]. It consists of applying a direct positive (anodal) or negative (cathodal) 1–2 mA current to the scalp. This stimulation supports the depolarization or hyperpolarization of neurons, thus leading them closer to, or farther away from firing, acting on synaptic transmission or synaptic plasticity [21,23]. Further, tDCS has been used alternatively to (or sometimes concurrently with) dopaminergic drug therapy, because the latter can lose its efficacy during the natural course of the disease, in particular regarding its benefit on postural and gait disorders. Gait is now considered a higher level of cognitive function that involves the integration of attention, planning, memory and other motor, perceptual and cognitive processes. In fact, walking and balance constitute a combination of automatic movement processes, afferent information processing, and intentional adjustments that require a delicate balance between various interacting neuronal systems. In PD, to compensate the loss of motor task, cognitive resources as attention and executive function performed by the dorsolateral pre-frontal cortex (DLPFC) plays a critical role in the relief of gait disorder [24]. In addition, previous studies have shown that anodal tDCS stimulation to either the motor area (M1) or dorsolateral prefrontal cortex (DLPFC) had a significant impact on the motor, non-motor, and balance functional outcomes in PD patients. In fact, brain activation patterns in M1 and DLPFC are extremely involved in successful locomotion performance in patients with PD [21,25–27]. Further, the effectiveness of tDCS for alleviating gait and postural instability seems promising [28–31], however, evidence of its benefit remains unclear and controversial [23,32] because different tDCS protocols and target areas of scalp have been considered, leading to conflicting evidence on MDS-UPDRS scores [23,28].

Our work aims to objectively quantify the motor performance improvements, if any, due to tDCS treatment in a population of patients with PD and gait disturbances. To this aim, we used wearables to measure specific motor tasks, and analyzed the related results by means of the standardized response mean (SRM) index, comparing them with those obtained by the clinical evaluation.

2. Materials and Methods

2.1. Subjects

Ten PD patients (Table 1) with postural and gait disturbances were recruited at Tor Vergata University Hospital, Rome, Italy. Idiopathic PD was diagnosed according to the MDS clinical diagnostic criteria for PD [13], and patients were enrolled at Hoehn & Yahr disease stages between 1.5

and 4, and with MDS-UPDRS III scores related to a gait higher than 1. Exclusion criteria were age (younger than 30 or older than 85), dementia (mini mental status evaluation, MMSE, score < 24 [33]), therapy changes in the last three months, orthopedic comorbidities, other neurological disorders, and therapy with drugs possibly interfering with motor function (e.g., antipsychotics).

Table 1. Patients' information.

Age	77.2 ± 6.3 y
Gender	7 M, 3 F
Disease duration	10.37 ± 3.8 y
MDS-UPDRS II	15.6 ± 3.66
MDS-UPDRS III	35.2 ± 5.63
Hoehn & Yahr	2.9 ± 0.16
Levodopa equivalent daily dose	771.7 ± 213.58 mg

This study was conducted in agreement with the ethical principles of the Helsinki declaration. Informed consent was obtained from each participant and ethical approval was obtained by the local committee (RS 190/18). Patients consented to participate and did not change the therapy during the study, from T0 to T2 (Figure 2), in order to minimize any alteration of motor performance due to dopaminergic therapy variations.

2.2. Motor Tests

We requested each participant to perform six motor tasks which, according to clinical standards, are relevant for a comprehensive evaluation of balance and gait. Tasks included stance feet together (SFT), tandem stance (TS), the pull test (PT), timed up and go test (TUG), stop and go test (S&G), and narrow walking test (NW). In particular, SFT and TS are useful to test balance; PT corresponds to the item 3.12 of MDS-UPDRS III to test postural response; TUG, S&G and NW are used to assess mobility and gait. Wearables were placed by means of Velcro strips on segments of the body, according to the particular test, as schematized in Figure 1. The descriptions of the tests and corresponding placements of the wearable sensors are specified in the following.

2.2.1. Stance Feet Together (SFT) and Tandem Stance (TS)

In SFT and TS tests, the patient has to stand and maintain the posture for 30 s. More particularly, in the SFT with feet side-by-side and close together, in TS with feet in tandem position (i.e., one ahead, aligned and close to the other). The wearables were placed on the posterior trunk at the level of T5 and on the external parts of the calf segments of both legs.

2.2.2. Pull Test (PT)

The subject, comfortably standing upright with shoulders to the examiner, is rapidly and vigorously pushed backward on his/her shoulders so as to be forced to make one, or more, steps backwards, recovering his/her balance. The sensors were placed as for SFT and TS.

2.2.3. Timed Up and Go (TUG)

The subject starts seated on a straight-backed chair with arms across the chest, then gets up, walks straight 6 m, turns around, walks straight back and, turning on his/her-self, sits down returning to the initial condition. The sensors were placed on the patient's pelvis at the level of L5, posterior trunk at the level of T5, on the external parts of thighs and calf segments of both lower limbs, arms, and forearms.

2.2.4. Stop and Go (S&G)

The subject walks for six meters in a straight line, turns around, walks six meters back while the examiner tells him/her to stop and go for 6 times. The sensors were placed on the patient's pelvis at L5 level, posterior trunk at T5 level, on the external parts of thighs and calf segments of both lower limbs. The time, when the examiner tells the patient to stop was recorded.

2.2.5. Narrow Walking (NW)

The subject walks 6 m straight, but passing through a 70 cm narrow door in the middle of the path. The sensors were placed on the patient's pelvis at L5 level, posterior trunk at T5 level, on the external parts of thighs, and calf segments of both lower limbs. The time, the time when the patient passes through the door was recorded.

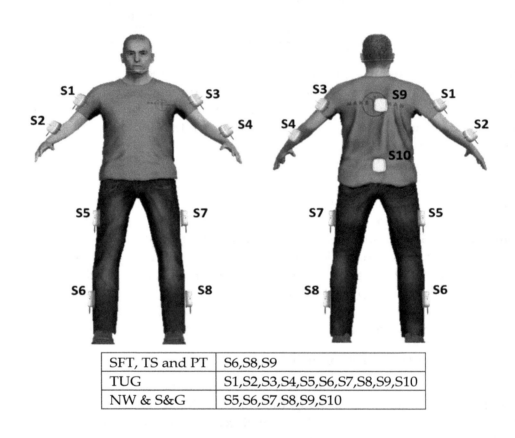

SFT, TS and PT	S6,S8,S9
TUG	S1,S2,S3,S4,S5,S6,S7,S8,S9,S10
NW & S&G	S5,S6,S7,S8,S9,S10

Figure 1. Sensors, labeled from S1 to S10, as located on the body of the patients. Different motor tests resulted with a different number of used sensors.

2.3. tDCS Stimulation

Direct current (DC) was delivered to stimulate the left dorsolateral-prefrontal cortex (DLPFC) by means of a tDCS low-intensity stimulator (BrainStim, EMS Srl, Bologna, Italy). Two saline-soaked electrodes (35 cm^2) were placed on F4 (according to the 10–20 international EEG nomenclature) and on the right forearm, respectively. The stimulation was of 2mA DC (0.057 mA/cm^2 in density) delivered for 20 min (30 s step-up ramp, 30 s step-down ramp), repeated ten times, obtaining one session/day, for five consecutive days. Such a stimulation session was followed by two non-stimulation days, and again by another five days of long stimulation (Figure 2). During each tDCS application, patients were at rest without any concurrent motor tasks.

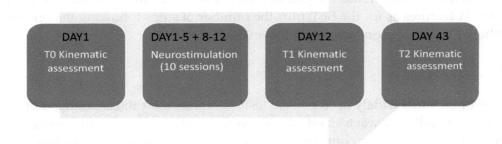

Figure 2. Flow diagram showing the study design and stimulation protocol.

2.4. Wearable Electronics

Different technologies can furnish data in terms of gait and balance performances. We can refer, for instance, to pressure sensors embedded into the floor and electro-goniometers, etc., with the optical-based systems considered as the gold standard because of their high accuracy. However, optical-based systems have some important drawbacks, such as the necessities of a free line of sight, time-consuming calibration procedures, necessity of skilled personnel and, above all, a very high cost. Wearable electronics have none of those drawbacks, and have been demonstrated to perform with the appropriate accuracy for our purposes [34,35].

Wearable electronics constitute a network of validated inertial measurement units (IMUs) termed Movit (by Captiks Srl, Rome Italy) [7,34,35], each housing a 3-axis accelerometer (±8 g) and a 3-axis gyroscope (±2000°/s), synchronized to a personal computer receiver, with a 50 Hz data transfer rate. A proprietary application, termed Motion Studio, processes and stores data.

The number of used IMUs and the position of patients' bodies (by means of elastic bands) varied according to the particular motor tasks performed. Measured data consist of accelerations, angular velocities, and joint angles, computed from the related quaternions via Euler decomposition. In turn, the quaternions are generated using a Kalman filter on data coming from the accelerometers and the gyroscopes, sampled at 200 Hz. By means of a patented calibration procedure, the spatial orientations of the dressed IMUs are represented on a computer screen as a human avatar, which replicates patient movements, with his/her joint angles gathered with a forward kinematic procedure in a parent-child hierarchy.

2.5. Features

For each task, we obtained several features, as reported in Table 2 and described in the following paragraphs.

2.5.1. Stance Feet Together (SFT) and Tandem Stance (TS)

Eleven features from the sensor located on the trunk were taken into consideration: range of accelerations, angular velocities and angles of the trunk in the medial-lateral (ML), anterior-posterior (AP) and vertical (V) directions; Jerk and Sway Area. In particular, Jerk, gathered from the accelerometers, represents the time derivative of acceleration [36], and is used as an empirical measure of the smoothness of the movements [37,38]. The Sway Area is the area of the ellipse that encompasses 95% of the values of medial lateral and anterior posterior accelerations around their mean values.

2.5.2. Pull Test (PT)

The PT test is useful to evaluate the postural responses to an unexpected external perturbation. We extracted the 11 features as for the SFT, plus the number of steps following the pushing as resulted from data gathered by the sensors placed on the ankles.

2.5.3. Time Up and Go (TUG)

TUG is one of the most widely used clinical tests and allows for the assessment of several aspects of gait. Parkinsonian gait is characterized by a slowed speed, decreased arm swing, shuffling steps, and difficulty to turn [39]. TUG is composed by four phases: the sit-to-stand phase (patient gets up from the sitting position with arms across the chest), the walking phase (patient walks for 6 m forth and back), the turning phase (the patient turns 180°), and the turn-to-sit phase (the patient turns and sit back on the chair). Each phase is segmented considering data gathered by the IMU on the trunk. We detected the sit-to-stand and turn-to-sit phases considering the interval between the two local minimum values before and after a local maximum of the accelerometer data, in the AP direction, corresponding to the flexion/extension movement of trunk. The turning phase is identified using thresholds on the trunk angle in the vertical direction (the turning component looks as a positive or negative ramp, depending on the direction of the turn). Further details on the segmentation of TUG test are reported in [7].

From these segmentations, 24 features were computer, as described in Table 2, including:

1. Temporal gait characteristics, such as number of steps, step duration, stance duration and swing duration;
2. Features related to upper and lower limb movements, such as the range of motion of arms and legs (Flex Arm, Flex Leg), the average angular velocity (Average Vel) of arms, forearms, legs and thighs, and the asymmetry between right and left limbs (Asym Arm, Asym Leg);
3. Turning parameters, such as the angular velocity of the trunk (Peak Turning Vel), the turning velocity (Turning Vel) and the number of steps (Steps Turning).

2.5.4. Stop and Go (S&G) & Narrow Walking (NW)

Parkinsonian gait problems are often triggered by some circumstances such as spaces with a narrow passage (e.g., a door), unexpected visual or auditory stimuli, stressful situations, cognitive load anxiety and difficulty in starting and stopping [39]. The results are a decreasing step length and step time, decreasing velocity, and increasing variability of step length and time [40,41]. The S&G and NW tests are used to provide evidence for these symptoms. We computed seven features for each task.

For the S&G test, we computed the duration of steps, stance and swing, as well as the angular velocity of the leg of the first steps at the beginning of gait, thus, after each stop signal of the examiner and the variability of the temporal step variables (CV Step, CV Stance, CV Swing).

For the NW test, we computed the same features but extracted them during the 3 s when the patient was passing through the door.

Table 2. Extracted Features from each motor test.

Task	Feature	Description
SFT, TS, PT	Jerk	Time derivative of acceleration in ML and AP directions [42]
	Sway Area	The ellipse that encompasses 95% of the values of ML and AP acceleration around their mean values [42]
	Range	The range of acceleration and angular velocity signals in all the three directions (6 features in total)
PT	# of Steps	The number of steps performed by the subject following the push
TUG	TUG phases duration	Include TUG time (duration of the entire test), sit-to-stand time, walk time, turning time and turn-to-sit time
	# of Steps	Number of steps during the walking phase.
	Gait metrics	Include mean and coefficient of variation of step duration, stance duration, and swing duration
	Flex Arm, Flex Leg	The angular flexion range of arms and legs
	Asym Arm, Asym Leg	Difference in angular flexion range between the faster and slower arm/leg divided by the larger value (lv%)
	Average Vel	The average angular velocity of arm, forearm and thigh along the medial lateral axis during the walking phase
	Turning Vel	The range of turning (180°) divided by turning time
	Peak Turning Vel	The maximum achieved angular velocity of the trunk rotation in the vertical axis during the turning phase
	Steps Turning	The number of steps during the turning phase
	Average Vel SitStand	The average angular velocity of trunk during sit-to-stand in in the anterior posterior plane
S&G	Gait metrics	Mean and coefficient of variation of duration of step, stance and swing computed on first four steps at the beginning of gait, after each stop signal of the examiner
	Step velocity	The angular velocity of legs computed on first four steps at the beginning of gait, after each stop signal of the examiner
NW	Gait metrics	Mean and coefficient of variation of duration of step, stance and swing computed on the 3 s time with patient passing through the door.
	Step velocity	The angular velocity of legs computed on the 3 s time with the patient passing through the door

2.6. Clinical and Wearables-Based Evaluations

Motor test performances of each of the ten PD patients just before the stimulation protocol (T0 time), just soon after the protocol (T1 time), and 1 month after (T2 time) were evaluated in order to quantify the effect of the tDCS and its persistence, if any.

The evaluations were performed both as standard clinical ones and by the analysis of data gathered through the wearable electronics.

All patients were evaluated by a movement disorder specialist, with general neurological examination, clinical tests, and questionnaires. Clinical tests consisted in the administration of MDS unified Parkinson's disease rating scale (MDS-UPDRS) and the Berg balance scale (BBS) [43], a clinical five-point ordinal scale that assess balance. Each patient was also evaluated with the freezing of gait questionnaire (FOG-Q) [44], a 6-item questionnaire used to assess gait disturbance severity in patients with PD, and the Hoehn and Yahr scale (H&Y) [45], a commonly used system for describing the progress of symptoms.

To evaluate the responsiveness of a treatment, we considered two aspects. First, we assessed the ability of wearable features to detect change over a particular time frame. Then, we evaluated the relationship between a change in the feature values and the external measure (e.g., the clinical score).

The standardized response mean (SRM) [46] was used to assess the responsiveness to the tDCS therapy. A reason for choosing SRM is because, differently from the paired t-test, it has no dependence on sample size [47]. The SRM expresses the ratio of TT:SDC, where TT is the mean change between T1 and T0 and between T2 and T1, and SDC the standard deviation of the change. Empirically, an SRM value of 0.20 represents a small, 0.50 a moderate, and 0.80 a large responsiveness, respectively.

We used Spearman's rank correlation coefficient to investigate the relation between the clinical scores and the features. Stance feet together (SFT) and tandem stance (TS) tasks were used to evaluate the static balance, assessed by the clinicians using the BBS scale. Features extracted from SFT and TS are compared with the BBS score. PT features were correlated to the corresponding UPDRS III item 3.12 score (PT is part of UPDRS III tasks). Features extracted from gait related tasks (TUG; ST and NW) were correlated with the UPDRS III gait item score (3.10). The significance level was set at 0.05.

3. Results

Table 3 shows the mean, standard deviation values, and SRM of the clinical evaluation results. Tables 4–9 report the motor features of SFT, TS, PT, TUG, S&G and NW tests, and correlation analysis between the features and the corresponding clinical evaluation.

Table 3. Clinical evaluation.

Clinical Evaluation	T0 Mean ± SD	T1 Mean ± SD	T2 Mean ± SD	SRM (T0 vs. T1)	SRM (T0 vs. T2)	SRM (T1 vs. T2)
MDS-UPDRS II	15.6 ± 3.67	13.9 ± 3.21	14.3 ± 3.23	−0.53	−0.42	0.23
MDS-UPDRS III	35.2 ± 5.64	30.5 ± 6.8	30.4 ± 3.47	−0.67	−1.15	−0.01
Gait item (3.10)	2.20 ± 0.60	1.60 ± 0.49	1.50 ± 0.50	−0.90	−0.90	−0.33
PT item (3.12)	1.80 ± 0.75	1.20 ± 0.75	1.60 ± 0.49	−0.65	−0.23	0.82
FOGQ	13.4 ± 3.69	12.5 ± 3.47	12.4 ± 2.11	−0.62	−0.33	−0.04
BBS	42.3 ± 12.35	47.2 ± 7.97	49.3 ± 6.96	0.79	0.82	0.50

Table 4. Stance feet together (SFT): feature values at T0, T1, T2; values of SRM comparing times; correlation with BBS score.

Feature (SFT)	T0 Mean ± SD	T1 Mean ± SD	T2 Mean ± SD	SRM (T0 vs. T1)	SRM (T0 vs. T2)	SRM (T1 vs. T2)	Correlation with BBS
Jerk	0.08 ± 0.03	0.07 ± 0.03	0.07 ± 0.03	−0.22	−0.72	−0.15	−0.38 *
Sway Area	0.32 ± 0.22	0.32 ± 0.3	0.32 ± 0.26	−0.01	−0.01	0.01	−0.22
Range Acc V	0.66 ± 0.53	0.61 ± 0.42	0.5 ± 0.34	−0.13	−0.53	−0.39	−0.60 *
Range Acc ML	0.56 ± 0.16	0.59 ± 0.28	0.59 ± 0.24	0.12	0.18	0.05	−0.46 *
Range Acc AP	0.99 ± 0.35	0.92 ± 0.38	0.9 ± 0.37	−0.14	−0.22	−0.07	−0.17
Range Gyr V	7.76 ± 3.45	10.71 ± 5.77	9.04 ± 5.13	0.53	0.24	−0.28	−0.48 *
Range Gyr ML	11.66 ± 5.78	10.95 ± 6.81	9.88 ± 4.87	−0.08	−0.32	−0.20	−0.55 *
Range Gyr AP	4.55 ± 2.35	5.05 ± 4.05	4.32 ± 2.49	0.13	−0.10	−0.27	−0.44 *

* p value < 0.05.

Table 5. Tandem stance (TS): features values at T0, T1, T2; values of SRM comparing times; correlation with BBS score.

Feature (TS)	T0 Mean ± SD	T1 Mean ± SD	T2 Mean ± SD	SRM (T0 vs. T1)	SRM (T0 vs. T2)	SRM (T1 vs. T2)	Correlation with BBS
Jerk	0.78 ± 1.32	0.21 ± 0.14	0.42 ± 0.45	−0.41	−0.33	0.44	−0.43 *
Sway Area	3.05 ± 4.44	1 ± 0.75	1.14 ± 1.28	−0.43	−0.41	0.13	−0.37 *
Range Acc V	2.79 ± 2.4	1.42 ± 1.36	1.32 ± 1.23	−0.47	−0.62	−0.11	−0.45 *
Range Acc ML	2.73 ± 2.45	1.73 ± 1.48	2.52 ± 2.45	−0.33	−0.08	0.29	−0.51 *
Range Acc AP	3.04 ± 2.88	1.87 ± 0.82	1.77 ± 1.19	−0.39	−0.43	−0.08	−0.35 *
Range Gyr V	40.01 ± 27.54	26.24 ± 12.28	40.06 ± 41.53	−0.42	0.00	0.35	−0.54 *
Range Gyr ML	58.97 ± 73.46	20.48 ± 13.44	29.28 ± 30.11	−0.47	−0.37	0.29	−0.53 *
Range Gyr AP	27.67 ± 26.98	14.68 ± 10.79	15.18 ± 10.01	−0.42	−0.46	0.04	−0.52 *

* p value < 0.05.

Table 6. Pull test (PT): feature values at T0, T1, T2; values of SRM comparing times; correlation with UPDRS item 3.12 (PT) score.

Feature (PT)	T0 Mean ± SD	T1 Mean ± SD	T2 Mean ± SD	SRM (T0 vs. T1)	SRM (T0 vs. T2)	SRM (T1 vs. T2)	Correlation with PT Item
Number of Steps	4.5 ± 1.8	4.2 ± 1.25	4.2 ± 2.27	−0.15	−0.09	0.00	−0.10
Jerk	11.03 ± 13.43	13.87 ± 18.82	13.64 ± 13.88	0.28	0.40	−0.02	−0.22
Sway Area	99.28 ± 140.03	83.99 ± 91.55	66.66 ± 63.16	−0.22	−0.38	−0.38	−0.27
Range Acc V	15.05 ± 6.23	14.92 ± 5.95	15.71 ± 5.95	−0.02	0.10	0.16	−0.45 *
Range Acc ML	16.33 ± 8.07	15.46 ± 6.17	15.89 ± 8.59	−0.11	−0.06	0.05	−0.28
Range Acc AP	11.52 ± 6.59	13.85 ± 8.27	12.33 ± 6.14	0.34	0.14	−0.23	−0.23
Range Gyr V	238.32 ± 209.22	246.18 ± 166.59	207.18 ± 104.41	0.08	−0.16	−0.27	−0.32
Range Gyr ML	456.96 ± 241.32	340.59 ± 230.85	402.52 ± 228.77	−0.34	−0.22	0.31	−0.47 *
Range Gyr AP	114.13 ± 111.22	91.72 ± 30.45	80.3 ± 31.42	−0.19	−0.33	−0.27	−0.16

* p-value < 0.05.

Table 7. TUG: feature values at T0, T1, T2; values of SRM comparing times; correlation with UPDRS item 3.10 (Gait) score.

Feature (TUG)	T0 Mean ± SD	T1 Mean ± SD	T2 Mean ± SD	SRM (T0 vs. T1)	SRM (T0 vs. T2)	SRM (T1 vs. T2)	Correlation with Gait Item
Tug Time	32.19 ± 10.24	28.27 ± 9.7	26.8 ± 6.49	−0.48	−0.93	−0.24	0.55 *
Sit-to-Stand Time	3.03 ± 2.64	1.94 ± 0.99	2.12 ± 0.89	−0.41	−0.39	0.13	0.28
Walk Time	20.58 ± 6.96	17.92 ± 6.02	17.81 ± 4.62	−0.52	−0.78	−0.04	0.56 *
Turning Time	3.9 ± 1.71	3.92 ± 2.24	3.09 ± 0.89	0.01	−0.68	−0.44	0.53 *
Turn-to-Sit Time	4.67 ± 1.66	4.48 ± 1.16	3.78 ± 1.2	−0.11	−0.48	−0.67	0.23
Number of Steps	40.13 ± 10.3	37.78 ± 11.76	38.3 ± 9.38	−0.05	−0.57	−0.21	0.49 *
Step duration	1.17 ± 0.08	1.14 ± 0.11	1.15 ± 0.1	−0.34	−0.24	0.21	0.24
Stance	57.94 ± 3.53	55.9 ± 7.88	57.56 ± 3.31	−0.23	−0.30	0.18	0.20
Swing	42.26 ± 3.62	43.97 ± 7.52	42.44 ± 3.31	0.20	0.20	−0.17	−0.22
CV step	0.07 ± 0.03	0.06 ± 0.03	0.09 ± 0.08	−0.24	0.17	0.54	0.47 *
CV Stance	0.08 ± 0.04	0.36 ± 0.89	0.08 ± 0.03	0.30	−0.09	−0.29	0.12
CV Swing	0.13 ± 0.1	0.11 ± 0.08	0.1 ± 0.04	−0.17	−0.27	−0.08	0.21
Flex Leg	23.41 ± 4.43	23.37 ± 7.39	23.91 ± 6.32	−0.01	0.09	0.10	−0.54 *
Flex Arm	30.38 ± 13.57	28.53 ± 18.85	28.1 ± 14.63	−0.13	−0.22	−0.05	0.28
Asym Leg	12.68 ± 6.62	17.03 ± 20.31	16.22 ± 13.22	0.19	0.22	−0.05	0.20
Asym Arm	40.06 ± 27.2	43.99 ± 22.93	40.81 ± 22.05	0.15	0.04	−0.22	−0.07
Average Vel Thigh	38.08 ± 6.56	43.61 ± 8.07	41.66 ± 7.55	0.62	0.49	−0.31	−0.60 *
Average Vel Leg	72.72 ± 17.24	89.6 ± 17.35	88.24 ± 16.19	0.83	0.83	−0.15	−0.52 *
Average Vel Arm	24.42 ± 12.82	25.41 ± 11.03	23.57 ± 9.24	0.14	−0.10	−0.27	0.11
Average Vel Forearm	38.82 ± 17.6	40.26 ± 21.41	34.79 ± 10.74	0.11	−0.28	−0.34	0.06
Turning Vel	51.82 ± 14.09	58.92 ± 23.8	62.47 ± 14.75	0.32	0.93	0.22	−0.53 *
Peak Turning Vel	91.12 ± 18.8	105.04 ± 30.13	101.76 ± 26.65	0.61	0.60	−0.19	−0.25
Steps Turning	5 ± 1	6.5 ± 3.67	5.6 ± 2.65	0.39	0.31	−0.22	0.48 *
Average Vel Sit Stand	27.27 ± 7.96	34.42 ± 11.1	33.37 ± 10.46	0.93	0.61	−0.09	−0.43 *

* p-value < 0.05.

Table 8. Stop and go (S&G): feature values at T0, T1, T2; values of SRM comparing times; correlation with UPDRS item 3.10 (gait) score.

Feature (S&G)	T0 Mean ± SD	T1 Mean ± SD	T2 Mean ± SD	SRM (T0 vs. T1)	SRM (T0 vs. T2)	SRM (T1 vs. T2)	Correlation with Gait Item
Step duration	1.44 ± 0.38	1.33 ± 0.29	1.34 ± 0.17	−0.21	−0.31	0.04	−0.42 *
Stance	0.99 ± 0.39	0.91 ± 0.33	0.86 ± 0.21	−0.14	−0.35	−0.13	−0.18
Swing	0.45 ± 0.06	0.42 ± 0.07	0.48 ± 0.08	−0.44	0.34	0.86	−0.22
Step velocity	179.34 ± 46.87	184.93 ± 60.03	174.42 ± 47.18	0.08	−0.10	−0.24	−0.08
CV step	0.15 ± 0.12	0.1 ± 0.06	0.1 ± 0.06	−0.35	−0.34	0.05	0.02
CV Stance	0.31 ± 0.22	0.24 ± 0.18	0.33 ± 0.16	−0.21	0.06	0.48	−0.13
CV Swing	0.17 ± 0.04	0.18 ± 0.05	0.17 ± 0.05	0.13	0.04	−0.14	0.07

* p-value < 0.05.

Table 9. Narrow walking (NW): feature values at T0, T1, T2; values of SRM comparing times; correlation with UPDRS item 3.10 (gait) score.

Feature (NW)	T0 Mean ± SD	T1 Mean ± SD	T2 Mean ± SD	SRM (T0 vs. T1)	SRM (T0 vs. T2)	SRM (T1 vs. T2)	Correlation with Gait Item
Step duration	1.18 ± 0.09	1.09 ± 0.08	1.11 ± 0.09	−1.60	−0.91	0.77	0.25
Stance	0.65 ± 0.12	0.63 ± 0.08	0.65 ± 0.07	−0.17	0.02	0.49	0.05
Swing	0.5 ± 0.03	0.46 ± 0.05	0.47 ± 0.04	−1.58	−0.90	0.50	−0.01
Step velocity	266.98 ± 40.93	297.96 ± 50.31	284.76 ± 39.79	1.56	0.92	−0.66	−0.44*
CV step	0.1 ± 0.05	0.07 ± 0.03	0.08 ± 0.04	−0.59	−0.23	0.27	−0.02
CV Stance	0.14 ± 0.07	0.12 ± 0.04	0.14 ± 0.08	−0.27	−0.01	0.21	0.04
CV Swing	0.13 ± 0.06	0.09 ± 0.03	0.11 ± 0.04	−0.74	−0.37	0.60	0.35*

* p-value < 0.05.

3.1. Clinical Evaluation

MDS-UPDRS sections two and three, BBS, and FOG-Q (Table 3) demonstrated moderate responsiveness to tDCS at the end of the treatment. The effect appears stable after one month with some improvement in BBS and MDS-UPDRS Section 2 score.

3.2. Stance Feet Together (SFT) and Tandem Stance (TS)

Jerk demonstrated a decrement, but only in a small percentage, in SFT (Table 4) and TS (Table 5) in both T1 and T2. During TS, Sway Area, range of the accelerations and angular velocities in the three directions decreased in T1 with a responsiveness around 0.4. The effect is stable at T2 compared to T1 with low improvements in some features.

The BBS score correlates significantly with almost all the features extracted from SFT and TS such as Jerk, Sway area (only TS, r = −0.37) and range of the accelerations and angular velocities. So, features highly reflect the clinical evaluation in this case.

3.3. Pull Test (PT)

During the PT, the obtained results (Table 6) showed an unchanged number of steps after tDCS treatment, a small increment of Jerk, and a small reduction of Sway Area at the end of the treatment and one month after.

Regarding the clinical evaluation, only few features (Range Acc V, r = −0.45; Range Gyr ML, r = −0.47) correlated with the UPDRS PT sub score.

3.4. Time Up and Go (TUG)

It was found that tDCS showed a moderate effect on the duration of sit-to-stand and walking phase in T1 and T2, as compared to the baseline (Table 7). A lower duration of the Turning phase is present only at T2. In correlation with a lower duration of the walking phase, our results show a reduction of the number of steps and stance duration. No changes were found in features related to the upper limbs. Conversely, the velocity of the lower extremities meaningfully increased. Finally, patients increased the velocity to turn and sit at T1 and T2, with comparison to the baseline values.

The UPDRS gait item score correlates significantly with several features extracted from TUG. Significant correlations regard the features representing the duration of the TUG phases (namely tug time, walk time and turning time). So, patients that take time to complete TUG have higher score on gait item. Weak correlation was for the temporal gait characteristics with the exception of number of steps and CV step. Gait item correlates significantly with features related to lower limb movements (Flex Leg, Average Vel Thigh, and Average Vel Leg) and the turning phase (Turning Vel, Steps Turning).

3.5. Stop and Go (S&G) & Narrow Walking (NW)

Both S&G (Table 8) and NW (Table 9) tests show a shorter duration of the step and swing phase and decreased variability of step duration in both T1 and T2 with respect to the baseline. The velocity remained unchanged in S&G but increased in NW. Large responsiveness is found in NW related to step duration, swing duration, velocity, and all the temporal step variability features.

One feature from S&G (step duration, $r = -0.42$) and two features from NW (Step Velocity, $r = -0.44$; CV Swing, $r = 0.35$) are significantly related to the UPDRS gait item.

4. Discussion

The response to dopaminergic drug replacement therapy in PD may lose its effectiveness during the course of the disease. Postural and gait disturbances, in particular, are symptoms that are difficult to treat with currently available pharmacological therapies.

Recent studies suggest a potential positive impact of tDCS on gait and balance in PD patients, symptoms of the late stage of PD, poorly responding to the classic dopaminergic treatment.

Our work focused on objectively quantifying the effect of tDCS on gait and postural stability from measured data gathered by wearable electronics used during motor tests of Parkinson's disease patients.

Within this context, the obtained results demonstrate the impact of wearable electronics with respect to standard clinical evaluation, allowing for interesting insights on the range of change on motor performance following the therapy. In fact, wearable electronics can evidence key elements of postural instability or gait abnormalities, both for evaluating the progression in PD and even to identify the disease at early stages [7,48–50]. Accordingly, in this study, specific motor tests were considered to assess the effects of tDCS therapy on balance and gait disturbances, taking into account the effects on measured motor features, soon after the delivery and one month later.

For balance assessment, three different motor tests were adopted to evaluate the equilibrium in three different conditions: SFT for static balance, TS to assess the balance when a low perturbation is introduced, and PT to assess postural responses to an unexpected perturbation. According to the kinematic assessment, Jerk is the only feature that presents a significant variation in SFT, TS and PT, suggesting that it is a highly sensitive measure of balance. This confirms the finding reported in previous studies, wherein Jerk was suggested as a valid biomarker of PD [7,49].

For gait assessment, the TUG test was useful to evaluate the slower speed, decreased arm swing, shuffling steps and difficulty to turn. Further S&G and NW tests were useful to evaluate step time, velocity, and variability of steps, due to the difficulty to start/stop and pass through a narrow door.

Our results show a reduction of step and stance duration and an increment of lower limb velocity during TUG, S&G and NW tests. These achievements confirm the findings reported in other works, which evidenced some improvement of hypokinetic gait in PD after tDCS treatment [29,30,51].

The effect is more evident in NW test, where we observed a large responsiveness to tDCS. The reason why PD patients tend to decrease step time and velocity when approaching a narrowed space is not completely understood [39], however tDCS in some way improves this aspect. We evidenced an improvement of gait in turning and standing tasks during TUG test too, when patients increased the velocity to turn and sit after the stimulation protocol. In particular, changes in turning are one of the early motor deficiencies in PD, as previously reported [50]. The wearable impact in analyzing this complex motor task is relevant. In fact, clinical evaluation alone demonstrated an amelioration in gait and pull test items but was not able to disclose which features of these two motor functions improved. Being able to thoroughly phenotype patients' motor performances is crucial to understanding the effect of a therapeutic intervention and to allow for speculation with respect to its dynamics.

In order to provide clinical validity for our approach, we investigated the relation between the clinical scores, given by the examiners, and the measured features. Clinical vs. wearables outcomes demonstrated general significant results (Tables 4–9). In particular, a higher correlation was found between features extracted from static balance tasks (SFT and TS) and BBS scores and between TUG features and UPDRS gait item scores.

Not all of the features presented a perfect correlation with clinical rating, and this is also expected since these measures should be more sensitive than clinical scales, mostly due to the fact that clinical examination is based on a rating scale with only a few steps, while wearables produce a density scale with a high number of steps [52]. For example, in the TUG test, the duration of the performance is a significant parameter for both the classical clinical exam and "technology-based assessment". Conversely, the average velocity of lower limbs was significantly and accurately measured only by the wearable sensors. The same consideration applies for the other features extracted from the balance and gait tests. These results are in accordance with a recent work [7], evidencing that several features extracted by sensors were able to detect subtle abnormalities in early stage PD patients where the corresponding clinical score, obtained by visual examination, was considered normal for the majority of subjects.

It could be argued that a better sensitivity can be clinically irrelevant, detecting differences too small to have a real impact on a patient's life and functioning. Alternatively, it allows investigators to better phenotype motion alterations and their changes after a therapy, and to objectively measure the benefit from a standard intervention, in view of its customization and relevant optimization.

We are aware of some limitations of the present study. First, tDCS was adopted for patients under other medical treatments that had already been adjusted for the optimal dose. We did not use a test-retest design, thus we cannot exclude variability due to participants' physical or mental conditions, or to drug response fluctuations. To minimize the effects of the aforementioned limitations, we performed the study at the same time of the day for every patient, and no modification to the therapy was allowed in the three months preceding the study and during its course. The study cannot exclude a placebo effect. Moreover, we performed the experiment on a small sample size. Indeed, further studies, on larger cohorts, are mandatory in order to confirm our findings.

5. Conclusions

Our study aimed to demonstrate the advantages of outcomes from technology-based measures in clinical trials. These advantages are particularly important for revealing the effectiveness of tDCS protocols in late stage PD patients. This is because the benefit of tDCS remains unclear and controversial, thus the outcomes from electronic wearables can help the clinical rating of the tDCS effectiveness. In particular, our results provide evidence of the wearable electronic impact, as a complementary tool to the standard clinical evaluation.

The adoption of wearables furnished a number of motor features, some of them with a good correlation with standard clinical assessment, others adding information not evident to human eyes.

Nonetheless, even if wearables can provide motor features for an insight of each patient's motor performances, they remain rarely adopted in clinical trials. We believe that relevant reasons for this can be ascribed to the lack of an integrated platform that can be easily used by nurses and clinicians, and a lack of regulatory approval and appropriate cost–benefit ratios [15,52]. However, the idea to develop and integrate technologies into the assessment of therapy effectiveness has become so evident that several academic centers and companies have started to bring them to the market.

Author Contributions: conceptualization, writing—review and editing, M.R., G.D.L., A.P., F.G. and G.S.; methodology and investigation, M.R., G.D.L., A.P., S.S., M.A., C.S. and G.S.; software, M.R.; formal analysis and data curation, M.R. and G.D.L.; validation, M.R., G.D.L., A.P., F.G. and G.S.; writing—original draft preparation, M.R., and G.D.L.; supervision, A.P., F.G. and G.S.

Acknowledgments: We acknowledge the support given by Luca Pietrosanti in measurements.

References

1. Saggio, G.; Lazzaro, A.; Sbernini, L.; Carrano, F.M.; Passi, D.; Corona, A.; Panetta, V.; Gaspari, A.L.; Di Lorenzo, N. Objective surgical skill assessment: An initial experience by means of a sensory glove paving the way to open surgery simulation? *J. Surg. Educ.* **2015**, *72*, 910–917. [CrossRef] [PubMed]

2. Saggio, G.; Santosuosso, G.L.; Cavallo, P.; Pinto, C.A.; Petrella, M.; Giannini, F.; Di Lorenzo, N.; Lazzaro, A.; Corona, A.; D'Auria, F.; et al. Gesture recognition and classification for surgical skill assessment. In Proceedings of the IEEE International Symposium on Medical Measurements and Applications, Bari, Italy, 30–31 May 2011.

3. Sbernini, L.; Quitadamo, L.R.; Riillo, F.; Di Lorenzo, N.; Gaspari, A.L.; Saggio, G. Sensory-Glove-Based Open Surgery Skill Evaluation. *IEEE Trans. Hum.-Mach. Syst.* **2018**, *48*, 213–218. [CrossRef]

4. Lukowicz, P.; Kirstein, T.; Tröster, G. Wearable systems for health care applications. *Methods Inf. Med.* **2004**, *43*, 232–238. [PubMed]

5. Park, S.; Jayaraman, S. Enhancing the Quality of Life Through Wearable Technology. *IEEE Eng. Med. Biol. Mag.* **2003**, *22*, 41–48. [CrossRef] [PubMed]

6. Darwish, A.; Hassanien, A.E. Wearable and implantable wireless sensor network solutions for healthcare monitoring. *Sensors* **2011**, *11*, 5561–5595. [CrossRef]

7. Ricci, M.; Di Lazzaro, G.; Pisani, A.; Mercuri, N.B.; Giannini, F.; Saggio, G. Assessment of motor impairments in early untreated Parkinson's disease patients: The wearable electronics impact. *IEEE J. Biomed. Health. Inform.* **2019**. [CrossRef]

8. Piro, N.E.; Baumann, L.; Tengler, M.; Piro, L. Telemonitoring of patients with Par-kin son's disease using inertia sensors. *Appl. Clin. Inform.* **2014**, *5*, 503–511.

9. Giuberti, M.; Ferrari, G.; Contin, L.; Cimolin, V.; Azzaro, C.; Albani, G.; Mauro, A. Assigning UPDRS scores in the leg agility task of parkinsonians: Can it be done through BSN-based kinematic variables? *IEEE Internet Things J.* **2015**, *2*, 41–51. [CrossRef]

10. Dai, H.; Zhang, P.; Lueth, T.C. Quantitative assessment of parkinsonian tremor based on an inertial measurement unit. *Sensors* **2015**, *15*, 25055–25071. [CrossRef]

11. Weiss, A.; Sharifi, S.; Plotnik, M.; van Vugt, J.P.P.; Giladi, N.; Hausdorff, J.M. Toward automated, at-home assessment of mobility among patients with Parkinson disease, using a body-worn accelerometer. *Neurorehabil. Neural Repair* **2011**, *25*, 810–818. [CrossRef]

12. Rovini, E.; Maremmani, C.; Cavallo, F. How wearable sensors can support parkinson's disease diagnosis and treatment: A systematic review. *Front. Neurosci.* **2017**, *11*, 555. [CrossRef] [PubMed]

13. Postuma, R.B.; Berg, D.; Stern, M.; Poewe, W.; Olanow, C.W.; Oertel, W.; Obeso, J.; Marek, K.; Litvan, I.; Lang, A.E.; et al. MDS clinical diagnostic criteria for Parkinson's disease. *Mov. Disord.* **2015**, *30*, 1591–1601. [CrossRef] [PubMed]

14. Christopher, G.G. MDS-UPDRS. *Off. Work. Doc.* **2008**, *23*, 2129–2170. [CrossRef]

15. Artusi, C.A.; Mishra, M.; Latimer, P.; Vizcarra, J.A.; Lopiano, L.; Maetzler, W.; Merola, A.; Espay, A.J. Integration of technology-based outcome measures in clinical trials of Parkinson and other neurodegenerative diseases. *Park. Relat. Disord.* **2018**, *46*, S53–S56. [CrossRef] [PubMed]

16. Goetz, C.G.; Tilley, B.C.; Shaftman, S.R.; Stebbins, G.T.; Fahn, S.; Martinez-Martin, P.; Poewe, W.; Sampaio, C.;

Stern, M.B.; Dodel, R.; et al. Movement Disorder Society-sponsored revision of the Unified Parkinson's Disease Rating Scale (MDS-UPDRS): Scale presentation and clinimetric testing results. *Mov. Disord.* **2008**, *23*, 2129–2170. [CrossRef]

17. Lipsmeier, F.; Taylor, K.I.; Kilchenmann, T.; Wolf, D.; Scotland, A.; Schjodt-Eriksen, J.; Cheng, W.Y.; Fernandez-Garcia, I.; Siebourg-Polster, J.; Jin, L.; et al. Evaluation of smartphone-based testing to generate exploratory outcome measures in a phase 1 Parkinson's disease clinical trial. *Mov. Disord.* **2018**, *33*, 1287–1297. [CrossRef] [PubMed]

18. Parkinson's KinetiGraph®system. Available online: https://www.globalkineticscorporation.com/the-pkg-system/ (accessed on 15 September 2019).

19. What is Wearable Technology and How Can It Help People with Parkinson's Disease? Available online: https://www.apdaparkinson.org/article/wearable-technology-in-parkinsons/ (accessed on 15 September 2019).

20. Roche Technology Measures Parkinson's Disease Fluctuations. Available online: https://www.roche.com/media/store/roche_stories/roche-stories-2015-08-10.htm (accessed on 15 September 2019).

21. Fregni, F.; Boggio, P.S.; Santos, M.C.; Lima, M.; Vieira, A.L.; Rigonatti, S.P.; Silva, M.T.A.; Barbosa, E.R.; Nitsche, M.A.; Pascual-Leone, A. Noninvasive cortical stimulation with transcranial direct current stimulation in Parkinson's disease. *Mov. Disord.* **2006**, *21*, 1693–1702. [CrossRef]

22. Brunoni, A.R.; Nitsche, M.A.; Bolognini, N.; Bikson, M.; Wagner, T.; Merabet, L.; Edwards, D.J.; Valero-Cabre, A.; Rotenberg, A.; Pascual-Leone, A.; et al. Clinical research with transcranial direct current stimulation (tDCS): Challenges and future directions. *Brain Stimul.* **2012**, *5*, 175–195. [CrossRef]

23. Elsner, B.; Kugler, J.; Pohl, M.; Mehrholz, J. Transcranial direct current stimulation (tDCS) for idiopathic Parkinson's disease. *Cochrane Database Syst. Rev.* **2016**, *2016*. [CrossRef]

24. Snijders, A.H.; Takakusaki, K.; Debu, B.; Lozano, A.M.; Krishna, V.; Fasano, A.; Aziz, T.Z.; Papa, S.M.; Factor, S.A.; Hallett, M. Physiology of freezing of gait. *Ann. Neurol.* **2016**, *80*, 644–659. [CrossRef]

25. Dagan, M.; Herman, T.; Harrison, R.; Zhou, J.; Giladi, N.; Ruffini, G.; Manor, B.; Hausdorff, J.M. Multitarget transcranial direct current stimulation for freezing of gait in Parkinson's disease. *Mov. Disord.* **2018**, *33*, 642–646. [CrossRef] [PubMed]

26. Vitorio, R.; Stuart, S.; Rochester, L.; Alcock, L.; Pantall, A. fNIRS response during walking—Artefact or cortical activity? A systematic review. *Neurosci. Biobehav. Rev.* **2017**, *83*, 160–172. [CrossRef] [PubMed]

27. Stuart, S.; Vitorio, R.; Morris, R.; Martini, D.N.; Fino, P.C.; Mancini, M. Cortical activity during walking and balance tasks in older adults and in people with Parkinson's disease: A structured review. *Maturitas* **2018**, *113*, 53–72. [CrossRef] [PubMed]

28. Hadoush, H.; Al-Jarrah, M.; Khalil, H.; Al-Sharman, A.; Al-Ghazawi, S. Bilateral anodal transcranial direct current stimulation effect on balance and fearing of fall in patient with Parkinson's disease. *NeuroRehabilitation* **2018**, *42*, 63–68. [CrossRef] [PubMed]

29. Manenti, R.; Brambilla, M.; Rosini, S.; Orizio, I.; Ferrari, C.; Borroni, B.; Cotelli, M. Time up and go task performance improves after transcranial direct current stimulation in patient affected by Parkinson's disease. *Neurosci. Lett.* **2014**, *580*, 74–77. [CrossRef] [PubMed]

30. Yotnuengnit, P.; Bhidayasiri, R.; Donkhan, R.; Chaluaysrimuang, J.; Piravej, K. Effects of Transcranial Direct Current Stimulation Plus Physical Therapy on Gait in Patients with Parkinson Disease: A Randomized Controlled Trial. *Am. J. Phys. Med. Rehabil.* **2018**, *97*, 7–15. [CrossRef]

31. Lattari, E.; Costa, S.S.; Campos, C.; de Oliveira, A.J.; Machado, S.; Maranhao Neto, G.A. Can transcranial direct current stimulation on the dorsolateral prefrontal cortex improves balance and functional mobility in Parkinson's disease? *Neurosci. Lett.* **2017**, *636*, 165–169. [CrossRef]

32. Lefaucheur, J.P.; Antal, A.; Ayache, S.S.; Benninger, D.H.; Brunelin, J.; Cogiamanian, F.; Cotelli, M.; De Ridder, D.; Ferrucci, R.; Langguth, B.; et al. Evidence-based guidelines on the therapeutic use of transcranial direct current stimulation (tDCS). *Clin. Neurophysiol.* **2017**, *128*, 56–92. [CrossRef]

33. O'Neill, D. The Mini—Mental Status Examination. *J. Am. Geriatr. Soc.* **1991**, *39*, 733. [CrossRef]

34. Ricci, M.; Terribili, M.; Giannini, F.; Errico, V.; Pallotti, A.; Galasso, C.; Tomasello, L.; Sias, S.; Saggio, G. Wearable-based electronics to objectively support diagnosis of motor impairments in school-aged children. *J. Biomech.* **2019**, *83*, 243–252. [CrossRef]

35. Alessandrini, M.; Micarelli, A.; Viziano, A.; Pavone, I.; Costantini, G.; Casali, D.; Paolizzo, F.; Saggio, G. Body-worn triaxial accelerometer coherence and reliability related to static posturography in unilateral

vestibular failure. *Acta Otorhinolaryngol. Ital.* **2017**, *37*, 231–236. [PubMed]

36. Flash, T.; Hogan, N. The coordination of arm movements: An experimentally confirmed mathematical model. *J. Neurosci.* **1985**, *5*, 1688–1703. [CrossRef] [PubMed]

37. Chen, T.Z.; Xu, G.J.; Zhou, G.A.; Wang, J.R.; Chan, P.; Du, Y.F. Postural sway in idiopathic rapid eye movement sleep behavior disorder: A potential marker of prodromal Parkinsons disease. *Brain Res.* **2014**, *1559*, 26–32. [CrossRef] [PubMed]

38. Mancini, M.; Horak, F.B.; Zampieri, C.; Carlson-Kuhta, P.; Nutt, J.G.; Chiari, L. Trunk accelerometry reveals postural instability in untreated Parkinson's disease. *Park Relat. Disord.* **2011**, *17*, 557–562. [CrossRef] [PubMed]

39. Beck, E.N.; Martens, K.A.E.; Almeida, Q.J. Freezing of gait in Parkinson's disease: An overload problem? *PLoS ONE* **2015**, *10*, e0144986. [CrossRef] [PubMed]

40. Morris, M.E.; Iansek, R.; Matyas, T.A.; Summers, J.J. Stride length regulation in Parkinson's disease: Normalization strategies and underlying mechanisms. *Brain* **1996**, *119*, 551–568. [CrossRef]

41. Hausdorff, J.M.; Cudkowicz, M.E.; Firtion, R.; Wei, J.Y.; Goldberger, A.L. Gait variability and basal ganglia disorders: Stride-to-stride variations of gait cycle timing in Parkinson's disease and Huntington's disease. *Mov. Disord.* **1998**, *13*, 428–437. [CrossRef]

42. Mancini, M.; Salarian, A.; Carlson-Kuhta, P.; Zampieri, C.; King, L.; Chiari, L.; Horak, F.B. ISway: A sensitive, valid and reliable measure of postural control. *J. Neuroeng. Rehabil.* **2012**, *9*, 1–8. [CrossRef]

43. Li, S. The balance scale. *Nature* **2010**, *464*, 804. [CrossRef]

44. Giladi, N.; Shabtai, H.; Simon, E.S.; Biran, S.; Tal, J.; Korczyn, A.D. Construction of freezing of gait questionnaire for patients with Parkinsonism. *Park Relat. Disord.* **2000**, *6*, 165–170. [CrossRef]

45. Martinez-Martin, P. Hoehn and Yahr Staging Scale. *Encycl. Mov. Disord.* **2010**, *1*, 23–25.

46. Nahler, G.; Nahler, G. standardized response mean (SRM). In *Dictionary of Pharmaceutical Medicine*; Springer: Vienna, Austria, 2009; p. 173.

47. Husted, J.A.; Cook, R.J.; Farewell, V.T.; Gladman, D.D. Methods for assessing responsiveness: A critical review and recommendations. *J. Clin. Epidemiol.* **2000**, *53*, 459–468. [CrossRef]

48. Horak, F.B.; Mancini, M. Objective biomarkers of balance and gait for Parkinson's disease using body-worn sensors. *Mov. Disord.* **2013**, *28*, 1544–1551. [CrossRef] [PubMed]

49. Mancini, M.; Carlson-Kuhta, P.; Zampieri, C.; Nutt, J.G.; Chiari, L.; Horak, F.B. Postural sway as a marker of progression in Parkinson's disease: A pilot longitudinal study. *Gait Posture* **2012**, *36*, 471–476. [CrossRef] [PubMed]

50. Salarian, A.; Zampieri, C.; Horak, F.B.; Carlson-Kuhta, P.; Nutt, J.G.; Aminian, K. Analyzing 180° turns using an inertial system reveals early signs of progression of Parkinson's disease. In Proceedings of the 31st Annual International Conference of the IEEE Engineering in Medicine and Biology Society: Engineering the Future of Biomedicine, Minneapolis, MN, USA, 3–6 September 2009; pp. 224–227.

51. Von Papen, M.; Fisse, M.; Sarfeld, A.S.; Fink, G.R.; Nowak, D.A. The effects of 1 Hz rTMS preconditioned by tDCS on gait kinematics in Parkinson's disease. *J. Neural Transm.* **2014**, *121*, 743–754. [CrossRef] [PubMed]

52. Espay, A.J.; Hausdorff, J.M.; Sánchez-Ferro, Á.; Klucken, J.; Merola, A.; Bonato, P.; Paul, S.S.; Horak, F.B.; Vizcarra, J.A.; Mestre, T.A.; et al. A roadmap for implementation of patient-centered digital outcome measures in Parkinson's disease obtained using mobile health technologies. *Mov. Disord.* **2019**, *34*, 657–663. [CrossRef]

14

Apheresis in Autoimmune Encephalitis and Autoimmune Dementia

Rosa Rössling [1,2] **and Harald Prüss** [1,2,*]

[1] Department of Neurology and Experimental Neurology, Charité–Universitätsmedizin Berlin, Charitéplatz 1, 10117 Berlin, Germany; rosa.roessling@charite.de
[2] German Center for Neurodegenerative Diseases (DZNE) Berlin, 10117 Berlin, Germany
*   Correspondence: harald.pruess@charite.de

Abstract: Autoimmune encephalitis (AE) is a rapidly progressive inflammatory neurological disease. Underlying autoantibodies can bind to neuronal surfaces and synaptic proteins resulting in psychiatric symptoms, focal neurological signs, autonomic dysfunction and cognitive decline. Early and effective treatment is mandatory to reduce clinical symptoms and to achieve remission. Therapeutic apheresis, involving both plasma exchange (PE) and immunoadsorption (IA), can rapidly remove pathogenic antibodies from the circulation, thus representing an important first-line treatment in AE patients. We here review the most relevant studies regarding therapeutic apheresis in AE, summarizing the outcome for patients and the expanding clinical spectrum of treatment-responsive clinical conditions. For example, patients with slowly progressing cognitive impairment suggesting a neurodegenerative dementia can have underlying autoantibodies and improve with therapeutic apheresis. Findings are encouraging and have led to the first ongoing clinical studies assessing the therapeutic effect of IA in patients with anti-neuronal autoantibodies and the clinical presentation of dementia. Therapeutic apheresis is an established and well tolerated option for first-line therapy in AE and, potentially, other antibody-mediated central nervous system diseases.

Keywords: autoimmune encephalitis; limbic encephalitis; NMDAR (N-Methyl-D-Aspartat); antibody; paraneoplastic; apheresis; plasma exchange; immunoadsorption

1. Introduction

Autoimmune encephalitis (AE) is a rapidly progressive inflammatory neurological disease with subacute onset. Patients may present with behavioral changes and altered mental status as well as reduced levels of consciousness and new focal neurological signs or epileptic seizures [1]. Furthermore, deficits in working or short-term memory frequently occur.

AE comprises both, antibody-mediated and paraneoplastic, i.e., cytotoxic T-cell-mediated, encephalitides. Clinical presentation is diverse and depends on the specific underlying antibody (Table 1). As more and more novel antibodies and new clinical phenotypes are being identified, the incidence is rising and currently estimated at 5–10 per 100,000 inhabitants per year [1]. Age and gender preferences are often specific for a given antibody. In some cases, the exact target of novel antibodies is not known yet. In other cases, even if the underlying antigen is known, the pathogenic relevance still awaits scientific clarification.

1.1. Antibody-Mediated AE

The most common and best-known form of antibody-mediated AE is NMDA (N-Methyl-D-Aspartat) receptor (NMDAR) encephalitis, defined by cerebrospinal fluid (CSF) IgG antibodies targeting the NMDA type glutamate receptor. Patients present with subacute onset of psychiatric symptoms, autonomic instability, focal neurological signs and behavioral changes as well as new-onset epileptic seizures and reduced levels of consciousness. Other AE-defining autoantibodies bind directly to excitatory transmitter receptors besides NMDAR (such as AMPA (α-amino-3-hydroxy-5-methyl-4-isoxazolepropionic acid) receptors), inhibitory transmitter receptors (GABAB (gamma-aminobutyric acid B), GABAA (gamma-aminobutyric acid A), glycine receptors), ion channel subunits and cell adhesion molecules (Caspr2 (contactin-associated protein 2), IgLON5) or soluble synaptic proteins (LGI1 (leucine-rich, glioma inactivated protein 1).

Autoimmune dementia might be considered a sub-form of AE with predominant cognitive deficits. Cognitive impairment is a common feature in AE. For instance, patients with encephalitis caused by LGI1 antibodies showed markedly impaired verbal and visuo-spatial memory as well as a significantly reduced hippocampal volume. A severe clinical course correlated with more pronounced structural damage of the hippocampus and correspondingly a worse overall memory performance [2]. As patients show good response to immunotherapy, especially in the early stage of disease, prompt and sufficiently "aggressive" treatment including apheresis is highly important. Interestingly, the cognitive deficits in LGI1 encephalitis can come in isolation and lead to the working diagnosis of a primary neurodegenerative disease such as Alzheimer's. Increasing awareness and the search for autoantibodies such as LGI1 are needed and can result in the early identification of dementia patients with an immunotherapy-responsive phenotype [3,4].

1.2. Paraneoplastic AE

In contrast to the neuronal surface antibodies, antibodies in classical paraneoplastic neurological syndromes (PNS) bind to intracellular antigens (such as Hu, Ri, Yo or Ma2 antibodies) and therefore do not cause the neurotoxicity directly; they rather serve as valuable biomarkers for an underlying tumor, often small cell lung cancer and gynecological tumors. The neuronal damage in these cases is, rather, caused by cytotoxic T-cells with oligoclonal T-cell receptor expansion and autoreactivity against neuronal structures. Among the antibodies targeting intracellular antigens, GAD (glutamic acid decarboxylase) and amphiphysin antibodies are an exception as they are not necessarily associated with a tumor and seem to be pathogenically relevant despite their intracellular antigen location [5].

Table 1. Most important antibodies and clinical syndromes.

Antigen	Clinical Presentation	Age/Gender	Tumor Type
	Antibodies against neurotransmitter receptors [6]		
NMDAR [7]	Schizophreniform psychosis, perioral dyskinesia, epileptic seizures, coma, dystonia, hypoventilation	All ages, peak in childhood and youth, 75% women	Ovarian teratoma
GABAaR	Epileptic seizures, schizophreniform syndrome, refractory status epilepticus and epilepsia partialis continua	Younger adults; m > f (1.5:1)	Hodgkin lymphoma
GABAbR	LE with frequent epileptic seizures	Older adults f = m	50% lung cancer (SCLC)
AMPAR	LE, Epileptic seizures, memory deficits, psychosis	Older Adults f > m (2.3:1)	In 70% lung/breast cancer
mGluR5	LE, Ophelia syndrome (depression, agitation, hallucination, memory deficits, personality changes)	Young adults, m > f (1.5:1)	Hodgkin lymphoma
GlycinR	PERM (progressive encephalomyelitis with rigidity and myoclonus), SPS, cognitive deficits	Older adults f = m	Thymoma (<10%)
DPPX	LE with tremor, myoclonus, hallucinations, therapy refractory diarrhea	Older adults f < m (1:2.3)	Not known

Table 1. *Cont.*

Antigen	Clinical Presentation	Age/Gender	Tumor Type
	Antibodies against ion channel subunits or cell adhesion molecules [8,9]		
LGI1	Facio-brachial dystonic seizures (FBDS), amnesia, psychosis, LE, hyponatremia	Adults > 40 years, m > f (2:1)	Rare
Caspr2	LE, neuro-myotonia, Morvan syndrome, can slowly progress over up to 1 year;similar to LGI1, but no hyponatremia	Elderly m > f (9:1)	Thymoma possible
IgLON5	REM- and non-REM sleep disorders, sleep apnea, stridor, dysarthria, dysphagia, dysautonomia, movement disorders, dementia	Older adults, f = m	Not known
	Antibodies against intracellular (onconeural) antigens [10,11]		
Hu (ANNA-1)	Encephalomyelitis, brainstem encephalitis, LE, Denny-Brown syndrome	Large variability, depending on tumor type	>90%, SCLC
Ri (ANNA-2)	OMS, CS, encephalomyelitis		>90%, Ovary, breast cancer
Yo (PCA-1)	CS		>90%, Ovary cancer
Ma2	LE, CS, diencephalic/hypothalamic involvement		>90%, Testicular, lung cancer
CV2 (CRMP5)	Encephalomyelitis, LE, CS		>90%, SCLC, thymoma
Amphiphysin	SPS		>90%, Breast, SCLC
GAD	SPS, LE, ataxia	Middle aged, f > m (4:1)	Tumor association rare

LE: limbic encephalitis, SPS: Stiff-person syndrome, OMS: Opsoclonus-myoclonus syndrome, CS: cerebellar syndrome, SCLC: small cell lung cancer, PCD: paraneoplastic cerebellar degeneration.

1.3. Therapy for AE

At this point, there is no clear evidence-based treatment standard for AE. Established treatment strategies for first-line therapy of AE include high-dose corticosteroids (three to five days course of 1000 mg intravenous methylprednisolone), intravenous immunoglobulins (IVIG) (2 g/kg body weight over three to five days), as well as therapeutic apheresis. Cyclophosphamide and the CD20-antibody rituximab (1000 mg, with the first two administrations at day 1 and day 15 followed by six months intervals) might be added in case of persisting or relapsing symptoms and as a long term maintenance therapy. Most centers favor a low threshold for rituximab initiation given its good safety profile and potential effect in preventing relapses. Many other treatments have been used with variable success, including mycophenolate mofetil, methotrexate or azathioprine. It is broadly agreed that immunotherapy needs to be started as early as possible after symptom onset to be most effective. Nevertheless, marked recovery can be seen in some patients with antibody-mediated AE in whom therapy is only started months after disease onset. The choice of adequate therapy depends on the clinical syndrome and the underlying antibody. However, comparative treatment studies in patients with AE are sparse and focus on the most common forms of AE, such as NMDAR encephalitis.

In paraneoplastic AE with antibodies targeting intracellular proteins, rituximab, intravenous immunoglobulins and therapeutic apheresis often have only little effect as the antibodies are not directly pathogenic. Here, neuronal damage is caused by cytotoxic T-cells. Evidence of a tumor requires prompt and complete removal in order to withdraw the auto-antigen expressed by the tumor that triggers the production of autoantibodies. Nevertheless, despite advanced immunotherapy and tumor removal, in many cases neuronal damage in paraneoplastic AE progresses.

Therapeutic apheresis and the removal of autoantibodies is a major therapeutic option in AE. The pathophysiological binding of antibodies to their antigens can thereby be reduced.

2. Search Strategy

To conduct the review, we followed the PRISMA (Preferred Reporting Items for Systematic Reviews and Meta-Analyses) guidelines and screened the articles independently for their respective eligibility [12].

2.1. Inclusion Criteria

We included all articles about patients with autoimmune encephalitis—antibody-mediated as well as paraneoplastic—treated with plasma exchange or immunoadsorption. Treatment regimen, such as concomitant immunotherapy, as well as details about the apheresis itself (plasma exchange (PE) or immunoadsorption (IA), number of courses) had to be specified in the article. Further, outcome measures, such as the modified Rankin Scale (mRS) or structured neuropsychological assessment had to be provided. The mRS ranges from zero (no symptoms) to six (death from the disease), and a change of ±1 mRS point is considered as clinically significant improvement or deterioration. Cut-off for independent living is at ≤2 mRS points.

2.2. Search Strategy

The following strategy was used to find previous literature and trials (Figure 1): MEDLINE (medical literature analysis and retrieval system online) was searched for articles published up until 30 June 2020 in English or German. The Medical Subject Headings (MeSH) terms used were "autoimmune encephalitis" and "apheresis" (37 hits), "plasma exchange" (104 hits) or "immunoadsorption" (12 hits). Furthermore, the references of the included articles were screened for potential additional articles.

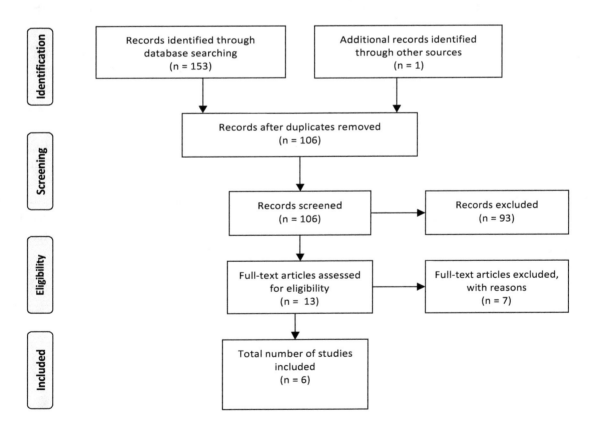

Figure 1. Preferred Reporting Items for Systematic Reviews and Meta-Analyses (PRISMA) flow diagram of the reviewed literature.

3. Results

3.1. Therapeutic Apheresis in Autoimmune Encephalitides

Therapeutic apheresis is an important treatment option in a range of inflammatory central nervous system diseases [13]. It has been proven to be beneficial in primary demyelinating disease as well as in encephalitis caused by antibodies targeting neuronal proteins [14] (Table 2).

Therapeutic apheresis has been shown to be safe and effective leading to measurable laboratory and clinical improvement in several inflammatory diseases of the central and peripheral nervous system, including myasthenia gravis, Guillain-Barré syndrome and multiple sclerosis. Apheresis is recommended by the German Society of Neurology as escalation treatment of severe courses of AE. Patients should be treated with apheresis at least five times every other day. In cases with predominant CSF antibodies seven to ten treatment courses are usually needed for relevant reduction of CSF antibody titers. Before receiving therapeutic apheresis, patients mostly show either severe clinical symptoms on hospital admission or an insufficient response to therapy with high-dose cortisone or IVIG.

Much has been learned from acquired myasthenia gravis, which represents a "model disease" for the much later discovered forms of autoantibody-mediated AE. It could first be demonstrated that removal of the disease-defining acetylcholine receptor antibodies using plasma-exchange led to marked symptom improvement [15]. Antibodies in antibody-mediated AE are mostly directed against neuronal surface antigens. Emerging studies have demonstrated that clinical symptoms relate directly to pathogenic autoantibodies. For example, isolated human monoclonal autoantibodies from patients with NMDAR encephalitis targeted the NR1 subunit of the NMDAR and were alone sufficient to induce morphological and electrophysiological changes in the neurons, and to lead to synaptic dysfunction by downregulation of NMDAR [16]. Thus, the pathogenic effect is caused by the antibodies themselves, indicating that removal of these antibodies can disrupt the disease-causing mechanisms.

Therapeutic apheresis has been shown to improve clinical symptoms in different antibody-mediated diseases. According to the American Society for apheresis (ASFA) guidelines PE and IA are strongly recommended for different antibody-mediated encephalitis forms ranging from low to moderate evidence. In contrast, the therapeutic role of apheresis is not yet established for paraneoplastic neurological syndromes and individual decision-making is necessary [23]. In NMDAR encephalitis, recovery and symptom remission often correlate with a reduction of antibodies, in particular with a decline in CSF titers. In this way, antibody titers can serve as intra-individual disease biomarkers and support treatment decisions [24]. Efficacy of therapeutic apheresis relates to the extracorporeal elimination of circulating serum antibodies, redistribution of antibodies from the extracellular space and a number of secondary immunomodulatory changes. The inflammatory processes during AE are likely to involve a leakier blood-brain barrier, which might support further redistribution of autoantibodies from the central nervous system into the blood [25].

Table 2. Overview of studies on therapeutic apheresis in autoimmune encephalitis (AE).

Author	Year	Journal	Study Type	AE Type	Sample Size	Procedure	Outcome Measurement	Results	Ref.
DeSena AD	2015	J Clin Aph	Retrospective	NMDAR	10	PE	Modified Rankin scale (mRS)	Steroids alone not as effective as steroids followed by PE	[17]
Ehrlich S	2012	Nervenarzt	Retrospective	Antibody-mediated, paraneoplastic	30	PE, IA	mRS	Improvement of mRS after PE or IA	[18]
Heine J	2016	J Neurol	Prospective	NMDAR, LGI1, Caspr2, GAD, mGluR5, Hu	21	PE, IA	mRS	Improvement of mRS in 60% of patients	[19]
Hempel P	2016	Ther Apher Dial	Prospective	agAAB	8	IA	Neuropsychological test	Stabilized cognitive performance after 4-day treatment	[20]
Köhler W	2014	Eur J Neurol	Retrospective	NMDAR, GABA, LGI1, GAD	13	IA	mRS	Improvement of mRS in 11/13 patients	[21]
Onugoren MD	2016	Neurol Neuroimmunol Neuroinflamm	Retrospective	LGI1, Caspr2, NMDAR, GAD	19	IA	mRS	Improvement of mRS in patients with LGI1, Caspr2, NMDAR, no improvement in patients with GAD	[22]

3.2. Therapeutic Procedure for Apheresis

Therapeutic apheresis offers two different procedures. On the one hand is plasma exchange (PE), where a defined plasma volume is removed and replaced by human albumin or fresh frozen plasma. On the other hand is immunoadsorption (IA), a procedure that more specifically removes immunoglobulins and immune complexes by passing the plasma over an adsorber column, allowing reinfusion of the patients' own plasma. Two different IA procedures were used in the reviewed articles: either a regenerative double column system or a disposable tryptophan column. Tolerability and therapeutic effects do not show relevant differences between PE and IA in recent studies [14,19,26]. Related to the procedure is a rare risk of pathogen transmission in PE due to substitution with donor-derived blood components, which is not existent in IA [19]. However, angiotensin-converting enzyme inhibitors need to be paused for a minimum of 48 h prior to IA, otherwise there exists a risk of IA-associated bradykinin-release syndrome. Main side effects are not caused by the apheresis directly, but are rather related to the necessary central venous catheter. They include bleedings, hematoma, infections, thrombosis or damage caused by the puncture [22].

Usually a minimum of five sessions of apheresis is performed. When patients show a CSF predominant antibody, more sessions are generally needed in order to eliminate the antibody in the central nervous system. Most studies included in this review describe a central venous catheter in an internal jugular vein as vascular access. Only Hempel et al. use a peripheral vein to perform IA and in order to treat patients as outpatients. However, they report significant patient drop-out due to a failure of repeatedly accessing the vein [20].

The treated plasma volumes can be calculated using Sprenger's formula [27]. Depending on the protocol, a total of 1.5–2.2 plasma volume is processed in PE, whereas in IA 2000–2500 mL plasma per session are treated [19,22]. Patients treated with PE receive a replacement solution, such as 4% human albumin or fresh frozen plasma. Treatments take place every other day, although the first two to three sessions can be conducted on consecutive days in selected cases. Due to the central venous catheter, anticoagulation is necessary to minimize the risk of thrombosis.

3.3. Initiation of Therapy with Apheresis and Prior Treatment

The specific mechanism of antibody removal has been shown to be a more beneficial treatment of NMDAR encephalitis than intravenous methylprednisolone alone. In a retrospective study 2/14 patients showed significant clinical improvement following steroids, whereas 9/14 patients who received additional PE improved in the mRS during the third and fifth cycle of apheresis [17]. This is likely to be related to the high therapeutic specificity and therefore efficacy of therapeutic apheresis compared to intravenous immunoglobulins (IVIG) or high-dose corticosteroids. Early diagnosis and prompt start of a sufficiently "aggressive" therapy are mandatory for symptom reduction and long-term remission. Interestingly, a study by Heine et al. showed that treatment delay was not associated with a significantly worsened outcome [19], whereas Onugoren et al. found that, in patients with irreversible damage of brain structures, such as fixed hippocampal sclerosis, no clinical improvement could be achieved by IA [22].

Many patients with AE treated with apheresis receive prior treatment with high-dose steroids or IVIG. The decision for treatment with apheresis is often only made after unsuccessful or incomplete recovery after these other therapies. It has been shown that both patients who did and patients who did not receive prior treatment benefitted from apheresis [19]. In all studies analysed, a substantial part of the patients (up to more than half) received apheresis as initial treatment.

In the study by Onugoren et al. all patients except one out of 19 were treated with high-dose prednisolone (median dose 4.9 g) in parallel to IA [22]. It is reported that in some patients immunosuppressive therapy with steroids is continued on a maintenance dose [18]. Especially, patients with antibodies to LGI1 respond well to continued treatment with steroids [8,9].

Apheresis in patients with AE is most established in the acute phase of the disease. However, repeated apheresis might also be applied in refractory disease with clinical signs of AE and constant detection of high antibody titers. Yet in one study, repeated IA after 4.5 months (median) in six patients with antibodies against NMDAR, LGI1, Caspr2 and GAD that responded insufficiently to a first series of IA, did not show any further clinical improvement measured by mRS [22].

In case of an underlying malignancy, tumor removal is essential for improving further disease course.

3.4. Effects of Treatment with Apheresis in Patients with AE

A better outcome in patients with NMDAR encephalitis was strongly associated with an early start of immunotherapy (less than 40 days after symptom onset) [28]. Response rate in general is considerably higher when therapy initiation is started early [29] and includes improvement in state-of-the-art imaging and neuropsychological assessments [30].

According to a prospective study, symptoms that responded best to apheresis include apathy, aphasia, stupor, sleep disorders, agitation, myoclonus and dystonia, sensory neuropathy, apraxia and seizures [19]. In another study, in the majority of patients the modified Rankin Scale (mRS) improved by ≥1 point. It is of note that no patient worsened during apheresis in these studies.

Treatment efficacy is more pronounced in patients with antibodies against cell surface antibodies (NMDAR, LGI1, Caspr2, mGluR5) or in patients with intracellular synaptic antibodies (GAD), whereas no positive treatment effect was observed in patients with paraneoplastic intracellular antigens (anti-Hu) [19,22]. Marked reduction of serum antibodies occurred during the first five sessions of IA, but titers dropped further when apheresis was continued. Five days after IA a median decrease in titers of 97% and 64% was noted for serum and CSF, respectively. Interestingly, the decrease further continued until the next follow-up (median time after IA 3.9 months) [22]. In a retrospective study, all cerebral magnetic resonance imaging (MRI) changes in 17 patients with NMDAR encephalitis decreased [18].

Marked and rapid effects of apheresis can be seen in patients with epileptic seizures concerning seizure frequency. This was seen for patients with LGI1 and Caspr2 antibodies, where five out of seven patients became seizure free immediately after initiation of therapy with IA [22]. This treatment effect results in reduction or even complete removal of antiepileptic drugs.

Several case reports point to the efficacy of PE in drug-resistant status epilepticus caused by AE in children and adults. Both convulsive and non-convulsive status have been described as being responsive to apheresis. In patients with abnormal electroencephalogram (EEG) prior to apheresis, EEG normalization was observed after 5 cycles of PE. EEG improvement correlated with decrease in antibody titers [31,32].

Treatment of severe AE complicated by status epilepticus or autonomic instability might need to take place on an intensive care unit. On the ICU, benefit from immunotherapy, including apheresis, strongly depends on medical complications associated with a prolonged ICU stay [33].

In patients with predominantly psychiatric symptoms related to treatable autoimmunity, corticosteroids are often hesitantly used given the potential side effect of steroid-induced psychosis. Overall, notable neuropsychiatric side effects can occur in up to 6% of patients who receive steroids [34]; however, in antibody-mediated AE the clinical improvement with immunotherapy quickly outrivals any steroid-related effects on psychiatric symptoms according to our experience.

In paraneoplastic AE with antibodies targeting intracellular proteins, therapeutic effects of rituximab, IVIG and therapeutic apheresis are usually limited as the antibodies are not directly pathogenic, but neuronal damage is caused by cytotoxic T-cells [19,26]. Furthermore, diagnosis in paraneoplastic disease is often delayed and substantial irreversible neuronal cell damage has already occurred at the time of therapy initiation. Discontinuation of therapy should be considered in patients in whom brain damage has progressed to an advanced stage in MRI after three to six months despite intensified immunotherapy.

After therapeutic apheresis with both PE and IA, a transient spurious intrathecal immunoglobulin synthesis of all three subclasses (IgG, IgA, IgM) can be observed. The transient intrathecal Ig fractions and increased IgG index are due to dropped serum IgG levels following apheresis. This "intrathecal pseudo-synthesis" regularly occurs in the first two days after apheresis in a majority of patients [35]. Thus, one needs to consider these abnormalities for interpretation of CSF results from lumbar puncture shortly after apheresis in order to prevent false diagnostic assumptions.

3.5. Future Treatment Options for Apheresis

Clinical indications for therapeutic apheresis in AE might expand to less recognized antibody-mediated conditions in the near future. We could recently demonstrate that asymptomatic mothers of a child requiring psychiatric in-patient diagnostics carried low-level pathogenic human NR1 antibodies more frequently than control mothers having a healthy child [36]. To better understand this possible connection, we developed a murine model of pregnancy-related materno-fetal antibody transfer. Here, human monoclonal NR1 antibodies diaplacentally transferred to the offspring, enriched in the fetal circulation and brain, caused neurotoxic effects during neonatal development, inducing brain network changes, and led to neuropathological disorders in the offspring persisting into adulthood [36]. Given the relatively high frequency of NR1 autoantibodies in the healthy human population, the findings indicate a novel disease principle with high clinical relevance for lifelong neuropsychiatric morbidity in the affected children [37]. Most importantly, these pathologies are potentially treatable with apheresis in asymptomatic mothers, but further studies are needed to better understand the frequency of autoantibodies, the susceptible window during pregnancy and the contribution of genetic and further risk factors. Further, this seems not to be limited to the NMDAR, as other maternal anti-neuronal autoantibodies may similarly cause neurodevelopmental disorders in the offspring, such as with antibodies against Caspr2 [38].

The use of therapeutic apheresis has been shown to be safe in pregnant women, both for mother and fetus. A recent Italian study evaluated the use of apheresis during pregnancy. Among 48 pregnant women receiving apheresis one had suspected autoimmune encephalitis. Adverse events occurred in 2.1% of all patients analysed, which is reported to be lower than the Italian average. Peripheral veins are preferred as a vascular access during pregnancy to avoid the risks associated with a central venous catheter [39].

3.6. Apheresis in Children with AE

Children with autoimmune disorders such as antibody-mediated AE can also be treated with therapeutic apheresis. PE was retrospectively evaluated in 22 children. All children had been treated with IVIG and/or steroids before PE. Each patient received a median number of six PE sessions. No PE-related mortality was observed and adverse events occurred in 2.2%, which is the expected average. Adverse events consisted of hypotension and urticaria. In total, three pediatric patients with antibody-mediated encephalitis were treated with PE, two patients improved and one patient showed partial recovery with persistent neurological deficits after three-year follow-up. One patient with paraneoplastic encephalitis did not benefit from PE and was lost to follow-up [40]. Another prospective observational study evaluated 535 children with acquired demyelinating syndrome or encephalitis treated with steroids, IVIG or PE. Here, pediatric patients with autoimmune encephalitis other than acute disseminated encephalomyelitis (ADEM) had the highest frequency of poor outcome. However, the individual treatment decisions were not specified [41].

3.7. Autoimmune Dementia and Treatment with Apheresis

Compared to 'classic' AE with subacute onset of neuropsychiatric as well as behavioral symptoms, antibody-associated dementias are a more slowly progressing group of diseases where decline in working and short-term memory as well as visuo-spatial deficits are the most prominent features. Detection of high-level autoantibodies in patients with dementia is rare, but autoimmune dementias represent a form of cognitive decline that is potentially treatable. A Mayo clinic study reported improvement of cognition in 64% of patients with suspected autoimmune dementia after immunomodulatory treatment [29]. An underlying autoimmune mechanism and response to immunotherapy is more likely when patients do not fulfill routine criteria for established neurodegenerative dementia forms, but rather present with subacute onset, psychiatric symptoms, fluctuating disease course, shorter delay to treatment, seropositivity for a specific autoantibody and inflammatory CSF [29].

In a retrospective study analyzing 286 CSF and serum samples of patients with different dementia forms, 16% of the serum samples had NMDAR IgA, IgM or IgG antibodies compared to 4.3% in a healthy control group [42]. Besides the spectrum of known and established pathogenic antibodies, there might be an even broader range of autoantibodies for which pathogenicity has not yet been confirmed. It is unclear from these studies whether anti-neuronal autoantibodies develop secondarily to neurodegeneration or whether they primarily contribute to and drive the disease. It is highly possible that neurodegeneration leads to the presentation of autoantigens from dying neurons with consecutive establishment of a specific autoimmune response. In this way, formed autoantibodies may contribute to synaptic dysfunction, further accelerate cognitive decline or contribute to clinical symptoms such as behavioral abnormalities commonly present in dementia patients.

Another recent target in dementia patients are autoantibodies against G protein-coupled receptors. In a small trial analyzing the effect of IA in patients with mild to moderate dementia and agonistic autoantibodies (agAAB) against α-adrenergic receptors, treatment with four cycles of IA not only caused disappearance of autoantibodies, but resulted in stabilization of the cognitive and mental condition during the follow-up period of 12–18 months [20]. Another study that is currently recruiting (ClinicalTrials.gov Identifier: NCT03132272) investigates the effects of IA in patients with Alzheimer's disease positive for agAAB. The group aims to demonstrate discontinuation of the vascular remodeling and slowing of cognitive decline following IA treatment.

Apheresis not only has an acute effect on disease activity but can be used for longer lasting immunomodulation. In case of uncertainty of the immunological findings, first-line therapy including steroids or apheresis may serve as a diagnostic test to support the autoimmune etiology [43]. In our experience, however, short-term treatment (such as intravenous high-dose steroids for three to five days) cannot demonstrate clinical improvement in autoimmune dementia in most cases, thus requiring longer administration for four to six weeks (e.g., daily 0.5 mg/kg prednisone).

Based on the new developments in this field, the ongoing identification of dementia-associated autoantibodies and the concern about overlooking treatable etiologies, we now offer diagnostic antibody testing in serum and CSF to every patient with suspected dementia in our memory clinic at the department of neurology at Charité. In this way we increasingly identify patients with a working diagnosis of Alzheimer's, frontotemporal dementia or atypical dementia who have new or established autoantibodies against neuronal and glial proteins, as exemplarily shown in the case vignette of an 81-year-old gentleman (Box 1).

Detection of antibodies against neurochondrin (Figure 2) in this patient led to immunotherapy with IA. The observed clinical improvement prompted B-cell depleting therapy with rituximab that led to long-term stabilization.

The patient participates in an ongoing clinical trial (DRKS00016017) analyzing the role of anti-neuronal and anti-glial surface antibodies in cognitive disorders and potential improvement following IA. The study aims to identify dementia patients who harbor autoantibodies against structures of the central nervous system using cell-based assays for detection of established autoantibodies as well as screening assays using indirect immunofluorescence on unfixed murine brain sections. Autoantibody-positive patients with cognitive decline can enroll in the study and receive therapeutic apheresis (Figure 3). Treatment includes five to six IA sessions over a 12-day course. Cognitive performance is evaluated prospectively and compared to historic controls. Patients further undergo structural und functional MRI before and after IA. CSF analysis evaluates the reduction of autoantibody levels over the course of IA and the potential utility of further biomarkers of neurodegeneration, such as micro-RNAs.

Box 1. Clinical case of autoimmune dementia.

An 81-year-old dementia patient presented to our outpatient memory clinic at the department of Neurology at Charité—Universitätsmedizin Berlin with deficits in working and short term memory as well as difficulties in concentration. Symptoms began nine months prior to presentation with increasing loss of orientation for place and time, confusion and reported visual hallucinations. Brain MRI at symptom onset was unremarkable apart from microangiopathic lesions in the left temporoparietal lobe (Figure 2A). Basic CSF analysis showed markedly increased protein. Symptoms improved after several weeks without specific therapy, but anterograde memory deficit persisted. During the following months, two episodes with re-appearance of confusion occurred, but lasted only for days.

In our center, the patient showed a persisting dysexecutive syndrome with amnestic and visuo-constructive deficits and apraxia. No other neurological deficits were observed. Montreal cognitive assessment showed mild cognitive impairment with a score of 21 out of 30. A second CSF analysis revealed normal cell count, but still increased protein of 1288 mg/L (normal <450 mg/L). No infectious cause was found. Extensive search for anti-neuronal autoantibodies in serum and CSF including indirect immunofluorescence staining on rodent brain sections detected neurochondrin IgG antibodies in the CSF (Figure 2B).

The diagnosis of AE with oligosymptomatic memory deficits was established. A three-day course of intravenous methylprednisolone with 1 g/day led to improved gait, but no impact on cognition was observed. Because of the persisting memory deficits, two months later five sessions of IA were administered every other day and resulted in reduction of CSF neurochondrin antibody titers (Figure 2C). The patient reported vertigo during IA, but vital signs were unremarkable at all times. After IA, the patient described improved concentration; his wife reported better organization of daily life and his ability to care for himself again. In the Bristol Activities of Daily Living Scale the patient improved from 20 points to 9 points.

The patient's autoantibodies targeted neurochondrin, a leucine-rich protein expressed not only in the brain, but also in bones and cartilage. As neurochondrin is located intracellularly, the pathogenicity of neurochondrin antibodies is unclear and they might only be a biomarker of autoimmunity including T-cell-mediated neurotoxicity [44]. Neurochondrin expression is highest in cerebellar Purkinje cells, brainstem, lateral parts of the central amygdala nuclei and the hippocampal pyramidal cells. Antibodies against neurochondrin bind robustly to the hippocampus, cerebellum and amygdala, while binding to the striatum, thalamus and cerebral cortex is less pronounced [45]. Patients described so far presented with rapidly progressing cerebellar ataxia, brainstem signs and neuropsychiatric symptoms.

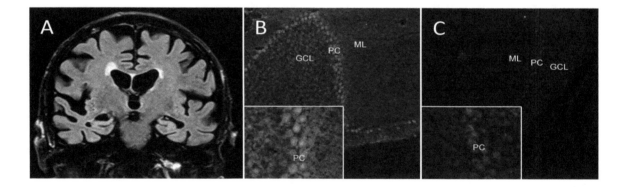

Figure 2. Autoantibodies against neurochondrin. (**A**) MRI T2/FLAIR (fluid-attenuated inversion recovery) of the 81-year-old dementia patient was largely unremarkable apart from few microangiopathic lesions in the left temporoparietal lobe. (**B**) Indirect immunofluorescence of murine cerebellum sections demonstrated CSF IgG antibodies against neurochondrin (GCL, granule cell layer; PC, Purkinje cells; ML, molecular layer). (**C**) Following immunotherapy with five sessions of IA, antibody titers in CSF were markedly reduced.

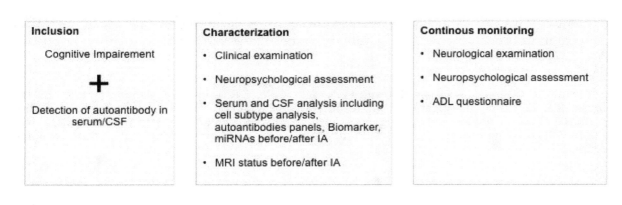

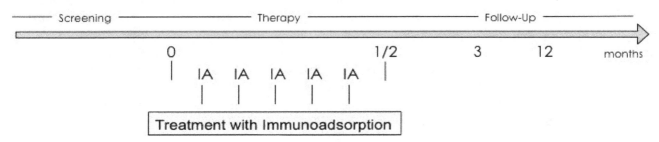

Figure 3. Immunoadsorption in autoantibody-positive patients with cognitive impairment—trial protocol. Patients with confirmed autoantibodies against central nervous system antigens and progressing cognitive impairment receive immunotherapy with five sessions of IA together with detailed neuropsychological, MRI and CSF biomarker assessment. Follow-up monitoring includes two visits after three and 12 months.

3.8. Closing Remarks and Outlook

Predictors for beneficial outcome after treatment with apheresis in patients with AE include start of the treatment early in the disease before substantial irreversible brain damage has occurred. Nevertheless, after longer periods from symptom onset to therapy initiation, apheresis can also result in symptom improvement. Immunotherapy with steroids or IVIG prior to apheresis does not seem to have an effect on the overall outcome. Especially in patients with severe disease courses apheresis is a major treatment option and should be initiated early, possibly together with other immune therapies.

For selected patient groups such as children and pregnant women as well as patients requiring ICU treatment, the safety and efficacy of apheresis could also be shown.

According to all studies reviewed, the ASFA guidelines and the recommendations given by the German Society of Neurology, no benefit of apheresis in patients with onco-neuronal antibodies could be shown. Here, results are inconsistent, with most patients showing no therapeutic effect after apheresis, or even further deterioration, but in single patients clinical improvement could sometimes be seen. A clear treatment response to apheresis, both, PE and IA, is established in patients with antibodies against surface antigens or synaptic antigens. In the articles screened for this review, there was no difference in outcome of patients treated with PE or IA. Therapeutic apheresis is a valuable option within the complex multimodal immune therapy of AE. The benefit of treating patients with antibody-mediated AE with apheresis by far outweighs the possible side effects that were not severe and were mainly associated with the central venous catheter. Furthermore treatment with apheresis may be complicated by the necessity of an ICU setting and poor patient cooperation.

Although predominant humoral autoimmunity seems to be rare in dementia patients and requires further study, the search for autoantibodies in these patients allows the detection of potentially treatable dementia forms and holds the potential to prevent further cognitive decline in selected patients. Thus, therapeutic apheresis is not only an important first-line therapy in patients with AE but may be increasingly considered in further patients who are positive for autoantibodies against neuronal structures. This already includes patients with cognitive decline but may in the future expand to novel clinical indications ranging from antibody-associated psychosis to autoantibody-positive pregnant women.

Author Contributions: Conceptualization, R.R. and H.P.; methodology, R.R. and H.P.; validation, R.R. and H.P.; formal analysis, R.R. and H.P.; investigation, R.R.; resources, H.P.; data curation, R.R.; writing—original draft preparation, R.R.; writing—review and editing, H.P.; visualization, R.R. and H.P.; supervision, H.P.; project administration, H.P.; funding acquisition, H.P. All authors have read and agreed to the published version of the manuscript.

References

1. Graus, F.; Titulaer, M.J.; Balu, R.; Benseler, S.; Bien, C.G.; Cellucci, T.; Cortese, I.; Dale, R.C.; Gelfand, J.M.; Geschwind, M.; et al. A clinical approach to diagnosis of autoimmune encephalitis. *Lancet Neurol.* **2016**, *15*, 391–404. [CrossRef]
2. Finke, C.; Prüss, H.; Heine, J.; Reuter, S.; Kopp, U.A.; Wegner, F.; Bergh, F.T.; Koch, S.; Jansen, O.; Münte, T.; et al. Evaluation of cognitive deficits and structural hippocampal damage in encephalitis with leucine-rich, glioma-inactivated 1 antibodies. *JAMA Neurol.* **2017**, *74*, 50. [CrossRef] [PubMed]
3. Reintjes, W.; Romijn, M.D.; Hollander, D.; Ter Bruggen, J.P.; Van Marum, R.J. Reversible dementia: Two nursing home patients with voltage-gated potassium channel antibody-associated limbic encephalitis. *J. Am. Med. Dir. Assoc.* **2015**, *16*, 790–794. [CrossRef] [PubMed]
4. Marquetand, J.; Lessen, M.; Bender, B.; Reimold, M.; Elsen, G.; Stoecker, W.; Synofzik, M. Slowly progressive LGI1 encephalitis with isolated late-onset cognitive dysfunction: A treatable mimic of Alzheimer's disease. *Eur. J. Neurol.* **2016**, *23*, 28–29. [CrossRef]
5. Saiz, A.; Blanco, Y.; Sabater, L.; González, F.; Bataller, L.; Casamitjana, R.; Ramió-Torrentà, L.; Graus, F. Spectrum of neurological syndromes associated with glutamic acid decarboxylase antibodies: Diagnostic clues for this association. *Brain* **2008**, *131*, 2553–2563. [CrossRef]
6. Dalmau, J.; Graus, F. Antibody-mediated encephalitis. *N. Engl. J. Med.* **2018**, *378*, 840–851. [CrossRef]
7. Dalmau, J.; Armangué, T.; Planagumà, J.; Radosevic, M.; Mannara, F.; Leypoldt, F.; Geis, C.; Lancaster, E.; Titulaer, M.J.; Rosenfeld, M.R.; et al. An update on anti-NMDA receptor encephalitis for neurologists and psychiatrists: Mechanisms and models. *Lancet Neurol.* **2019**, *18*, 1045–1057. [CrossRef]
8. Gaig, C.; Graus, F.; Compta, Y.; Högl, B.; Bataller, L.; Brüggemann, N.; Giordana, C.; Heidbreder, A.; Kotschet, K.; Lewerenz, J.; et al. Clinical manifestations of the anti-IgLON5 disease. *Neurology* **2017**, *88*, 1736–1743. [CrossRef]
9. Irani, S.R.; Alexander, S.; Waters, P.; Kleopa, K.A.; Pettingill, P.; Zuliani, L.; Peles, E.; Buckley, C.; Lang, B.; Vincent, A. Antibodies to Kv1 potassium channel-complex proteins leucine-rich, glioma inactivated 1 protein and contactin-associated protein-2 in limbic encephalitis, Morvan's syndrome and acquired neuromyotonia. *Brain* **2010**, *133*, 2734–2748. [CrossRef]
10. Graus, F.; Delattre, J.Y.; Antoine, J.C.; Dalmau, J.; Giometto, B.; Grisold, W.; Honnorat, J.; Smitt, P.S.; Vedeler, C.; Verschuuren, J.; et al. Recommended diagnostic criteria for paraneoplastic neurological syndromes. *J. Neurol. Neurosurg. Psychiatry* **2004**, *75*, 1135–1140. [CrossRef]
11. Gultekin, S.H.; Rosenfeld, M.R.; Voltz, R.; Eichen, J.; Posner, J.B.; Dalmau, J. Paraneoplastic limbic encephalitis: Neurological symptoms, immunological findings and tumour association in 50 patients. *Brain* **2000**, *123*, 1481–1494. [CrossRef] [PubMed]
12. Moher, D.; Liberati, A.; Tetzlaff, J.; Altman, U.G. Preferred reporting items for systematic reviews and meta-analyses: The PRISMA statement. *PLoS Med.* **2009**, *6*, e1000097. [CrossRef] [PubMed]
13. Sorgun, M.H.; Erdogan, S.; Bay, M.; Ayyıldız, E.; Yücemen, N.; Iihan, O.; Yücesan, C.; Ayyildiz, E. Therapeutic plasma exchange in treatment of neuroimmunologic disorders: Review of 92 cases. *Transfus. Apher. Sci.* **2013**, *49*, 174–180. [CrossRef] [PubMed]
14. Weinshenker, B.G.; O'Brien, P.C.; Petterson, T.M.; Noseworthy, J.H.; Lucchinetti, C.F.; Dodick, D.W.; Pineda, A.A.; Stevens, L.N.; Rodriguez, M. A randomized trial of plasma exchange in acute central nervous system inflammatory demyelinating disease. *Ann. Neurol.* **1999**, *46*, 878–886. [CrossRef]
15. Pinching, A.J.; Peters, D.K. Remission of myasthenia gravis following plasma-exchange. *Lancet* **1976**, *308*, 1373–1376. [CrossRef]

16. Kreye, J.; Wenke, N.K.; Chayka, M.; Leubner, J.; Murugan, R.; Maier, N.; Jurek, B.; Ly, L.-T.; Brandl, D.; Rost, B.R.; et al. Human cerebrospinal fluid monoclonal N-methyl-D-aspartate receptor autoantibodies are sufficient for encephalitis pathogenesis. *Brain* **2016**, *139*, 2641–2652. [CrossRef]

17. DeSena, A.D.; Noland, D.K.; Matevosyan, K.; King, K.; Phillips, L.; Qureshi, S.S.; Greenberg, B.M.; Graves, D. Intravenous methylprednisolone versus therapeutic plasma exchange for treatment of anti-n-methyl-d-aspartate receptor antibody encephalitis: A retrospective review. *J. Clin. Apher.* **2015**, *30*, 212–216. [CrossRef]

18. Ehrlich, S.; Fassbender, C.; Blaes, C.; Finke, C.; Günther, A.; Harms, L.; Hoffmann, F.; Jahner, K.; Klingel, R.; Kraft, A.; et al. Therapeutische Apherese bei autoimmuner Enzephalitis. *Der Nervenarzt* **2013**, *84*, 498–507. [CrossRef]

19. Heine, J.; Ly, L.-T.; Lieker, I.; Slowinski, T.; Finke, C.; Prüss, H.; Harms, L. Immunoadsorption or plasma exchange in the treatment of autoimmune encephalitis: A pilot study. *J. Neurol.* **2016**, *263*, 2395–2402. [CrossRef]

20. Hempel, P.; Heinig, B.; Jerosch, C.; Decius, I.; Karczewski, P.; Kassner, U.; Kunze, R.; Steinhagen-Thiessen, E.; Bimmler, M. Immunoadsorption of agonistic autoantibodies against α1-adrenergic receptors in patients with mild to moderate dementia. *Ther. Apher. Dial.* **2016**, *20*, 523–529. [CrossRef]

21. Kohler, W.; Ehrlich, S.; Dohmen, C.; Haubitz, M.; Hoffmann, F.; Schmidt, S.; Klingel, R.; Kraft, A.; Neumann-Haefelin, T.; Topka, H.; et al. Tryptophan immunoadsorption for the treatment of autoimmune encephalitis. *Eur. J. Neurol.* **2014**, *22*, 203–206. [CrossRef] [PubMed]

22. Onugoren, M.D.; Golombeck, K.S.; Bien, C.; Abu-Tair, M.; Brand, M.; Bulla-Hellwig, M.; Lohmann, H.; Münstermann, D.; Pavenstädt, H.; Thölking, G.; et al. Immunoadsorption therapy in autoimmune encephalitides. *Neurol. Neuroimmunol. Neuroinflamm.* **2016**, *3*, e207. [CrossRef] [PubMed]

23. Padmanabhan, A.; Connelly-Smith, L.; Aqui, N.; Balogun, R.A.; Klingel, R.; Meyer, E.; Pham, H.P.; Schneiderman, J.; Witt, V.; Wu, Y.; et al. Guidelines on the use of therapeutic apheresis in clinical practice—evidence-based approach from the writing committee of the american society for apheresis: The eighth special issue. *J. Clin. Apher.* **2019**, *34*, 171–354. [CrossRef] [PubMed]

24. Gresa-Arribas, N.; Titulaer, M.J.; Torrents, A.; Aguilar, E.; McCracken, L.; Leypoldt, F.; Gleichman, A.J.; Balice-Gordon, R.; Rosenfeld, M.R.; Lynch, D.; et al. Antibody titres at diagnosis and during follow-up of anti-NMDA receptor encephalitis: A retrospective study. *Lancet Neurol.* **2013**, *13*, 167–177. [CrossRef]

25. Dalmau, J.; Gleichman, A.J.; Hughes, E.G.; Rossi, J.E.; Peng, X.; Lai, M.; Dessain, S.K.; Rosenfeld, M.R.; Balice-Gordon, R.; Lynch, D.R. Anti-NMDA-receptor encephalitis: Case series and analysis of the effects of antibodies. *Lancet Neurol.* **2008**, *7*, 1091–1098. [CrossRef]

26. Fassbender, C.; Klingel, R.; Köhler, W. Immunoadsorption for autoimmune encephalitis. *Atheroscler. Suppl.* **2017**, *30*, 257–263. [CrossRef]

27. Sprenger, K.B.G.; Huber, K.; Kratz, W.; Henze, E. Nomograms for the prediction of patient's plasma volume in plasma exchange therapy from height, weight and hematocrit. *J. Clin. Apher.* **1987**, *3*, 185–190. [CrossRef]

28. Irani, S.R.; Vincent, A. NMDA receptor antibody encephalitis. *Curr. Neurol. Neurosci. Rep.* **2011**, *11*, 298–304. [CrossRef]

29. Flanagan, E.P.; McKeon, A.; Lennon, V.A.; Boeve, B.F.; Trenerry, M.R.; Tan, K.M.; Drubach, D.A.; Josephs, K.A.; Britton, J.W.; Mandrekar, J.N.; et al. Autoimmune dementia: Clinical course and predictors of immunotherapy response. *Mayo Clin. Proc.* **2010**, *85*, 881–897. [CrossRef]

30. Finke, C.; Kopp, U.A.; Pajkert, A.; Behrens, J.R.; Leypoldt, F.; Wuerfel, J.T.; Ploner, C.J.; Prüss, H.; Paul, F. Information, P.E.K.F.C. structural hippocampal damage following anti-n-methyl-d-aspartate receptor encephalitis. *Biol. Psychiatry* **2016**, *79*, 727–734. [CrossRef]

31. Bektaş, Ö.; Yılmaz, A.; Kendirli, T.; Şıklar, Z.; Deda, G.; Yilmaz, A.; Kendirli, T. Hashimoto encephalopathy causing drug-resistant status epilepticus treated with plasmapheresis. *Pediatr. Neurol.* **2012**, *46*, 132–135. [CrossRef] [PubMed]

32. Pari, E.; Rinaldi, F.; Premi, E.; Codella, M.; Rao, R.; Paghera, B.; Panarotto, M.B.; De Maria, G.; Padovani, A. A follow-up 18F-FDG brain PET study in a case of Hashimoto's encephalopathy causing drug-resistant status epilepticus treated with plasmapheresis. *J. Neurol.* **2014**, *261*, 663–667. [CrossRef] [PubMed]

33. Mittal, M.K.; Rabinstein, A.A.; Hocker, S.E.; Pittock, S.J.; Wijdicks, E.F.M.; McKeon, A. Autoimmune

encephalitis in the ICU: Analysis of phenotypes, serologic findings, and outcomes. *Neurocritical Care* **2015**, *24*, 240–250. [CrossRef] [PubMed]

34. Dubovsky, A.N.; Arvikar, S.; Stern, T.A.; Axelrod, L. The neuropsychiatric complications of glucocorticoid use: Steroid psychosis revisited. *Psychosomatics* **2012**, *53*, 103–115. [CrossRef]

35. Berger, B.; Hottenrott, T.; Leubner, J.; Dersch, R.; Rauer, S.; Stich, O.; Prüss, H. Transient spurious intrathecal immunoglobulin synthesis in neurological patients after therapeutic apheresis. *BMC Neurol.* **2015**, *15*, 1–6. [CrossRef]

36. Jurek, B.; Chayka, M.; Kreye, J.; Lang, K.; Kraus, L.; Fidzinski, P.; Kornau, H.; Dao, L.; Wenke, N.K.; Long, M.; et al. Human gestational N -methyl- d -aspartate receptor autoantibodies impair neonatal murine brain function. *Ann. Neurol.* **2019**, *86*, 656–670. [CrossRef]

37. Dahm, L.; Ott, C.; Steiner, J.; Stepniak, B.; Teegen, B.; Saschenbrecker, S.; Hammer, C.; Borowski, K.; Begemann, M.; Lemke, S.; et al. Seroprevalence of autoantibodies against brain antigens in health and disease. *Ann. Neurol.* **2014**, *76*, 82–94. [CrossRef]

38. Coutinho, E.; Jacobson, L.; Pedersen, M.G.; Benros, M.E.; Nørgaard-Pedersen, B.; Mortensen, P.B.; Harrison, P.J.; Vincent, A. CASPR2 autoantibodies are raised during pregnancy in mothers of children with mental retardation and disorders of psychological development but not autism. *J. Neurol. Neurosurg. Psychiatry* **2017**, *88*, 718–721. [CrossRef]

39. Colpo, A.; Marson, P.; Pavanello, F.; Tison, T.; Gervasi, M.T.; Zambon, A.; Ruffatti, A.; De Silvestro, G.; Hoxha, A. Therapeutic apheresis during pregnancy: A single center experience. *Transfus. Apher. Sci.* **2019**, *58*, 652–658. [CrossRef]

40. Özkale, M.; Erol, I.; Özkale, Y.; Kozanoğlu, I. Overview of therapeutic plasma exchange in pediatric neurology: A single-center experience. *Acta Neurol. Belg.* **2018**, *118*, 451–458. [CrossRef]

41. Armangue, T.; Olivé-Cirera, G.; Martínez-Hernandez, E.; Sepulveda, M.; Ruiz-Garcia, R.; Muñoz-Batista, M.; Ariño, H.; González-Álvarez, V.; Felipe-Rucián, A.; Martínez-González, M.J.; et al. Associations of paediatric demyelinating and encephalitic syndromes with myelin oligodendrocyte glycoprotein antibodies: A multicentre observational study. *Lancet Neurol.* **2020**, *19*, 234–246. [CrossRef]

42. Doss, S.; Wandinger, K.-P.; Hyman, B.T.; Panzer, J.A.; Synofzik, M.; Dickerson, B.; Mollenhauer, B.; Scherzer, C.R.; Ivinson, A.J.; Finke, C.; et al. High prevalence of NMDA receptor IgA/IgM antibodies in different dementia types. *Ann. Clin. Transl. Neurol.* **2014**, *1*, 822–832. [CrossRef] [PubMed]

43. Flanagan, E.P.; Drubach, D.A.; Boeve, B.F. Autoimmune dementia and encephalopathy. *Handb. Clin. Neurol.* **2016**, *133*, 247–267. [CrossRef] [PubMed]

44. Miske, R.; Gross, C.C.; Scharf, M.; Golombeck, K.S.; Hartwig, M.; Bhatia, U.; Schulte-Mecklenbeck, A.; Bönte, K.; Strippel, C.; Schöls, L.; et al. Neurochondrin is a neuronal target antigen in autoimmune cerebellar degeneration. *Neurol. Neuroimmunol. Neuroinflamm.* **2016**, *4*, e307. [CrossRef]

45. Weisenhorn, D.M.V.; Floss, T.; Wurst, W.; Istvánffy, R. Expression of neurochondrin in the developing and adult mouse brain. *Dev. Genes Evol.* **2004**, *214*, 206–209. [CrossRef]

15

Is a Wearable Sensor-Based Characterisation of Gait Robust Enough to Overcome Differences Between Measurement Protocols? A Multi-Centric Pragmatic Study in Patients with Multiple Sclerosis

Lorenza Angelini [1,2,*], Ilaria Carpinella [3], Davide Cattaneo [3], Maurizio Ferrarin [3], Elisa Gervasoni [3], Basil Sharrack [4], David Paling [5], Krishnan Padmakumari Sivaraman Nair [2,4] and Claudia Mazzà [1,2]

[1]   Department of Mechanical Engineering, University of Sheffield, Sheffield S1 3JD, UK;
       c.mazza@sheffield.ac.uk
[2]   Insigneo Institute for in silico Medicine, University of Sheffield, Sheffield S1 3JD, UK; siva.nair@nhs.net
[3]   IRCCS Fondazione Don Carlo Gnocchi, 20121 Milan, Italy; icarpinella@dongnocchi.it (I.C.);
       dcattaneo@dongnocchi.it (D.C.); mferrarin@dongnocchi.it (M.F.); egervasoni@dongnocchi.it (E.G.)
[4]   Academic Department of Neuroscience, Sheffield NIHR Neuroscience BRC, Sheffield Teaching Hospital
       NHS Foundation Trust, Sheffield S10 2JF, UK; basil.sharrack@nhs.net
[5]   Sheffield Institute of Translational Neuroscience, Sheffield Teaching Hospitals NHS Foundation Trust,
       Sheffield S10 2JF, UK; david.paling@nhs.net
*   Correspondence: L.Angelini@sheffield.ac.uk

Abstract: Inertial measurement units (IMUs) allow accurate quantification of gait impairment of people with multiple sclerosis (pwMS). Nonetheless, it is not clear how IMU-based metrics might be influenced by pragmatic aspects associated with clinical translation of this approach, such as data collection settings and gait protocols. In this study, we hypothesised that these aspects do not significantly alter those characteristics of gait that are more related to quality and energetic efficiency and are quantifiable via acceleration related metrics, such as intensity, smoothness, stability, symmetry, and regularity. To test this hypothesis, we compared 33 IMU-based metrics extracted from data, retrospectively collected by two independent centres on two matched cohorts of pwMS. As a worst-case scenario, a walking test was performed in the two centres at a different speed along corridors of different lengths, using different IMU systems, which were also positioned differently. The results showed that the majority of the temporal metrics (9 out of 12) exhibited significant between-centre differences. Conversely, the between-centre differences in the gait quality metrics were small and comparable to those associated with a test-retest analysis under equivalent conditions. Therefore, the gait quality metrics are promising candidates for reliable multi-centric studies aiming at assessing rehabilitation interventions within a routine clinical context.

Keywords: multiple sclerosis; gait metrics; wearable sensors; test-retest reliability; sampling frequency; accelerometry; autocorrelation; harmonic ratio; six-minute walk

1. Introduction

Multiple sclerosis (MS) is a chronic demyelinating disease of the central nervous system affecting 2.3 million people worldwide [1]. MS is the major non-traumatic cause of disability in young and middle-aged adults [2], with a significant negative impact on independence and social participation [3]. Walking impairment is one of the most common functional deficits due to MS, even in the early stages of the disease [4]. Importantly, nearly 70% of people with MS (pwMS) reported that walking difficulty is the most challenging aspect of their condition [5].

Given the high impact of gait impairment on pwMS, different rehabilitation interventions focused on improving locomotion are currently applied to improve the quality of life in this population [6]. The effects of these interventions, together with the progression of the disease, are usually assessed in clinical practice using clinical scales, such as the expanded disability status scale (EDSS) [7] or timed tests, such as the timed up and go test (TUG) [8], the timed 25-foot walk test (T25FW) [9], and the 6-minute walk test (6MWT) [10]. Although widely used, these tests suffer from some limitations. Firstly, they assess only the time taken to execute the test (e.g., TUG and T25FW) or the distance travelled in a given time (6 min for the 6MWT), without providing objective measures of the different components and characteristics of the task that could be useful to describe *how* the performance is possibly impaired [11]. Secondly, these clinical tests have a relatively limited sensitivity to change [9,12,13] and a flooring effect [9,14] that makes it difficult to detect possible alterations in minimally impaired pwMS [15–17].

Instrumental methods may partly overcome these limitations by providing additional quantitative information for a more complete characterisation of walking, which can be useful to tailor the rehabilitative intervention and objectively assess its effects [11,18]. In particular, wearable inertial measurement units (IMUs), including accelerometers, gyroscopes, and magnetometers, represent cost-effective tools to perform objective assessments of walking in pwMS outside movement analysis labs [19,20], and even during free-living and community contexts [21,22]. IMUs have been widely used to analyse different locomotor tasks in pwMS, such as straight-line over ground [17,23–27] and treadmill walking [28], standing up, walking, turning, and sitting down (e.g., the TUG) [15,29], walking with head turns and over/around obstacles [30,31], walking while texting [32], and stairway walking [33]. During these tests, several parameters have been extracted from IMUs, including spatio-temporal parameters [15,24,27,28,31,32,34], indexes of gait variability and stability [17,23,24,26,31,33], trunk sway metrics [15,23,30,34], and angular variables [15,25,27,34]. Nonetheless, what does not yet clearly emerge from current literature on pwMS is which of these could be more reliably adopted within the clinical context.

Besides the issue of identifying among the above metrics those that are more capable of characterising the disease progression, hence providing similar results for patients with similar clinical conditions, and that have the sensitivity to detect changes associated with clinical interventions, the clinical adoption of specific gait metrics also requires accounting for a number of pragmatic limitations associated with testing conditions. These include an understanding of which output is more robust to testing site characteristics (e.g., corridor lengths, lightening, noise, etc.), adopted measuring instruments and their configuration (e.g., brand, location on the body, sampling frequency) [35–37], type of gait test (e.g., a single pass, a 1-minute or a 6MWT), or instructions given to patients (e.g., self-selected or fast walking speed, use or not use of an assistive device) [28,38–45]. All these aspects are particularly difficult to standardise in a busy clinical environment and most likely occur in combination with each other.

The aim of this study was to identify those gait metrics that provide equivalent assessment of pwMS with similar characteristics in terms of age, gender, and gait disability, despite these being tested in different centres and in non-standardised conditions. Our hypothesis was that while pwMS might be able to adjust their gait in terms of spatio-temporal parameters in response to different testing conditions (e.g., if asked to increase their speed), they would not be able to control those aspects of gait more related to its overall quality and energetic efficiency [46,47]. As a result, metrics extracted directly from the acceleration signals and representative of intensity, smoothness, stability, symmetry, and regularity were expected to be more robust to differences in the test settings. To verify this hypothesis, we compared retrospective data from two matched cohorts of pwMS, which were collected by two independent hospitals using protocols that differed for: (i) brand, size, and sampling frequency of the IMUs; (ii) IMU positioning; (iii) subject instructing; (iv) length of the path. As a term of reference, we also compared differences in IMU-based metrics between the two centres (between-centre differences) to those observable between two sessions performed by the same centre (between-day test-retest reliability).

2. Materials and Methods

2.1. Participants

Two research centres, one located in Italy (centre A) and one in the United Kingdom (centre B), provided retrospective IMU data collected while pwMS walked back and forth for 6 min along a hospital corridor. The patients' level of disability was assessed with the EDSS scale, scored by an experienced neurologist. Patients were excluded if not free from any orthopaedic and/or musculoskeletal and neurological disorders other than MS that may have affected their gait and balance. Since there were no restrictions for MS subtypes, both patients with relapsing remitting MS who were relapse-free for 30 days prior to assessment (centre A) and patients with secondary progressive MS (centre B) were included in the study. Thirteen pwMS were selected from each data set to form two cohorts, with individual patients matched if having the same age, gender, EDSS score, and type of assistive device (Table 1). As a result of this matching, the sample size, percentage of females, EDSS score distribution, number of pwMS who required an assistive device, and type of assistive device used during the walking test were the same in the two centres. The average walking speed was calculated as the total distance walked during the test divided by the duration of the walking trial.

Table 1. Clinical characteristics of people with multiple sclerosis for centre A and centre B. Abbreviations: expanded disability status scale (EDSS); people with multiple sclerosis (pwMS); Mann-Whitney U (MWU) statistic; p-value (p); chi-square (X^2).

	Centre A (n = 13)	Centre B (n = 13)	Statistics
Age [years]	51 (35–63)	57 (34–64)	$U = 58, p = 0.18$
Gender [men/women]	3/10	3/10	$X^2(1) = 0.00, p = 1.00$
EDSS score (0–10)	4.5 (2.0–6.5)	4.5 (2.5–6.5)	$U = 83, p = 0.93$
Mild (2.0–2.5)	1	1	
Moderate (3.0–4.5)	6	6	
Severe (5.0–6.5)	6	6	
Assistive devices			
Walker	1 pwMS	1 pwMS	–
Cane	2 pwMS	2 pwMS	–
Walking speed [m/s]	1.1 (0.5–1.4)	0.7 (0.4–1.0)	$U = 31, p < 0.01$ *

Values are median (range) or numbers. * $p < 0.05$.

pwMS from centre B repeated the instrumented walking test on a second visit, which was held 7–14 days after the first test at the same time of the day. The testing procedures were also kept constant between the two sessions. These data were used to assess between-day test-retest reliability.

Institutional review boards or ethics committees at the institutions in each country approved the separate protocols (NRES Committee Yorkshire & The Humber-Bradford Leeds (reference 15/YH/0300) and Ethical Committee of Don Carlo Gnocchi Foundation, Milan, Italy, references 29-03-2017 and 13-02-2019). Written informed consent was provided by all subjects. Data were collected in accordance with the International Declaration of Helsinki.

2.2. Experimental Protocol

Acceleration and angular velocity data from three IMUs, located at the fifth lumbar vertebra and around the right and left ankles, were recorded in both centres while pwMS walked back and forth for 6 min along a straight corridor free of obstacles and other people. If needed, they could use an assistive device and take short resting breaks while standing. Each IMU was manually aligned along the anatomical antero-posterior (AP), medio-lateral (ML), and vertical (V) axes.

The differences between the experimental protocols followed by centre A and centre B were: (i) device manufacturers and sampling frequency used to record acceleration and angular velocity signals; (ii) ankle IMU position; (iii) length of the walkway; (iv) instructions given to participants (Figure 1). Specifically, Xsens IMUs (unit weight 16 g, unit size 47 mm × 30 mm × 13 mm; MTw, Xsens, NL) with a sampling frequency of 75 Hz were used in centre A and OPAL IMUs (unit weight 22 g, unit size 48.5 mm × 36.5 mm × 13.5 mm; OPAL, APDM Inc., Portland, OR, USA) with a sampling frequency of 128 Hz were used in centre B. The IMUs around both ankles were placed laterally in centre A and frontally in centre B. PwMS were requested to walk at their maximum speed along a 30-meter straight corridor in centre A and at preferred comfortable speed along a 10-meter straight corridor in centre B.

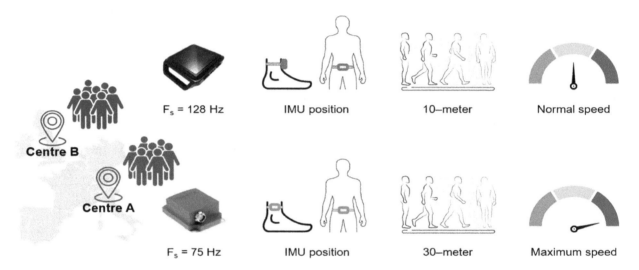

Figure 1. Experimental protocols followed by centre A (red) and centre B (blue).

2.3. Data Processing

Data processing routines were developed in Matlab® (MATLAB R2019b, MathWorks, Inc., Natick, MA, USA). A total of 33 IMU-based metrics were included in this analysis. IMU signals collected in centre B were down sampled from 128 Hz to 75 Hz to match data from centre A, and the influence of down sampling was investigated by comparing the outcome metrics from centre B as obtained before and after the down sampling. Data from the lumbar IMU were reoriented to a horizontal-vertical coordinate system [48] and filtered with a 10 Hz cut-off, zero phase, low-pass Butterworth filter.

The turning motion and resting breaks were detected and removed from IMU signals to isolate steady-state walking bouts, which were used to compute the metrics of interest. The approach proposed by Salarian, et al. [49] was adapted to determine 180° turns, which appear in the V component of the lumbar angular velocity, $\omega_z(t)$, as peaks of a given duration. The turning onset and offset were identified from the trunk rotation angle around the V axis, $\theta_z(t)$, obtained after integrating the $\omega_z(t)$ signal. The turning components were evidenced in $\theta_z(t)$ as steep positive or negative gradients, whereas walking components were evidenced as small oscillations round a flat line. Specifically, $\theta_z(t)$ was first smoothed using a weighted least-squares linear regression. Abrupt change points and their locations were then searched in $\theta_z(t)$ using a predefined Matlab® function based on the minimisation of a linear computational cost function [50]. Resting breaks were automatically detected by checking in 2-s window increments if: (i) the norm of the lumbar IMU angular velocity was less than 0.5 rad/s; (ii) the norm of the lumbar IMU acceleration was within ±10% of 9.81 m/s² [51]. A 2-s window was considered motionless if more than 50% of its samples fulfilled both criteria mentioned above.

Twelve gait metrics were extracted from the angular velocities recorded from the ankle IMUs and 21 were extracted from the lumbar IMU accelerations. Following the suggestions of Lord, et al. [52] and Buckley, et al. [53], these metrics were organised in independent gait domains (e.g., rhythm, variability, asymmetry, intensity, stability, smoothness, symmetry, and regularity).

Initial and final foot contact instances, referred to as gait events (GE), were identified for each steady-state walking bout as local minimum values of the ML angular velocity recorded from ankle IMUs of both legs [54]. These minima occur just before and after the instant of maximum ML angular velocity. Once the GE were determined, stride, step, swing and stance durations (representing rhythm domain) were separately estimated for left and right sides. Variability (i.e., within-subject combined standard deviation of left and right; variability domain) and asymmetry (i.e., absolute difference between the mean of left and right time series; asymmetry domain) of these metrics were also computed, applying the established formula in Galna, et al. [55] and Godfrey, et al. [56].

From processing the filtered acceleration signals in time and frequency domain, 21 additional metrics, referred to as gait quality metrics [57], were separately extracted for each acceleration component (AP, ML, and V): (i) intensity as the root mean square (RMS) of each acceleration component around its mean value [44]; (ii) stability as the ratio of the RMS in a given direction to the RMS vector magnitude [58]; (iii) smoothness as the RMS of the jerk [59]; (iv) symmetry represented by the harmonic ratio (HR), defined as the ratio of the sum of the amplitudes of the in-phase harmonics to the sum of the amplitudes of the out-of-phase harmonics [60,61]; (v) regularity as the ensemble of the following three metrics obtained from the unbiased normalised autocorrelation [62]:

$$Step\ regularity = 1st\ peak\ of\ (\frac{1}{N-|m|} \sum_{i=1}^{N-|m|} x(i) \cdot x(i+m)) \tag{1}$$

$$Stride\ regularity = 2nd\ peak\ of\ (\frac{1}{N-|m|} \sum_{i=1}^{N-|m|} x(i) \cdot x(i+m)) \tag{2}$$

$$Regularity\ index = \frac{|Stride\ regularity - Step\ regularity|}{mean(Stride\ regularity, Step\ regularity)} \tag{3}$$

All metrics were calculated for the part of signals corresponding to the middle eight steps of each pass along the corridor and then averaged over the whole trial. The choice of eight steps was due to the maximum number of steps which subjects in centre B could walk in completely straight condition. Since centre A adopted a three-times longer path, in order to process the same number of steps, only one walking bout in every three was included for centre B.

2.4. Statistical Analysis

Statistical analyses were performed in R version 3.4.3 [63]. Participant characteristics from centre A and centre B were compared using the independent Mann-Whitney U for age and EDSS scores and Pearson's chi-square for gender. Given the limited sample size and the non-normal distribution of most of the investigated metrics (as a result of the Shapiro-Wilk test), non-parametric tests were performed. The level of significance was taken at 5%. A Wilcoxon signed-rank test was performed to compare the centre B metrics obtained from IMU data sampled at 128 Hz and those down-sampled at 75 Hz.

Between-day test-retest reliability of the metrics was evaluated for centre B through the intra-class correlation coefficients (ICCs) with a 95% confidence interval (CI). ICCs were calculated using a two-way random-effect model and absolute agreement (ICC2,k) [64]. An ICC lower than 0.39 was classified as poor, an ICC between 0.40 and 0.59 as fair, an ICC between 0.60 and 0.74 as moderate, and an ICC greater than 0.75 as excellent [65]. The minimum detectable changes (MDCs), representing the smallest amount of change that can be considered above the bounds of the measurement error and/or within-subject variability, was also computed for each metric at the CI of 95%, according to Equation (4):

$$\text{MDC} = 1.96 \cdot \sqrt{2} \cdot \text{SEM} = 1.96 \cdot \sqrt{2} \cdot \text{SD} \cdot \sqrt{1 - \text{ICC}}, \tag{4}$$

where SEM is the standard error of the measurement and SD corresponds to the average of the standard deviations from test and re-test sessions [66].

A Wilcoxon signed-rank test was used to determine if there was a median difference in centre B metrics between the two sessions, whereas an independent Mann-Whitney U test was carried out to compare IMU-based metrics from centre A and centre B.

In all the above tests, if the *p*-value was lower than 0.05, the null hypothesis (e.g., the two population medians were identical) was rejected and the alternative hypothesis accepted. To avoid misinterpretation of the *p*-values and to account for a type II error, the effect size (*r*) for non-parametric tests was also calculated as follows:

$$r = z/\sqrt{N} \tag{5}$$

where z is the z-score and N is the size of the study (i.e., the number of total observations) on which z is based. Cohen [67] suggested thresholds of 0.1, 0.3, and 0.5 for small, medium, and large effect sizes, respectively.

Median, inter-quartile range, minimum, and maximum values were finally calculated for IMU-based metrics from centre A and centre B (both sessions).

3. Results

3.1. Effect of Sampling Frequency

The results of the comparison between the metrics calculated using the 128 Hz and 75 Hz sampling frequencies are reported in Table 2. The HR, representative of the symmetry domain, was the only metric that significantly differed between the two analyses.

Table 2. Effect of down-sampling of the acceleration and angular velocity signals on the investigated gait metrics. Abbreviations: sampling frequency (F_S), z-score (z), p-value (p), and effect size (r).

Domain	F_s of 128 Hz	F_s of 75 Hz	z	p	r
Rhythm [s]					
Stride duration	1.20 (1.01–1.74)	1.21 (1.01–1.74)	−0.82	0.41	−0.16
Step duration	0.60 (0.51–0.87)	0.60 (0.50–0.87)	0.00	1.00	0.00
Stance duration	0.75 (0.61–1.18)	0.75 (0.61–1.18)	−1.83	0.07	−0.36
Swing duration	0.44 (0.40–0.58)	0.44 (0.40–0.58)	−1.85	0.06	−0.36
Variability [ms]					
Stride duration	61 (32–100)	63 (32–98)	−1.55	0.12	−0.30
Step duration	46 (20–69)	45 (20–68)	−1.33	0.18	−0.26
Stance duration	65 (34–105)	65 (32–106)	−0.18	0.86	−0.04
Swing duration	29 (23–74)	30 (21–76)	−0.41	0.68	−0.08
Asymmetry [ms]					
Stride duration	2 (0–7)	2 (1–7)	−0.09	0.93	−0.02
Step duration	56 (0–238)	51 (0–242)	−1.49	0.14	−0.29
Stance duration	61 (3–149)	69 (2–130)	−1.58	0.11	−0.31
Swing duration	54 (1–155)	62 (0–138)	−1.33	0.18	−0.26

Table 2. *Cont.*

Domain	F_s of 128 Hz	F_s of 75 Hz	z	p	r
Intensity [m/s²]					
Antero-Posterior	1.10 (0.80–1.96)	1.10 (0.80–1.95)	−0.94	0.34	−0.19
Medio-Lateral	0.93 (0.65–1.41)	0.93 (0.65–1.41)	−1.44	0.15	−0.28
Vertical	1.37 (0.76–3.16)	1.38 (0.75–3.20)	−1.28	0.20	−0.25
Stability [–]					
Antero-Posterior	0.41 (0.37–0.61)	0.41 (0.37–0.61)	−0.30	0.77	−0.06
Medio-Lateral	0.34 (0.25–0.52)	0.34 (0.25–0.52)	−0.89	0.37	−0.18
Vertical	0.58 (0.36–0.62)	0.58 (0.36–0.63)	−0.29	0.77	−0.06
Smoothness [m/s³]					
Antero-Posterior	13.97 (8.86–30.75)	13.95 (8.93–30.82)	0.00	1.00	0.00
Medio-Lateral	13.92 (10.13–28.61)	13.87 (10.19–28.45)	−1.06	0.29	−0.21
Vertical	23.31 (11.06–48.81)	23.21 (10.89–49.38)	−0.75	0.45	−0.15
Symmetry (HR) [–]					
Antero-Posterior	2.94 (1.49–3.73)	2.89 (1.50–3.49)	−2.32	0.02 *	−0.45
Medio-Lateral	0.44 (0.32–0.56)	0.45 (0.32–0.56)	−2.19	0.03 *	−0.43
Vertical	3.01 (1.21–4.84)	2.94 (1.23–4.78)	−3.01	0.00 *	−0.59
Regularity [–]					
Step regularity					
Antero-Posterior	0.60 (0.20–0.85)	0.60 (0.20–0.84)	−1.70	0.09	−0.33
Medio-Lateral	−0.62 (−0.74−−0.37)	−0.60 (−0.73−−0.38)	−1.89	0.06	−0.37
Vertical	0.81 (0.32–0.95)	0.80 (0.32–0.94)	−1.44	0.15	−0.28
Stride regularity					
Anterior-Posterior	0.86 (0.50–0.93)	0.86 (0.50–0.92)	0.00	1.00	0.00
Medio-Lateral	0.77 (0.58–0.85)	0.75 (0.59–0.85)	−1.67	0.09	−0.33
Vertical	0.86 (0.34–0.95)	0.86 (0.34–0.95)	−1.80	0.07	−0.35
Regularity index					
Antero-Posterior	0.37 (0.04–0.82)	0.37 (0.04–0.83)	−1.10	0.27	−0.22
Medio-Lateral	−0.20 (−0.70−−0.08)	−0.20 (−0.66−−0.08)	−0.41	0.68	−0.08
Vertical	0.11 (0.02–0.59)	0.11 (0.02–0.59)	0.00	1.00	0.00

Values are median (range). * $p < 0.05$.

3.2. Between-Day Test-Retest Reliability

ICC, SEM, and MDC values for between-day assessment are shown in Table 3 for each metric estimated for pwMS from centre B who completed two testing visits. Overall, 17 out of 33 metrics revealed excellent test-retest reliability (ICC: 0.93–0.98; 95% CI: 0.76–0.93), 11 metrics showed moderate test-retest reliability (ICC: 0.88–0.92; 95% CI: 0.62–0.74), and only 5 metrics exhibited poor to fair test-retest reliability with ICC values between 0.72 and 0.86 and 95% CI between 0.13 and 0.52. The Wilcoxon signed-rank test showed no significant differences in any of the metrics between the two sessions (Figure 2 and Table 4).

Table 3. Intra-class correlation coefficients (ICC) with a 95% confidence interval (CI), standard error of the measurement (SEM), and minimum detectable change (MDC) for the investigated gait metrics.

Domains	ICC	95% CI		SEM	MDC
		Lower	Upper		
Rhythm [s]					
Stride duration	0.97	0.90	0.99	0.04	0.10
Step duration	0.97	0.90	0.99	0.02	0.05
Stance duration	0.96	0.86	0.99	0.03	0.09
Swing duration	0.97	0.91	0.99	0.01	0.03
Variability [ms]					
Stride duration	0.92	0.73	0.97	8	21
Step duration	0.92	0.74	0.98	5	13
Stance duration	0.94	0.80	0.98	6	18
Swing duration	0.95	0.85	0.99	4	11
Asymmetry [ms]					
Stride duration	**0.72**	**0.13**	**0.91**	**1**	**4**
Step duration	0.98	0.93	0.99	10	29
Stance duration	0.90	0.67	0.97	12	33
Swing duration	0.89	0.62	0.97	13	36
Intensity [m/s^2]					
Antero-Posterior	0.97	0.90	0.99	0.06	0.16
Medio-Lateral	0.98	0.93	0.99	0.04	0.11
Vertical	0.97	0.92	0.99	0.10	0.29
Stability [–]					
Antero-Posterior	0.93	0.78	0.98	0.02	0.05
Medio-Lateral	0.93	0.76	0.98	0.03	0.08
Vertical	0.91	0.69	0.97	0.03	0.09
Smoothness [m/s^3]					
Antero-Posterior	0.92	0.73	0.97	2.46	6.83
Medio-Lateral	0.93	0.79	0.98	1.55	4.29
Vertical	0.95	0.82	0.98	2.31	6.41
Symmetry (HR) [–]					
Antero-Posterior	0.95	0.85	0.99	0.14	0.38
Medio-Lateral	**0.75**	**0.15**	**0.92**	**0.04**	**0.10**
Vertical	0.92	0.74	0.98	0.21	0.59
Regularity [–]					
Step regularity					
Antero-Posterior	0.91	0.70	0.97	0.07	0.19
Medio-Lateral	**0.86**	**0.52**	**0.96**	**0.04**	**0.11**
Vertical	0.97	0.92	0.99	0.04	0.10
Stride regularity					
Antero-Posterior	0.88	0.64	0.96	0.05	0.13
Medio-Lateral	**0.85**	**0.50**	**0.96**	**0.04**	**0.10**
Vertical	0.93	0.77	0.98	0.04	0.10
Regularity index					
Antero-Posterior	**0.76**	**0.17**	**0.93**	**0.17**	**0.47**
Medio-Lateral	0.88	0.62	0.96	0.06	0.17
Vertical	0.89	0.63	0.97	0.09	0.24

Inertial measurement unit (IMU)-based gait metrics with poor to fair test-retest reliability are presented in bold.

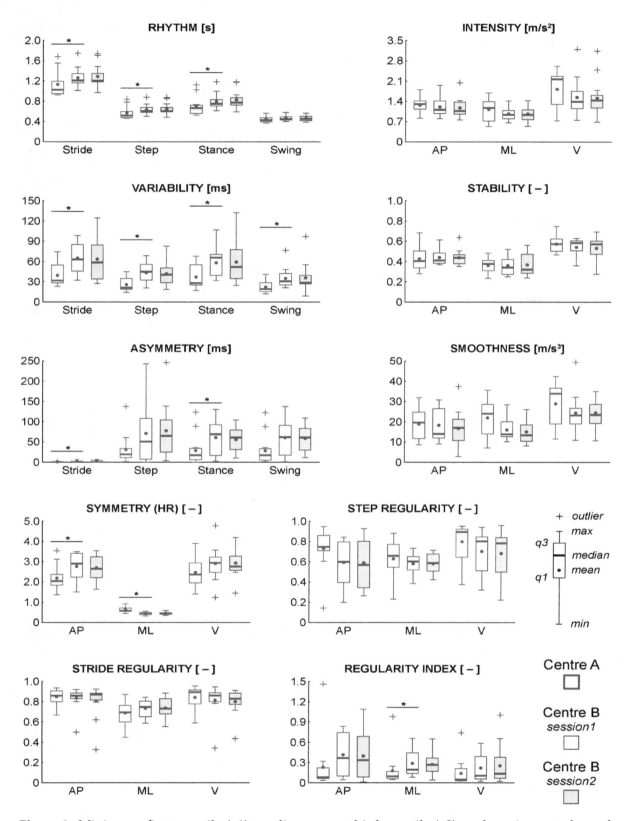

Figure 2. Minimum, first quartile (q1), median, mean, third quartile (q3), and maximum values of each IMU-based metrics relative to centre A (red) and centre B for between-day test-retest assessment (blue empty boxplots and blue filled boxplots). Values larger than q1 + 1.5(q3 + q1) or smaller than q1 − 1.5(q3 − q1) are considered outliers and are represented with crosses (+). * $p < 0.05$. Note that, for graphical convenience, the absolute values have been depicted for the step regularity and regularity index in the ML direction.

Table 4. Descriptive statistics for the investigated gait metrics from centre B (session1 and session2), including the z-score (z), *p*-value (*p*), and effect size (*r*).

Domain	Centre B (session1)	Centre B (session2)	z	p	r
Rhythm [s]					
Stride duration	1.21 (1.01–1.74)	1.20 (0.97–1.74)	−0.70	0.48	−0.14
Step duration	0.60 (0.50–0.87)	0.60 (0.48–0.87)	−0.56	0.58	−0.11
Stance duration	0.75 (0.61–1.18)	0.77 (0.59–1.18)	−1.57	0.12	−0.31
Swing duration	0.44 (0.40–0.58)	0.45 (0.38–0.56)	−1.99	0.05	−0.39
Variability [ms]					
Stride duration	63 (32–98)	58 (27–124)	−0.35	0.72	−0.07
Step duration	45 (20–68)	40 (18–83)	−0.35	0.72	−0.07
Stance duration	65 (32–106)	52 (24–132)	−0.03	0.97	−0.01
Swing duration	30 (21–76)	28 (9–97)	−0.53	0.60	−0.10
Asymmetry [ms]					
Stride duration	2 (1–7)	4 (0–7)	−1.34	0.18	−0.26
Step duration	51 (0–242)	65 (4–245)	−1.30	0.20	−0.25
Stance duration	69 (2–130)	61 (10–104)	−0.52	0.60	−0.10
Swing duration	62 (0–138)	61 (12–109)	−0.38	0.70	−0.08
Intensity [m/s^2]					
Antero-Posterior	1.10 (0.80–1.95)	1.07 (0.76–2.04)	−1.22	0.22	−0.24
Medio-Lateral	0.93 (0.65–1.41)	0.93 (0.53–1.42)	−0.08	0.94	−0.02
Vertical	1.38 (0.75–3.20)	1.43 (0.68–3.14)	−0.38	0.70	−0.08
Stability [–]					
Antero-Posterior	0.41 (0.37–0.61)	0.43 (0.35–0.64)	−0.28	0.78	−0.05
Medio-Lateral	0.34 (0.25–0.52)	0.32 (0.24–0.56)	0.00	1.00	0.00
Vertical	0.58 (0.36–0.63)	0.57 (0.28–0.69)	−0.27	0.79	−0.05
Smoothness [m/s^3]					
Antero-Posterior	13.95 (8.93–30.82)	17.11 (2.76–37.32)	−1.17	0.24	−0.23
Medio-Lateral	13.87 (10.19–28.45)	13.42 (8.04–26.07)	−1.24	0.22	−0.24
Vertical	23.21 (10.89–49.38)	23.43 (10.67–50.74)	−0.41	0.68	−0.08
Symmetry (HR) [–]					
Antero-Posterior	2.89 (1.50–3.49)	2.64 (1.62–3.54)	−0.31	0.75	−0.06
Medio-Lateral	0.45 (0.32–0.56)	0.46 (0.34–0.59)	−0.82	0.41	−0.16
Vertical	2.94 (1.23–4.78)	2.75 (1.45–4.19)	−0.51	0.61	−0.10
Regularity [–]					
Step regularity					
Antero-Posterior	0.60 (0.20–0.84)	0.57 (0.26–0.93)	−0.12	0.91	−0.02
Medio-Lateral	−0.60 (−0.73–−0.38)	−0.58 (−0.71–−0.42)	−0.07	0.94	−0.01
Vertical	0.80 (0.32–0.94)	0.78 (0.22–0.96)	−1.26	0.21	−0.25
Stride regularity					
Anterior-Posterior	0.86 (0.50–0.92)	0.87 (0.33–0.92)	−0.98	0.33	−0.19
Medio-Lateral	0.75 (0.59–0.85)	0.73 (0.55–0.88)	−0.03	0.97	−0.01
Vertical	0.86 (0.34–0.95)	0.83 (0.44–0.91)	−0.52	0.60	−0.10
Regularity index					
Antero-Posterior	0.37 (0.04–0.83)	0.34 (0.01–1.09)	−0.04	0.97	−0.01
Medio-Lateral	−0.20 (−0.66–−0.08)	−0.27 (−0.65–−0.04)	−0.14	0.89	−0.03
Vertical	0.11 (0.02–0.59)	0.14 (0.02–1.00)	−0.43	0.67	−0.08

Values are median (range). * $p < 0.05$.

3.3. Between-Centre Differences

As expected, the comparison between centre A and centre B via the independent Mann-Whitney U test highlighted significant differences for all the temporal metrics (Figure 2 and Table 5; rhythm domain), except for swing duration. Apart from asymmetry of step duration and asymmetry of swing duration, variability and asymmetry of the temporal metrics were significantly lower in centre A compared to centre B (Figure 2 and Table 5; variability and asymmetry domain). However, even though the difference in asymmetry of swing duration between the two centres was non-significant ($U = 48.0$; $p = 0.06$), a fairly moderate effect size was found for this specific metric ($r = 0.37$). Conversely, a consistency between the two centres was found for 18 out of 21 metrics extracted from acceleration signals (Figure 2 and Table 5; intensity, stability, smoothness, symmetry, and regularity domains). Only the differences in the regularity index in the ML direction and in the HR in the AP and ML directions were proved statistically significant between centre A and centre B (Figure 2 and Table 5).

Table 5. Descriptive statistics for the investigated gait metrics from centre A and centre B (session1), including the Mann-Whitney U (MWU) statistic, p-value (p), and effect size (r).

Domain	Centre A	Centre B	U	p	r
Rhythm [s]					
Stride duration	1.03 (0.92–1.68)	1.21 (1.01–1.74)	43.5	0.04 *	0.41
Step duration	0.51 (0.46–0.84)	0.60 (0.50–0.87)	44.0	0.04 *	0.41
Stance duration	0.66 (0.52–1.12)	0.75 (0.61–1.18)	40.0	0.02 *	0.45
Swing duration	0.43 (0.37–0.56)	0.44 (0.40–0.58)	57.0	0.17	0.28
Variability [ms]					
Stride duration	32 (23–74)	63 (32–98)	26.0	0.00 *	0.59
Step duration	21 (14–45)	45 (20–68)	27.5	0.00 *	0.57
Stance duration	28 (17–68)	65 (32–106)	30.0	0.01 *	0.55
Swing duration	19 (12–41)	30 (21–76)	33.0	0.01 *	0.52
Asymmetry [ms]					
Stride duration	1 (0–4)	2 (1–7)	45.0	0.04 *	0.40
Step duration	19 (1–138)	51 (0–242)	68.0	0.40	0.17
Stance duration	17 (0–123)	69 (2–130)	46.0	0.04 *	0.39
Swing duration	17 (1–122)	62 (0–138)	48.0	0.06	0.37
Intensity [m/s^2]					
Antero-Posterior	1.30 (0.81–1.80)	1.10 (0.80–1.95)	68.0	0.41	0.17
Medio-Lateral	1.17 (0.53–1.69)	0.93 (0.65–1.41)	62.0	0.26	0.23
Vertical	2.17 (0.73–2.62)	1.38 (0.75–3.20)	59.5	0.21	0.25
Stability [–]					
Antero-Posterior	0.40 (0.28–0.68)	0.41 (0.37–0.61)	69.0	0.44	0.16
Medio-Lateral	0.38 (0.23–0.48)	0.34 (0.25–0.52)	83.0	0.96	0.02
Vertical	0.57 (0.47–0.75)	0.58 (0.36–0.63)	72.5	0.55	0.12
Smoothness [m/s^3]					
Antero-Posterior	19.68 (8.56–31.85)	13.95 (8.93–30.82)	82.0	0.92	0.03
Medio-Lateral	24.01 (7.04–35.54)	13.87 (10.19–28.45)	52.5	0.11	0.32
Vertical	33.90 (11.56–42.39)	23.21 (10.89–49.38)	59.0	0.20	0.26
Symmetry (HR) [–]					
Antero-Posterior	2.04 (1.36–3.54)	2.89 (1.50–3.49)	43.5	0.04 *	0.41
Medio-Lateral	0.57 (0.44–0.91)	0.45 (0.32–0.56)	14.0	0.00 *	0.71
Vertical	2.35 (1.39–3.89)	2.94 (1.23–4.78)	52.5	0.11	0.32

Table 5. *Cont.*

Domain	Centre A	Centre B	U	p	r
Regularity [–]					
Step regularity					
Antero-Posterior	0.75 (0.14–0.95)	0.60 (0.20–0.84)	55.5	0.14	0.29
Medio-Lateral	−0.66 (−0.88−−0.23)	−0.60 (−0.73−−0.38)	63.0	0.28	0.22
Vertical	0.89 (0.37–0.95)	0.80 (0.32–0.94)	51.5	0.10	0.33
Stride regularity					
Anterior-Posterior	0.86 (0.67–0.93)	0.86 (0.50–0.92)	81.5	0.90	0.03
Medio-Lateral	0.69 (0.45–0.87)	0.75 (0.59–0.85)	63.0	0.28	0.22
Vertical	0.89 (0.59–0.96)	0.86 (0.34–0.95)	72.5	0.55	0.12
Regularity index					
Antero-Posterior	0.08 (0.03–1.46)	0.37 (0.04–0.83)	50.0	0.08	0.35
Medio-Lateral	−0.10 (−0.98−−0.05)	−0.20 (−0.66−−0.08)	40.5	0.03 *	0.44
Vertical	0.05 (0.02–0.74)	0.11 (0.02–0.59)	51.5	0.09	0.33

Values are median (range). * $p < 0.05$.

4. Discussion

This study aimed to identify comparable gait metrics as quantified from IMU data measured from two different hospital settings on two matched cohorts of pwMS (13 pwMS for each centre, Table 1), under the hypothesis that those metrics associated with the overall balance control and coordination of gait (i.e., gait quality metrics) would be robust, even when obtained from different experimental protocols. Reported results overall corroborated this assumption and showed that between-centre differences for most of these metrics were comparable to those obtained by the same centre in two different sessions.

The small sample size, resulting from the attempt of maximising the cohort match, is certainly a limitation of this study. It is worth noting, in fact, that while some of the investigated gait metrics in centre A (e.g., asymmetry of swing duration from asymmetry domain and regularity index from regularity domain) did not differ significantly from those in centre B, an observed medium effect size suggested the opposite might hold true (Table 5). This is indeed likely to be due to the small sample size and possibly due to the higher inter-subject variability observed in centre B.

Since MS is well known for heterogeneity of symptoms, high day-to-day fluctuations, and a large variability in its course [68], care must be taken before generalising our findings to all pwMS with different levels of gait impairment. Another limitation of this study might lie in the fact that patients recruited by the two centres differed in the subtypes of MS. Nonetheless, Dujmovic, et al. [69] showed that the altered gait pattern in pwMS did not depend on the disease phenotype. Additional studies are of course needed to further investigate this aspect.

The comparison between centre A and centre B implied down-sampling the data from the latter. As expected, this affected only the calculation of HR, which is the only metric based on frequency analysis. In particular, changing sampling frequency from 128 Hz to 75 Hz led to decreased values in the AP and V directions and increased values in the ML direction (Table 2). This is in line with what was previously reported by Riva, et al. [35].

Moderate to excellent between-day test-retest reliability was observed for 28 out of 33 IMU-based metrics with few exceptions, which exhibited poor to fair reliability (Table 3). Additionally, all the investigated metrics were not significantly different between the two sessions (Figure 2 and Table 4), even if some of these results (swing duration in particular) should be interpreted with care, due to the medium effect size. These findings confirmed that sensor-based gait analysis is a reliable tool in pwMS, as also reported in previous test-retest studies on pwMS [34].

Walking speed clearly affected the gait outcomes. In particular, the gait metrics representative of rhythm, variability, and asymmetry domains were evidently lower in centre A compared to centre

B (Figure 2 and Table 5) due to different instructions given to the participants in terms of walking speed (i.e., walk at maximum speed versus walk at self-selected speed). This finding is in agreement with previous studies on pwMS [28] and on people with other neurological conditions, such as Parkinson's disease [70], which observed a reduction of the above metrics with increasing walking speed. The shorter length of the walkway used in centre B could also have contributed to these differences. In fact, Storm, et al. [22] demonstrated that rhythm and variability metrics decreased when walking longer distances (e.g., lower stride duration and lower variability of stride duration). However, the data available for our study did not allow us to separate walking speed and path effects, and further studies should hence be performed to this purpose.

Unlike the temporal metrics, the gait quality metrics appeared to be robust with respect to the notable differences in the experimental gait protocols adopted by the two centres. Among these metrics, in fact, only differences in the regularity index in the ML direction and the HR (representative of symmetry domain) in the AP and ML directions were found to be statistically significant between centre A and centre B (Figure 2 and Table 5). Again, this specific result could be explained both by the different walking speed and by the different lengths of the walkway in the two centres. Indeed, an association between walking speed and HR has been previously showed, both in healthy young [43,44] and older subjects [39]. These authors observed that the HR increased at the self-selected comfortable walking speed and decreased at slower and faster speeds. A similar trend emerged from our analysis, except for the HR in the ML direction, but this specific metric should be handled with care due to its observed low test-retest reliability (Table 3). The low number of steps (i.e., eight steps) used for calculating the HR for each walking bout might also have contributed to reduce robustness and reliability of this metric [57,71]. However, this choice was imposed by the reduced length of the corridor in centre B. Testing the participants along a shorter path also implied a higher number of turns over the 6 min, resulting in a minor validity of the HR as showed in the research by Riva, et al. [35] and by Brach, et al. [40].

While further studies are of course needed to fully validate this hypothesis, our results suggest that, in agreement with what is already reported for other neurological diseases, such as Parkinson's disease [53], the gait quality metrics extracted from the upper body accelerations should not be considered as a simple reflection of gait spatio-temporal features and might bring complementary informative content in quantifying patients' gait ability. Additionally, these metrics have been recently shown to be sensitive to fatigue and pathology progression in pwMS [72] and, as such, they are promising candidates for quantification of disease progression and rehabilitation interventions in these patients.

5. Conclusions

In conclusion, this pragmatic study showed consistency in the gait metrics from two matched groups of pwMS, even when they were assessed in two different hospitals and under notably different gait testing conditions. The identification of such robust gait metrics opens the possibility of comparing retrospective data and paves the way for reliable multi-centre studies to be conducted in routine hospital settings rather than in specialised gait research laboratories. This is essential to allow an increase of sample size and statistical power of clinical trials in which rehabilitation interventions need to be quantitatively assessed.

Author Contributions: Conceptualisation, M.F. and C.M.; methodology, L.A., I.C., D.C., M.F. and C.M.; software, L.A.; formal analysis, L.A.; resources, D.C., E.G., B.S., D.P. and C.M.; writing-original draft preparation, L.A., I.C., M.F. and C.M.; writing-review and editing, L.A., I.C., D.C., M.F., E.G., B.S., D.P., K.P.S.N. and C.M.; visualisation, L.A.; funding acquisition, M.F., B.S., K.P.S.N. and C.M. All authors have read and agreed to the published version of the manuscript.

Acknowledgments: We would like to thank all participants for giving their time to support this research. This study was carried out at the NIHR Sheffield Clinical Research Facility (Sheffield, United Kingdom) and at the IRCCS Don Carlo Gnocchi Foundation (Milan, Italy). The authors would like to acknowledge William Hodgkinson, Craig Smith, and Jessy Moorman Dodd for the support in Sheffield's data collection.

References

1. Browne, P.; Chandraratna, D.; Angood, C.; Tremlett, H.; Baker, C.; Taylor, B.V.; Thompson, A.J. Atlas of Multiple Sclerosis 2013: A growing global problem with widespread inequity. *Neurology* **2014**, *83*, 1022–1024. [CrossRef]
2. Pugliatti, M.; Rosati, G.; Carton, H.; Riise, T.; Drulovic, J.; Vécsei, L.; Milanov, I. The epidemiology of multiple sclerosis in Europe. *Eur. J. Neurol.* **2006**, *13*, 700–722. [CrossRef]
3. Cattaneo, D.; Lamers, I.; Bertoni, R.; Feys, P.; Jonsdottir, J. Participation Restriction in People with Multiple Sclerosis: Prevalence and Correlations With Cognitive, Walking, Balance, and Upper Limb Impairments. *Arch. Phys. Med. Rehabil.* **2017**, *98*, 1308–1315. [CrossRef]
4. Martin, C.L.; Phillips, B.A.; Kilpatrick, T.J.; Butzkueven, H.; Tubridy, N.; McDonald, E.; Galea, M.P. Gait and balance impairment in early multiple sclerosis in the absence of clinical disability. *Mult. Scler. J.* **2006**, *12*, 620–628. [CrossRef]
5. LaRocca, N.G. Impact of Walking Impairment in Multiple Sclerosis. *Patient Patient-Cent. Outcomes Res.* **2011**, *4*, 189–201. [CrossRef]
6. Donzé, C. Update on rehabilitation in multiple sclerosis. *La Presse Med.* **2015**, *44*, e169–e176. [CrossRef]
7. Kurtzke, J.F. Rating neurologic impairment in multiple sclerosis. *Neurology* **1983**, *33*, 1444. [CrossRef]
8. Sebastião, E.; Sandroff, B.M.; Learmonth, Y.C.; Motl, R.W. Validity of the Timed Up and Go Test as a Measure of Functional Mobility in Persons with Multiple Sclerosis. *Arch. Phys. Med. Rehabil.* **2016**, *97*, 1072–1077. [CrossRef]
9. Phan-Ba, R.; Pace, A.; Calay, P.; Grodent, P.; Douchamps, F.; Hyde, R.; Hotermans, C.; Delvaux, V.; Hansen, I.; Moonen, G.; et al. Comparison of the timed 25-foot and the 100-meter walk as performance measures in multiple sclerosis. *Neurorehabil. Neural Repair.* **2011**, *25*, 672–679. [CrossRef]
10. Goldman, M.D.; Marrie, R.A.; Cohen, J.A. Evaluation of the six-minute walk in multiple sclerosis subjects and healthy controls. *Mult. Scler. J.* **2008**, *14*, 383–390. [CrossRef]
11. Horak, F.; King, L.; Mancini, M. Role of body-worn movement monitor technology for balance and gait rehabilitation. *Phys. Ther.* **2015**, *95*, 461–470. [CrossRef]
12. Kaufman, M.; Moyer, D.; Norton, J. The significant change for the Timed 25-Foot Walk in the Multiple Sclerosis Functional Composite. *Mult. Scler. J.* **2000**, *6*, 286–290. [CrossRef]
13. Kragt, J.J.; van der Linden, F.A.; Nielsen, J.M.; Uitdehaag, B.M.; Polman, C.H. Clinical impact of 20% worsening on Timed 25-foot Walk and 9-hole Peg Test in multiple sclerosis. *Mult. Scler. J.* **2006**, *12*, 594–598. [CrossRef]
14. Nieuwenhuis, M.M.; Van Tongeren, H.; Sorensen, P.S.; Ravnborg, M. The six spot step test: A new measurement for walking ability in multiple sclerosis. *Mult. Scler. J.* **2006**, *12*, 495–500. [CrossRef]
15. Spain, R.I.; St. George, R.J.; Salarian, A.; Mancini, M.; Wagner, J.M.; Horak, F.B.; Bourdette, D. Body-worn motion sensors detect balance and gait deficits in people with multiple sclerosis who have normal walking speed. *Gait Posture* **2012**, *35*, 573–578. [CrossRef]
16. Liparoti, M.; Della Corte, M.; Rucco, R.; Sorrentino, P.; Sparaco, M.; Capuano, R.; Minino, R.; Lavorgna, L.; Agosti, V.; Sorrentino, G.; et al. Gait abnormalities in minimally disabled people with Multiple Sclerosis: A 3D-motion analysis study. *Mult. Scler. Relat. Disord.* **2019**, *29*, 100–107. [CrossRef]
17. Pau, M.; Mandaresu, S.; Pilloni, G.; Porta, M.; Coghe, G.; Marrosu, M.G.; Cocco, E. Smoothness of gait detects early alterations of walking in persons with multiple sclerosis without disability. *Gait Posture* **2017**, *58*, 307–309. [CrossRef]
18. Muro-de-la-Herran, A.; Garcia-Zapirain, B.; Mendez-Zorrilla, A. Gait analysis methods: an overview of wearable and non-wearable systems, highlighting clinical applications. *Sensors* **2014**, *14*, 3362–3394. [CrossRef]
19. Vienne-Jumeau, A.; Quijoux, F.; Vidal, P.P.; Ricard, D. Wearable inertial sensors provide reliable biomarkers of disease severity in multiple sclerosis: A systematic review and meta-analysis. *Ann. Phys. Rehabil. Med.* **2019**. [CrossRef]

20. Vienne, A.; Barrois, R.P.; Buffat, S.; Ricard, D.; Vidal, P.P. Inertial Sensors to Assess Gait Quality in Patients with Neurological Disorders: A Systematic Review of Technical and Analytical Challenges. *Front. Psychology* **2017**, *8*, 817. [CrossRef]

21. Motl, R.W.; Pilutti, L.; Sandroff, B.M.; Dlugonski, D.; Sosnoff, J.J.; Pula, J.H. Accelerometry as a measure of walking behavior in multiple sclerosis. *Acta Neurol. Scand.* **2013**, *127*, 384–390. [CrossRef]

22. Storm, F.A.; Nair, K.P.S.; Clarke, A.J.; Van der Meulen, J.M.; Mazzà, C. Free-living and laboratory gait characteristics in patients with multiple sclerosis. *PLoS ONE* **2018**, *13*, e0196463. [CrossRef]

23. Huisinga, J.M.; Mancini, M.; St George, R.J.; Horak, F.B. Accelerometry reveals differences in gait variability between patients with multiple sclerosis and healthy controls. *Ann. Biomed. Eng.* **2013**, *41*, 1670–1679. [CrossRef]

24. Moon, Y.; Wajda, D.A.; Motl, R.W.; Sosnoff, J.J. Stride-Time Variability and Fall Risk in Persons with Multiple Sclerosis. *Mult. Scler. Int.* **2015**, *2015*, 7. [CrossRef]

25. Motta, C.; Palermo, E.; Studer, V.; Germanotta, M.; Germani, G.; Centonze, D.; Cappa, P.; Rossi, S.; Rossi, S. Disability and Fatigue Can Be Objectively Measured in Multiple Sclerosis. *PLoS ONE* **2016**, *11*, e0148997. [CrossRef]

26. Engelhard, M.M.; Dandu, S.R.; Patek, S.D.; Lach, J.C.; Goldman, M.D. Quantifying six-minute walk induced gait deterioration with inertial sensors in multiple sclerosis subjects. *Gait Posture* **2016**, *49*, 340–345. [CrossRef]

27. Psarakis, M.; Greene, D.A.; Cole, M.H.; Lord, S.R.; Hoang, P.; Brodie, M. Wearable technology reveals gait compensations, unstable walking patterns and fatigue in people with multiple sclerosis. *Phys. Meas.* **2018**, *39*, 075004. [CrossRef]

28. Moon, Y.; McGinnis, R.S.; Seagers, K.; Motl, R.W.; Sheth, N.; Wright, J.A., Jr.; Ghaffari, R.; Sosnoff, J.J. Monitoring gait in multiple sclerosis with novel wearable motion sensors. *PLoS ONE* **2017**, *12*, e0171346. [CrossRef]

29. Craig, J.J.; Bruetsch, A.P.; Lynch, S.G.; Huisinga, J.M. The relationship between trunk and foot acceleration variability during walking shows minor changes in persons with multiple sclerosis. *Clin. Biomech.* **2017**, *49*, 16–21. [CrossRef]

30. Corporaal, S.H.A.; Gensicke, H.; Kuhle, J.; Kappos, L.; Allum, J.H.J.; Yaldizli, Ö. Balance control in multiple sclerosis: Correlations of trunk sway during stance and gait tests with disease severity. *Gait Posture* **2013**, *37*, 55–60. [CrossRef]

31. Anastasi, D.; Carpinella, I.; Gervasoni, E.; Matsuda, P.N.; Bovi, G.; Ferrarin, M.; Cattaneo, D. Instrumented Version of the Modified Dynamic Gait Index in Patients with Neurologic Disorders. *PM&R* **2019**. [CrossRef]

32. Pau, M.; Corona, F.; Pilloni, G.; Porta, M.; Coghe, G.; Cocco, E. Texting while walking differently alters gait patterns in people with multiple sclerosis and healthy individuals. *Mult. Scler. Relat. Disord.* **2018**, *19*, 129–133. [CrossRef]

33. Carpinella, I.; Gervasoni, E.; Anastasi, D.; Lencioni, T.; Cattaneo, D.; Ferrarin, M. Instrumental Assessment of Stair Ascent in People with Multiple Sclerosis, Stroke, and Parkinson's Disease: A Wearable-Sensor-Based Approach. *IEEE Trans. Neural Syst. Rehabil. Eng.* **2018**, *26*, 2324–2332. [CrossRef]

34. Craig, J.J.; Bruetsch, A.P.; Lynch, S.G.; Horak, F.B.; Huisinga, J.M. Instrumented balance and walking assessments in persons with multiple sclerosis show strong test-retest reliability. *J. Neuroeng. Rehabil.* **2017**, *14*, 43. [CrossRef]

35. Riva, F.; Grimpampi, E.; Mazzà, C.; Stagni, R. Are gait variability and stability measures influenced by directional changes? *Biomed. Eng. Online* **2014**, *13*, 56. [CrossRef]

36. Brønd, J.C.; Arvidsson, D. Sampling frequency affects the processing of Actigraph raw acceleration data to activity counts. *J. Appl. Physiol.* **2015**, *120*, 362–369. [CrossRef]

37. England, S.A.; Granata, K.P. The influence of gait speed on local dynamic stability of walking. *Gait Posture* **2007**, *25*, 172–178. [CrossRef]

38. Brodie, M.A.D.; Menz, H.B.; Lord, S.R. Age-associated changes in head jerk while walking reveal altered dynamic stability in older people. *Exp. Brain Res.* **2014**, *232*, 51–60. [CrossRef]

39. Mazzà, C.; Iosa, M.; Pecoraro, F.; Cappozzo, A. Control of the upper body accelerations in young and elderly women during level walking. *J. Neuroengineering Rehabil.* **2008**, *5*, 30. [CrossRef]

40. Brach, J.S.; McGurl, D.; Wert, D.; Vanswearingen, J.M.; Perera, S.; Cham, R.; Studenski, S. Validation of a measure of smoothness of walking. *J. Gerontology. Ser. A Biol. Sci. Med. Sci.* **2010**, *66*, 136–141. [CrossRef]

41. Helbostad, J.L.; Moe-Nilssen, R. The effect of gait speed on lateral balance control during walking in healthy elderly. *Gait Posture* **2003**, *18*, 27–36. [CrossRef]

42. Rabuffetti, M.; Scalera, M.G.; Ferrarin, M. Effects of Gait Strategy and Speed on Regularity of Locomotion Assessed in Healthy Subjects Using a Multi-Sensor Method. *Sensors* **2019**, *19*, 513. [CrossRef] [PubMed]

43. Latt, M.D.; Menz, H.B.; Fung, V.S.; Lord, S.R. Walking speed, cadence and step length are selected to optimize the stability of head and pelvis accelerations. *Exp. Brain Res.* **2008**, *184*, 201–209. [CrossRef]

44. Menz, H.B.; Lord, S.R.; Fitzpatrick, R.C. Acceleration patterns of the head and pelvis when walking on level and irregular surfaces. *Gait Posture* **2003**, *18*, 35–46. [CrossRef]

45. Lowry, K.A.; Lokenvitz, N.; Smiley-Oyen, A.L. Age- and speed-related differences in harmonic ratios during walking. *Gait Posture* **2012**, *35*, 272–276. [CrossRef]

46. Pecoraro, F.; Mazzà, C.; Cappozzo, A.; Thomas, E.E.; Macaluso, A. Reliability of the intrinsic and extrinsic patterns of level walking in older women. *Gait Posture* **2007**, *26*, 386–392. [CrossRef]

47. Cappozzo, A. Analysis of the linear displacement of the head and trunk during walking at different speeds. *J. Biomech.* **1981**, *14*, 411–425. [CrossRef]

48. Moe-Nilssen, R. A new method for evaluating motor control in gait under real-life environmental conditions. Part 1: The instrument. *Clin. Biomech.* **1998**, *13*, 320–327. [CrossRef]

49. Salarian, A.; Horak, F.B.; Zampieri, C.; Carlson-Kuhta, P.; Nutt, J.G.; Aminian, K. iTUG, a Sensitive and Reliable Measure of Mobility. *IEEE Trans. Neural Syst. Rehabil. Eng.* **2010**, *18*, 303–310. [CrossRef]

50. Killick, R.; Fearnhead, P.; Eckley, I.A. Optimal Detection of Changepoints With a Linear Computational Cost. *J. Am. Stat. Assoc.* **2012**, *107*, 1590–1598. [CrossRef]

51. Palmerini, L.; Rocchi, L.; Mazilu, S.; Gazit, E.; Hausdorff, J.M.; Chiari, L. Identification of Characteristic Motor Patterns Preceding Freezing of Gait in Parkinson's Disease Using Wearable Sensors. *Front. Neurol.* **2017**, *8*, 394. [CrossRef] [PubMed]

52. Lord, S.; Galna, B.; Rochester, L. Moving forward on gait measurement: toward a more refined approach. *Movement Disorders* **2013**, *28*, 1534–1543. [CrossRef] [PubMed]

53. Buckley, C.; Galna, B.; Rochester, L.; Mazzà, C. Upper body accelerations as a biomarker of gait impairment in the early stages of Parkinson's disease. *Gait Posture* **2019**, *71*, 289–295. [CrossRef] [PubMed]

54. Salarian, A.; Russmann, H.; Vingerhoets, F.J.; Dehollain, C.; Blanc, Y.; Burkhard, P.R.; Aminian, K. Gait assessment in Parkinson's disease: toward an ambulatory system for long-term monitoring. *IEEE Trans. Biomed. Eng.* **2004**, *51*, 1434–1443. [CrossRef] [PubMed]

55. Galna, B.; Lord, S.; Rochester, L. Is gait variability reliable in older adults and Parkinson's disease? Towards an optimal testing protocol. *Gait Posture* **2013**, *37*, 580–585. [CrossRef]

56. Godfrey, A.; Del Din, S.; Barry, G.; Mathers, J.C.; Rochester, L. Instrumenting gait with an accelerometer: A system and algorithm examination. *Med. Eng. Phys.* **2015**, *37*, 400–407. [CrossRef]

57. Pasciuto, I.; Bergamini, E.; Iosa, M.; Vannozzi, G.; Cappozzo, A. Overcoming the limitations of the Harmonic Ratio for the reliable assessment of gait symmetry. *J. Biomech.* **2017**, *53*, 84–89. [CrossRef]

58. Sekine, M.; Tamura, T.; Yoshida, M.; Suda, Y.; Kimura, Y.; Miyoshi, H.; Kijima, Y.; Higashi, Y.; Fujimoto, T. A gait abnormality measure based on root mean square of trunk acceleration. *J. Neuroeng. Rehabil.* **2013**, *10*, 118. [CrossRef]

59. Fazio, P.; Granieri, G.; Casetta, I.; Cesnik, E.; Mazzacane, S.; Caliandro, P.; Pedrielli, F.; Granieri, E. Gait measures with a triaxial accelerometer among patients with neurological impairment. *Neurol. Sci.* **2013**, *34*, 435–440. [CrossRef]

60. Gage, S.H. Microscopy in America (1830–1945). *Trans. Am. Microsc. Soc.* **1964**, *83*, 1–125. [CrossRef]

61. Smidt, G.L.; Arora, J.S.; Johnston, R.C. Accelerographic analysis of several types of walking. *Am. J. Phys. Med. Rehabil.* **1971**, *50*, 285–300.

62. Moe-Nilssen, R.; Helbostad, J.L. Estimation of gait cycle characteristics by trunk accelerometry. *J. Biomech.* **2004**, *37*, 121–126. [CrossRef]

63. R Core Team. *R: A Language and Environment for Statistical Computing*; R Foundation for Statistical Computing: Vienna, Austria; Available online: http://cran.fhcrc.org/web/packages/dplR/vignettes/intro-dplR.pdf (accessed on 20 December 2019).

64. Li, L.; Zeng, L.; Lin, Z.-J.; Cazzell, M.; Liu, H. Tutorial on use of intraclass correlation coefficients for assessing intertest reliability and its application in functional near-infrared spectroscopy–based brain imaging. *J. Biomed. Opt.* **2015**, *20*, 050801. [CrossRef] [PubMed]

65. Cicchetti, D.V. Methodological Commentary The Precision of Reliability and Validity Estimates Re-Visited: Distinguishing Between Clinical and Statistical Significance of Sample Size Requirements. *J. Clin. Exp. Neuropsychology* **2001**, *23*, 695–700. [CrossRef]

66. Almarwani, M.; Perera, S.; VanSwearingen, J.M.; Sparto, P.J.; Brach, J.S. The test–retest reliability and minimal detectable change of spatial and temporal gait variability during usual over-ground walking for younger and older adults. *Gait Posture* **2016**, *44*, 94–99. [CrossRef]

67. Cohen, J. CHAPTER 3—The Significance of a Product Moment rs. In *Statistical Power Analysis for the Behavioral Sciences*; Available online: http://www.utstat.toronto.edu/~{}brunner/oldclass/378f16/readings/CohenPower.pdf (accessed on 20 December 2019).

68. Compston, A.; Coles, A. Multiple sclerosis. *Lancet* **2008**, *372*, 1502–1517. [CrossRef]

69. Dujmovic, I.; Radovanovic, S.; Martinovic, V.; Dackovic, J.; Maric, G.; Mesaros, S.; Pekmezovic, T.; Kostic, V.; Drulovic, J. Gait pattern in patients with different multiple sclerosis phenotypes. *Mult. Scler. Relat. Disord.* **2017**, *13*, 13–20. [CrossRef]

70. Cole, M.H.; Sweeney, M.; Conway, Z.J.; Blackmore, T.; Silburn, P.A. Imposed Faster and Slower Walking Speeds Influence Gait Stability Differently in Parkinson Fallers. *Arch. Phys. Med. Rehabil.* **2017**, *98*, 639–648. [CrossRef]

71. Riva, F.; Bisi, M.C.; Stagni, R. Gait variability and stability measures: Minimum number of strides and within-session reliability. *Comput. Biol. Med.* **2014**, *50*, 9–13. [CrossRef]

72. Shema-Shiratzky, S.; Gazit, E.; Sun, R.; Regev, K.; Karni, A.; Sosnoff, J.J.; Herman, T.; Mirelman, A.; Hausdorff, J.M. Deterioration of specific aspects of gait during the instrumented 6-min walk test among people with multiple sclerosis. *J. Neurol.* **2019**, *266*, 3022–3030. [CrossRef]

16

Plasma Exchange or Immunoadsorption in Demyelinating Diseases

Mark Lipphardt, Manuel Wallbach and Michael J. Koziolek *

Department of Nephrology and Rheumatology, University Medical Center Göttingen, Robert-Koch-Str. 40, D-37075 Goettingen, Germany; mark.lipphardt@med.uni-goettingen.de (M.L.); manuel.wallbach@med.uni-goettingen.de (M.W.)
* Correspondence: mkoziolek@med.uni-goettingen.de

Abstract: Multiple sclerosis (MS) is an inflammatory disease mainly affecting the central nervous system. In MS, abnormal immune mechanisms induce acute inflammation, demyelination, axonal loss, and the formation of central nervous system plaques. The long-term treatment involves options to modify the disease progression, whereas the treatment for the acute relapse has its focus in the administration of high-dose intravenous methylprednisolone (up to 1000 mg daily) over a period of three to five days as a first step. If symptoms of the acute relapse persist, it is defined as glucocorticosteroid-unresponsive, and immunomodulation by apheresis is recommended. However, several national and international guidelines have no uniform recommendations on using plasma exchange (PE) nor immunoadsorption (IA) in this case. A systematic review and meta-analysis was conducted, including observational studies or randomized controlled trials that investigated the effect of PE or IA on different courses of MS and neuromyelitis optica (NMO). One thousand, three hundred and eighty-three patients were included in the evaluation. Therapy response in relapsing-remitting MS and clinically isolated syndrome was 76.6% (95%CI 63.7–89.8%) in PE- and 80.6% (95%CI 69.3–91.8%) in IA-treated patients. Based on the recent literature, PE and IA may be considered as equal treatment possibilities in patients suffering from acute, glucocorticosteroid-unresponsive MS relapses.

Keywords: multiple sclerosis; plasma exchange; immunoadsorption

1. Introduction

Multiple sclerosis (MS) is a disease which is defined as an inflammatory condition affecting the central nervous system. Its main course of damage is due to abnormal immune mechanisms, resulting in acute inflammation, demyelination, axonal loss, and the formation of central nervous systemplaques consisting of inflammatory cells [1,2].

The epidemiology of MS differs greatly depending on the geographic regions with a prevalence from high levels in North America and Europe (>100/100,000 inhabitants) to low rates in Eastern Asia and sub-Saharan Africa (2/100,000 population). Women are generally more affected than men [3].

Symptoms that occur with the onset of MS are very unspecific, since MS can affect all regions of the central nervous system and can make it hard for a physician to make an early diagnosis. Symptoms of MS include vision problems with a decreased visual acuity (VA) and a prolonged visual evoked potential (VEP), weakness, fatigue, spasms, ataxia, cognitive dysfunction, or numbness [4]. The occurrence of an optic neuritis in its typical form is considered to be associated with MS. However, it is also regarded as a demyelinating clinically isolated syndrome (CIS) with the risk to convert to MS, especially in the white population [5]. With such a variety of symptoms a thorough medical history and examination is essential to make the right diagnosis of MS. Blood tests, lumbar punctures, magnetic resonance imaging, and evoked potential tests help in the process of differentiating between other diseases [6]. Based on the symptoms and the progression of the disease MS is divided in four types:

Relapsing-Remitting MS (RRMS), Secondary-Progressive MS (SPMS), Primary-Progressive MS (PPMS), and Progressive-Relapsing MS (PRMS).

MS can be characterized as a T-cell-driven disease with T helper (Th) cells, especially Th-1, Th-2, and Th-17 cells, as the main players in a various inflammatory cascade [7]. For instance, Th-1 cells are responsible for producing Interferon gamma (IFNγ) and tumor necrosis factor alpha (TNF-α) [8]. With the secretion of IFNy and TNF-α inflammation can be maintained by inhibiting Th-2 cell differentiation, since Th-2 cells produce anti-inflammatory cytokines like interleukin (IL)-4 and IL-13 [9,10]. Th-17 cells stimulate inflammation via secreting a vast number of various cytokines like IL-17, IL-21, IL-22, and IL-26 [11–13]. As a counterpart regulatory T (Treg) cells inhibit autoimmune responses [14]. In addition to that immunoglobulins (Ig) (especially IgG) are important in the pathogenesis of MS. Evidence of intrathecal Ig production and oligoclonal IgG bands contribute to the diagnosis of MS. Further differentiation shows various types of specific autoantibodies against myelin in subgroups of patients with MS, e.g., anti-myelin oligo-dendrocyte glycoprotein (anti-MOG) or anti-myelin basic protein (anti-MBP) [15]. Antibody-producing B-cells traveling between CNS, blood, and peripheral lymphatic organs clonally expanded B-cells and aggregated B-cells in meninges corroborate a pathophysiological role of B-cells and/or humoral immune answer in the pathogenesis of MS [16–19].

Based on the myelin protein loss, the geography and extension of plaques, the patterns of oligodendrocyte destruction, and the immunohistopathological evidence of complement activation Lucchinetti et al. described four different immunohistopathological patterns of demyelination in MS [20]. Patterns I and II showed close similarities to T-cell-mediated or T-cell plus antibody-mediated autoimmune encephalomyelitis. Patterns III and IV on the other hand were highly suggestive of a primary oligodendrocyte dystrophy.

Neuromyelitis optica (NMO) on the other hand is described as an idiopathic, severe, demyelinating disease of the central nervous system with the preference to affect the optic nerve and spinal cord. NMO has been considered as a variant of MS. However, with the analysis of clinical, laboratory, immunological, and pathological data the difference to MS is now acknowledged [21].

The treatment regime can be divided in treatment to modify the disease progression and treatment for the acute relapse. In the latter, the administration of high-dose intravenous methylprednisolone (up to 1000 mg daily) over a period of three to five days usually represents the first step in acute MS relapse treatment. A higher second high-dose intravenous methylprednisolone pulse with up to 2 g can be considered in unresponsive patients after an interval of 2 weeks [22–24]. Glucocorticoids may downregulate cellular cytotoxicity and lead to the death of activated B cells, but they will not modulate tissue destruction or conduction blockade by local antibody deposition [25]. If symptoms persist, the relapse is defined as glucocorticosteroid-unresponsive and immunomodulation by apheresis is recommended. However, several national and international guidelines have no uniform recommendations on using plasma exchange (PE) or immunoadsorption (IA) in this case. The American Society for Apheresis (ASFA) recommends PE for treatment to category II ("apheresis accepted as second-line therapy") and IA for treatment to category III ("optimum role of apheresis therapy is not established") [26]. The American Academy of Neurology also advises the use of PE for adjunctive treatment of relapsing forms of MS (Level B), while IA is not addressed [27,28]. The German guidelines are currently under reconstruction but formerly recommended both procedures as equivalent [29].

In this current issue, we review the use of IA and PE in treating, especially, the acute relapse of MS.

2. Effects of Apheresis Therapy

During PE, the patient's plasma, including all plasma proteins, is removed and substituted by human albumin solution or fresh frozen plasma. The concept of IA involves a selective elimination of plasma proteins, e.g., antibodies, while sparing other plasma proteins [30]. Both techniques include an extracorporeal circulation circuit with systemic and/or local anticoagulation, as well as the need of a vascular access. The latter can either be peripheral venous, if individual vascular situation allows it, or by a central venous catheter. In IA, a secondary circuit is established in which a defined physico-chemical interaction of selected plasma proteins with a defined matrix should theoretically guarantee selective removal of circulating pathogens. In praxis, a bandwidth of proteins are removed [31,32] which are responsible for therapeutic effects but also possible side effects of IA. These effects differ with regard to used matrix of the adsorber, which physicians should be aware.

The exact mechanism by which apheresis treatment works is actually not fully understood. MS patients may benefit by the immediate removal of plasma antibodies, immune complexes and cytokines, induction of a redistribution of antibodies from the extravascular space, and subsequent immunomodulatory changes [30]. Here, cell types with receptors for immunoglobulins (Fc receptors), such as monocytes, macrophages, and natural killer cells, are especially of interest [25]. Besides effects on humoral immune system, experimental data suggest a reduction of circulating autoantigens and regulatory proteins [32] and induction of a higher relative quantity of Treg to Th17 cells [33], as well as a silencing of cellular autoimmune response [32].

Early active MS lesions with an immunohistopathological type II pattern, which are selectively associated with Ig's and complement deposited along myelin sheaths, predict the best response to apheresis therapy in patients with steroid-unresponsive relapse [34], corroborating the hypothesis of effects on humoral immune response.

3. Plasma Exchange

3.1. Multiple Sclerosis (with Relapsing-Remitting and Progressive MS Sub-Sections)

The first study comparing the normal therapy regime with PE was performed by Khatri et al. in 1985 and included fifty-four patients with chronic progressive MS [35]. The results showed that patients with the additional PE have a higher improvement rate than patients with a "sham" PE. Following the study of Khatri et al., Weiner et al. enrolled 116 patients in a multicenter, randomized, double-blinded, controlled trial of 11 PE treatments in acute exacerbations of MS [36]. One of the main results showed patients treated with PE to have a significantly enhanced improvement after four weeks. In 1999, a study group of the Mayo Clinic conducted a randomized, sham-controlled, double-blinded study of PE in MS patients with severe neurological deficits after acute relapses, unresponsive to corticosteroids [37]. This study resulted in a moderate to greater improvement in neurological deficits in 42.1% of patients with true PE versus 5.9% of patients with sham PE. With the improved work with PE in the clinical setting, a variety of retrospective studies could demonstrate an improvement rate between 59–87.5% [38–40]. In a large study with 153 patients enrolled, Magana et al. identified 90 patients with moderate to marked functional neurological improvement within 6 months after treatment with PE [41].

An excellent and actual overview on apheresis in progressive MS forms is available in Reference [30]. So far, the ASFA recommends PE for treatment to category III: "Optimum role of apheresis therapy is not established. Decision making should be individualized" [26].

3.2. Clinically Isolated Syndrome

More recent studies set their focus not only on the relapsing-remitting and progressive MS sub-sections but also on the clinically isolated syndrome [42–44]. Therapy response rates ranged between 72–76%, therefore achieving a clinical response in the majority of patients.

3.3. Optic Neuritis

Studies analyzing the use of PE in the setting of for severe steroid unresponsive optic neuritis were performed by Ruprecht et al. and Deschamps et al. [45,46]. Ruprecht et al. al. demonstrated an improvement of visual acuity in 70% of patients. Out of these seven patients, three continued to improve with their visual acuity, two remained at a stable state, whereas two patients suffered from worsening symptoms during the follow-ups [46].

In the study performed by Deschamps et al., thirty-four patients with a remaining visual acuity of 0.1 were treated with PE. Afterwards, the median visual acuity was 0.8 [45].

Studies on PE are summarized in Table 1. However, the reader must be aware that the comparability of the studies is limited by the different technical implementation of PE. This varied in frequency, treated plasma volume, and total number of PEs. As a result, the ASFA defined a corridor of technical implementation that recommended treatment of 1–1.5-fold plasma volume per session for a number of 5 to 7 treatments over a period of 10 to 14 days [26].

Table 1. Studies on plasma exchange (PE) in treatment of relapsing-remitting multiple sclerosis (RRMS), clinically isolated syndrome (CIS), progressive MS, isolated optic neuritis, and neuromyelitis optica (NMO). EDSS = Expanded Disability Status Scale.

"Relapsing-Remitting Multiple Sclerosis" and "Clinically Isolated Syndrome"							
Citation	Year	*n*	Design	No. of Treatments	Treated Plasma Volume (mL)	Outcome	Limitation
[36]	1989	116	Double-blind, multi-center, randomized	11	n.a.	Significant improvement after 4 weeks	No plasmapheresis protocol specifications
[37]	1999	36	Double-blind	7	3000	Therapy response in 42% of patients	Patient collective with heterogenous MS-types
[39]	2005	13	Retrospective	5	3000	Therapy response in 71% of patients	Small number of subjects
[47]	2007	6	Retrospective	4	1.0-fold plasma volume	Therapy response in 100% of patients	Small number of subjects
[40]	2009	20	Retrospective	3–7	1.5-fold plasma volume	Therapy response in 76% of patients regarding visual acuity	Small number of subjects
[38]	2010	4	Retrospective	5	2750	Therapy response in 75% of patients	no placebo, Small number of subjects, the study was observational in character
[41]	2011	153	Retrospective	7	n.a.	Therapy response in 59% of patients	Patient collective with heterogenous MS-types
[48]	2013	15	Retrospective	≥7	1.0-fold plasma volume	Therapy response in 93.3% of patients	RRMS + CIS
[49]	2014	11	Retrospective	Median 7 (3–8)	3000 (2200–3500)	Therapy response in 91% of patients	CIS only
[43]	2015	90	Retrospective	3–8	1.0-fold plasma volume	Therapy response in 72% of patients	The lack of a control group
[50]	2016	16	Retrospective	n.a.	2000	Therapy response in 91% of patients regarding visual evoked potential	Small number of subjects and a higher expanded disability status scale in patients in the PE only group
[51]	2018	46	Retrospective	Mean 7.39 sessions	n.a.	Complete therapy response in 41% of patients and partial therapy response in 39% of patients	Patient collective with heterogenous MS-types
[44]	2019	42	Retrospective	4–11	Mean 2930 median 2000	Therapy response in 73% of patients	patients without sufficient follow-up data had a significantly higher patient age and longer duration of disease
[42]	2019	30	Double-blind, randomized, uni-center	On 5 days	0.69 ± 0.12-fold individual total plasma volume	Therapy response in 76% of patients	Lack of blinding and small number of subjects

Table 1. *Cont.*

"Progressive Multiple Sclerosis"							
Citation	Year	n	Design	No. of Treatments	Treated Plasma Volume (mL)	Outcome	Limitation
[52]	1983	18	Prospective, randomized	4–5	n.a.	Therapy response in 27.8% of patients	Small number of subjects, no plasmapheresis protocol specifications
[35]	1985	54	Double-blind controlled	20	n.a.	Therapy response in 54% of patients	No plasmapheresis protocol specifications
[53]	1994	24	Prospective	8	n.a.	Therapy response in 87.5% of patients	Small number of subjects, no plasmapheresis protocol specifications
[41]	2011	10	Retrospective	7	n.a.	Therapy response in 30% of patients	Small number of subjects
[54]	2015	6	open-label, single-center proof of concept study	4	2000–2500	Therapy response in 66.7% of patients	Small number of subjects

"Isolated Optic Neuritis"							
Citation	Year	n	Design	No. of Treatments	Treated Plasma Volume (mL)	Outcome	Limitation
[46]	2004	10	Retrospective	n.a.	n.a.	Therapy response in 70% of patients	Small number of subjects
[55]	2012	23	Retrospective	5	~3000	Therapy response in 70% of patients	heterogenous
[56]	2012	16	Retrospective	5	1.0-fold plasma volume	Therapy response in 87.5% of patients	Small number of subjects
[45]	2016	34	Retrospective	Median 5, range 5–10	1.5-fold body mass volume	Therapy response in 56% of patients regarding visual acuity	The lack of a control group

"Neuromyelitis Optica"							
Citation	Year	n	Design	No. of Treatments	Treated Plasma Volume (mL)	Outcome	Limitation
[57]	2007	6	Retrospective	3–5	2000–3000	Therapy response in 50% of patients	Small number of subjects
[58]	2011	5	Retrospective	≥5	1.0-fold plasma volume	Therapy response in 80% of patients	Small number of subjects
[41]	2011	26	Retrospective	7	n.a.	Therapy response in 42.3% of patients	Historical cohort study
[59]	2013	31	Retrospective	n.a.	n.a.	Therapy response in 65% of patients	No study controlled treatment regimes
[60]	2013	15	Retrospective	6	1.0–1.5-fold plasma volume	Therapy response in 78% of patients	Small number of subjects
[61]	2016	65	Retrospective	5–7	1.5-fold plasma volume	Therapy response in 65% of patients	Selection bias; use of EDSS scores as the primary outcome measure
[62]	2017	21	Retrospective	5	n.a.	Therapy response in 81% of patients	Use of EDSS scores as the primary outcome measure
[63]	2018	28	Retrospective	5	1000	Therapy response in 42.9% of patients	Use of EDSS scores as the primary outcome measure
[64]	2018	29	Retrospective	2–7	1.0-fold plasma volume	Therapy response in 82.8% of patients	Heterogenous treatment protocols
[65]	2018	9	Retrospective	7	1.0-fold plasma volume	Therapy response in 75% of patients	Small number of subjects

Table 1. *Cont.*

				"Neuromyelitis Optica"			
Citation	Year	*n*	Design	No. of Treatments	Treated Plasma Volume (mL)	Outcome	Limitation
[66]	2018	5	Retrospective	5 (3–7)	1.0-fold plasma volume	Therapy response in 80% of patients	Small number of subjects
[67]	2018	146	Retrospective	≥3	n.a.	Therapy response in 86% of patients	Heterogenous treatment protocols
[68]	2019	15	Retrospective	2–3	n.a	Therapy response in 100% of patients	Small number of subjects

4. Immunoadsorption

4.1. Multiple Sclerosis (with Relapsing-Remitting and Progressive MS Sub-Sections)

IA was firstly introduced in the treatment of MS by de Andres et al. in 2000 [69]. They managed a prompt and unequivocal clinical response with a parallel decrease in IgG, fibrinogen, and C3 complement plasma levels in all three patients treated with IA. In the following years, retrospective studies confirmed the initial results of de Andres et al., showing improvement rates from 85–88.3% in MS patients receiving an IA therapy [70,71].

4.2. Clinically Isolated Syndrome

Studies incorporating patients with clinically isolated syndrome showed marked to moderate clinical response with a total gain of function in 66–100% of patients after treatment with immunoadsorption [42,72].

4.3. Neuromyelitis Optica

The first prospective study investigating effects of IA therapy in patients with MS with steroid-refractory optical neuritis showed an improvement of the mean visual acuity in 8 from 11 patients at day 180 ± 10 after IA [32]. A more recent study confirmed the efficacy and good tolerance of IA in relapses of MS patients with failure to respond to a steroid pulse therapy adequately. Moreover, the study established IA as first-line relapse treatment during pregnancy and breastfeeding [73].

The most commonly used column was a tryptophane-linked polyvinyl alcohol adsorber, but also a Sepharose-conjugated sheep antibodies to human IgG, as well as protein A column, have been used. Table 2 gives an overview about IA-studies in acute relapses of MS.

5. Plasma Exchange vs. Immunoadsorption

5.1. Multiple Sclerosis (with Relapsing-Remitting and Progressive MS Sub-Sections)

Recently, studies have been designed to compare the efficacy of PE versus IA. The most impressive work is that of Dorst et al. [42]. Sixty-one patients with acute relapse of multiple sclerosis or clinically isolated syndrome and without complete clinical remission of symptoms after at least one cycle of high-dose intravenous methylprednisolone were randomly assigned to receive IA (*n* = 31) or PE (*n* = 30). In the IA group (using a protein A adsorber), the 2.0-fold individual total plasma volume was processed on day 1, and the 2.5-fold on days 2–5. In the PE group, 2 L of plasma (corresponding to the 0.69 ± 0.12-fold individual total plasma volume) were removed each day and substituted by 5% human albumin solution. The median improvement of Multiple Sclerosis Functional Composite after 4 weeks compared to baseline was 0.385 (interquartile range (IQR) 0.200–0.675; $p < 0.001$) in the IA group and 0.265 (IQR 0.100–0.408; $p < 0.001$) in the PE group. Improvement in the IA group was significantly larger ($p = 0.034$) compared to PE. Response rates after 4 weeks were 86.7% in the IA group and 76.7% in the PE group. One deep venous thrombosis occurred in each group. One limitation in interpretation of this study, however, is that the apheresis dose applied was quite different in the two treatment arms and the observation period was relatively short.

Hohenstein et al. reported the successful use of IA with regenerating adsorbers in MS patients as a single center experience [78]. Faissner et al. compared PE and IA directly and demonstrated in a grouped analysis of patients treated with combined PE/ IA, PE, or IA alone, that all groups presented with a better result of visual evoked potentials, providing a valid treatment option in steroid-refractory MS-relapses [50].

5.2. Clinically Isolated Syndrome

Dorst et al. [42] also enrolled patients suffering from a clinically isolated syndrome in their recent study. The results are discussed above.

5.3. Neuromyelitis Optica

In a small cohort study, Faissner et al. showed equivalent results treating patients with neuromyelitis optica spectrum disorder with IA instead of PE, constituting IA as a valid therapeutic option [77]. Studies of our own also indicate PE and IA to be of equal efficacy and treatment safety [44,79]. We assessed 140 adult patients treated with PE ($n = 73$) or IA ($n = 67$) in steroid refractory multiple sclerosis or neuromyelitis optica. During our studies, we became aware of the fact that differences in body-mass-index, duration of disease, number of treatments, vascular access and treated plasma volumes between IA - and PE cohorts are a main concern for possible bias in the assessment of IA and PE as a treatment for MS patients. We also performed a retrospective single-center cohort study of pediatric patients with inflammatory CNS demyelinating disorders showing excellent tolerance and favorable outcomes of PE and IA in all pediatric patients [31].

6. Meta-Analysis on Apheresis Effects on Demyelinating Diseases

6.1. Search Strategy and Inclusion Criteria

A systematic search was performed using Medline and Cochrane Library with combinations of the search terms "plasma exchange" OR "immunoadsorption" in combination with the terms "multiple sclerosis" OR "clinical isolated syndrome" OR "neuromyelitis optica" between 1980 and January 2020. Reports were screened independently for relevance based on title and abstract content by two authors (M.L. and M.J.K.). Randomized-controlled trials, as well as prospective cohort studies and retrospective studies and case series, were included if sufficient information on therapy response of PE or IA was provided. Studies with heterogeneous mixing MS, CIS, and/or NMO patients regarding therapy response were excluded if the treatment response was not specified separately in the individual indications. Moreover, case series with a case number less than five in the individual indication were also excluded. It should be mentioned as a limitation that there was no uniform definition of the term "therapy response" in the selected works and, with the exception of a few studies, the majority was retrospective data collection. The flow chart in Figure 1 summarizes the selection of studies in the meta-analysis.

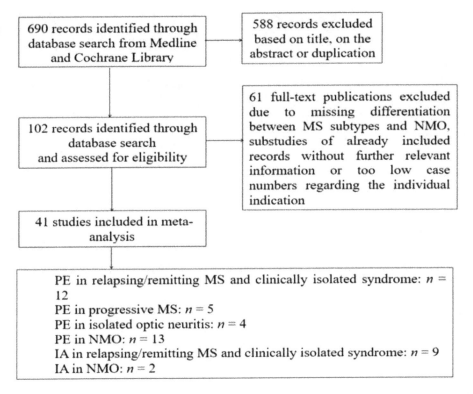

Figure 1. Flow chart of study selection. MS = multiple sclerosis, NMO = neuromyelitis optica, PE = plasma exchange, IA = immunoadsorption.

6.2. Statistical Analysis

Analysis was performed using RevMan V.5.3 (Nordic Cochrane Centre, Copenhagen, Denmark, the Cochrane Collaboration, 2014). Data were quantitatively synthesized by an inverse-variance-weighted meta-analysis using a random-effect model because of the presence of heterogeneity. The normal approximation interval (sqrt($p(1-p)/n$)) was used to generate the confidence interval for the therapy response rate. For studies where the normal approximation interval was zero, the confidence interval was set to one to calculate the random effect model. The 95% normal approximation confidence interval is provided in the meta-analyses.

7. Results

With the present search strategy and assessment of full-texts 690 studies, 40 observational and 1 randomized with a total of 1.383 patients could be analyzed. Figure 1 shows the flow chart of study selection.

Effects of PE can be summarized as follows: in relapsing-remitting MS and clinically isolated syndrome (12 studies and 398 patients) therapy response of 76.6% (95%CI 63.7–89.8%) (Figure 2A), in progressive MS (5 studies and 112 patients) therapy response of 53.9% (95%CI 29.5–78.4) (Figure 2B), in isolated optic neuritis (4 studies and 83 patients) therapy response of 71.5% (95%CI 56.4–86.6%) (Figure 2C), and in NMO (13 studies and 401 patients) therapy response of 72.5% (95%CI 61.0–83.9%) (Figure 2D).

Effects of IA can be summarized as follows: in relapsing-remitting MS and clinically isolated syndrome (9 studies and 352 patients), therapy response of 80.6% (95%CI 69.3–91.8%) (Figure 2E); and in NMO (2 studies and 37 patients), therapy response of 100% (95%CI 98.6–101.4%) (Figure 2F).

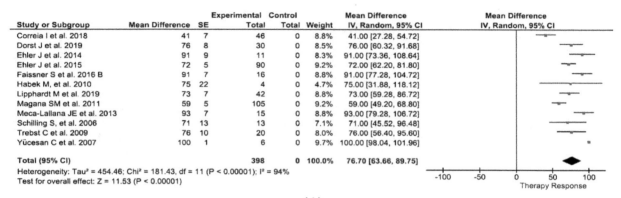

(A)

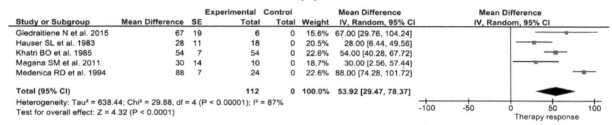

(B)

Study or Subgroup	Mean Difference	SE	Experimental Total	Control Total	Weight	Mean Difference IV, Random, 95% CI
Deschamps R et al. 2016	56	9	34	0	27.3%	56.00 [38.36, 73.64]
Merle H et al. 2012	88	8	16	0	29.7%	88.00 [72.32, 103.68]
Roesner S et al. 2012	70	10	23	0	25.1%	70.00 [50.40, 89.60]
Ruprecht K et al. 2004	70	14	10	0	17.9%	70.00 [42.56, 97.44]
Total (95% CI)			**83**	**0**	**100.0%**	**71.51 [56.41, 86.61]**

Heterogeneity: Tau² = 136.05; Chi² = 7.21, df = 3 (P = 0.07); I² = 58%
Test for overall effect: Z = 9.28 (P < 0.00001)

(C)

Study or Subgroup	Mean Difference	SE	PE Total	Control Total	Weight	Mean Difference IV, Random, 95% CI
Abboud H et al. 2016	65	6	65	0	9.2%	65.00 [53.24, 76.76]
Aungsmart S et al. 2017	81	9	21	0	8.2%	81.00 [63.36, 98.64]
Jiao Y et al. 2018	83	7	29	0	8.9%	83.00 [69.28, 96.72]
Kim SH et al. 2013	78	11	15	0	7.5%	78.00 [56.44, 99.56]
Kleiter I et al. 2018	86	3	146	0	10.0%	86.00 [80.12, 91.88]
Kumar R et al. 2018	80	18	5	0	5.2%	80.00 [44.72, 115.28]
Lim YM et al. 2013	65	9	31	0	8.2%	65.00 [47.36, 82.64]
Magana SM et al. 2011	42	10	26	0	7.9%	42.00 [22.40, 61.60]
Mori S et al. 2018	75	14	9	0	6.5%	75.00 [47.56, 102.44]
Song W et al. 2019	100	1	15	0	10.2%	100.00 [98.04, 101.96]
Srisupa-Olan T et al. 2018	43	9	28	0	8.2%	43.00 [25.36, 60.64]
Wang KC et al. 2011	80	18	5	0	5.2%	80.00 [44.72, 115.28]
Watanabe S et al. 2007	50	20	6	0	4.7%	50.00 [10.80, 89.20]
Total (95% CI)			**401**	**0**	**100.0%**	**72.45 [60.95, 83.94]**

Heterogeneity: Tau² = 336.10; Chi² = 147.35, df = 12 (P < 0.00001); I² = 92%
Test for overall effect: Z = 12.36 (P < 0.00001)

(D)

Figure 2. *Cont.*

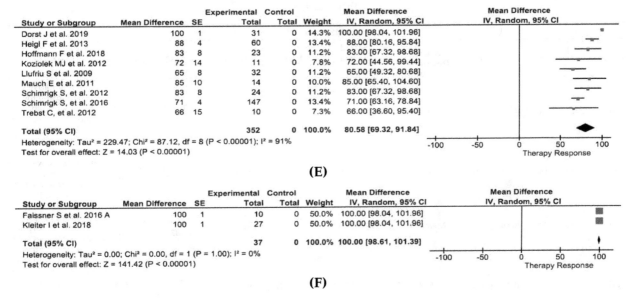

Study or Subgroup	Mean Difference	SE	Experimental Total	Control Total	Weight	Mean Difference IV, Random, 95% CI
Dorst J et al. 2019	100	1	31	0	14.3%	100.00 [98.04, 101.96]
Heigl F et al. 2013	88	4	60	0	13.4%	88.00 [80.16, 95.84]
Hoffmann F et al. 2018	83	8	23	0	11.2%	83.00 [67.32, 98.68]
Koziolek MJ et al. 2012	72	14	11	0	7.8%	72.00 [44.56, 99.44]
Llufriu S et al. 2009	65	8	32	0	11.2%	65.00 [49.32, 80.68]
Mauch E et al. 2011	85	10	14	0	10.0%	85.00 [65.40, 104.60]
Schimrigk S, et al. 2012	83	8	24	0	11.2%	83.00 [67.32, 98.68]
Schimrigk S, et al. 2016	71	4	147	0	13.4%	71.00 [63.16, 78.84]
Trebst C, et al. 2012	66	15	10	0	7.3%	66.00 [36.60, 95.40]
Total (95% CI)			**352**	**0**	**100.0%**	**80.58 [69.32, 91.84]**

Heterogeneity: Tau² = 229.47; Chi² = 87.12, df = 8 (P < 0.00001); I² = 91%
Test for overall effect: Z = 14.03 (P < 0.00001)

(E)

Study or Subgroup	Mean Difference	SE	Experimental Total	Control Total	Weight	Mean Difference IV, Random, 95% CI
Faissner S et al. 2016 A	100	1	10	0	50.0%	100.00 [98.04, 101.96]
Kleiter I et al. 2018	100	1	27	0	50.0%	100.00 [98.04, 101.96]
Total (95% CI)			**37**	**0**	**100.0%**	**100.00 [98.61, 101.39]**

Heterogeneity: Tau² = 0.00; Chi² = 0.00, df = 1 (P = 1.00); I² = 0%
Test for overall effect: Z = 141.42 (P < 0.00001)

(F)

Figure 2. The 95% normal approximation confidence interval is provided in the meta-analyses. The given SE correspond to normal approximation confidence interval (sqrt(p(1-p)/n)). (**A**) Effects of PE in RRMS and CIS. (**B**) Effects of PE in PMS. (**C**) Effects of PE in opticus neuritis. (**D**) Effects of PE in NMO. (**E**) Effects of IA in RRMS and CIS. (**F**) Effects of IA in NMO. RRMS = relapsing-remitting multiple sclerosis, CIS = clinically isolated syndrome, PMS = progressive multiple sclerosis, SE = standard error, IV = instrumental variables. Figure 2A: Correia et al. [51], Dorst et al. [42], Ehler et al. [49], Ehler at al. [43], Faissner et al. [50], Habek et al. [38], Lipphardt et al. [44], Magana et al. [41], Meca-Lallana et al. [48], Schilling et al. [39], Trebst et al. [40], Yücesan et al. [47]. Figure 2B: Giedraitiene et al. [54], Hauser et al. [52], Khatri et al. [35], Magana et al. [41], Medenica et al. [53]. Figure 2C: Deschamps et al. [45], Merle et al. [56], Roesner et al. [55], Ruprecht et al. [46]. Figure 2D: Abboud et al. [61], Aungsmart et al. [62], Jiao et al. [64], Kim et al. [60], Kleiter et al. [67], Kumar et al. [66], Lim et al. [59], Magana et al. [41], Mori et al. [65], Song et al. [68], Srisupa-Olan et al. [63], Wang et al. [58], Watanabe et al. [57]. Figure 2E: Dorst et al. [42], Heigl et al. [70], Hoffmann et al. [73], Koziolek et al. [32], Llufriu et al. [80], Mauch et al. [71], Schimrigk et al. [75], Schimrigk et al. [76], Trebst et al. [72]. Figure 2F: Faissner et al. [77], Kleiter et al. [67].

Table 2. Studies on immunoadsorption in treatment of relapsing-remitting multiple sclerosis (RRMS), clinically isolated syndrome (CIS) and neuromyelitis optica (NMO).

"RRMS" and "CIS"
Citation	Year	n	Design	No. of Treatments	Treated Plasma Volume (mL)	Matrix of Adsorber	Outcome	Limitation
[69]	2000	3	Retrospective	5–6	n.a.	n.a.	Therapy response in 100% of patients	small number of subjects
[74]	2005	12	Prospective	14	1.5-fold plasma volume	Sepharose-conjugated sheep antibodies to human immunoglobulin (IgG)	No significant therapy response	small number of subjects and patient collective with heterogenous MS-types
[71]	2011	14	Retrospective	5–6	n.a.	Tryptophan	Therapy response in 85% of patients	small number of subjects
[75]	2012	24	Retrospective	Mean 5 (range 3–6)	2000–2500	Tryptophan	Therapy response in 83% of patients	small number of subjects and patient collective with heterogenous MS-types
[72]	2012	10	Retrospective	5–7	2500	Tryptophan	Therapy response in 66% of patients	small number of subjects
[32]	2012	11	Prospective	5	2500	Tryptophan	Therapy response in 72% of patients	small number of subjects

Table 2. *Cont.*

Citation	Year	n	Design	No. of Treatments	Treated Plasma Volume (mL)	Matrix of Adsorber	Outcome	Limitation
					"RRMS" and "CIS"			
[70]	2013	60	Retrospective	6	2000	Tryptophan	Therapy response in 88% of patients	only qualitative data regarding the therapeutic success and clinical data on tolerability were available
[76]	2016	147	Retrospective	n.a.	2000–2500	Tryptophan	Therapy response in 71% of patients	Expanded Disability Status Scale was used to measure a change in relapse-related disability
[73]	2018	23	Retrospective	Mean 5.8	2031 ± 230	Tryptophan	Therapy response in 83% of patients	Lack of a control group; use of immunoadsorption was limited in some study centers
[44]	2019	32	Retrospective	5–7	2000–2500	Tryptophan	Therapy response in 65% of patients	patients without sufficient follow-up data had a significantly higher patient age and longer duration of disease
[42]	2019	31	Prospective, double-blind, randomized, uni-center	On 5 days	2.0-fold total plasma volume on day 1, and the 2.5-fold total plasma volume on day 2–5	protein A	Therapy response in 100% of patients	Lack of blinding and small number of subjects
					"NMO"			
[77]	2016	10	Retrospective	Mean 5.2 (3–7)	2000–2500	Tryptophan	Therapy response in 100% of patients	Small number of subjects
[67]	2018	27	Retrospective	≥3	n.a.	Tryptophan or Protein A	Therapy response in 100% of patients	Heterogenous treatment protocols

8. Safety Profile

8.1. General

Another important fact to consider is the treatment safety. The noted rates of side effects during those apheresis treatments are very heterogeneous. In the literature one can find complication rates from 4.2% until 25.6% [81–84]. In 2011, Köhler et al. postulated lower side effects using IA in patients suffering from myasthenia gravis [85]. They claim that a possible reason for the difference was due to the absence of albumin-substitution. Zoellner et al. designed a study to investigate the fibrinogen level and the occurrence of bleeding complications [86]. They demonstrated IA to have a lower degree of fibrinogen reduction as PE. Bleeding complications occurred in 1.3–3.1% of treatments. Schneider-Gold et al. reported allergic reactions, hypocoagulability, and bronchorespiratory infections with a significant higher frequency in the PE-only group as compared to the IA-only group or the both combined [87].

8.2. Multiple Sclerosis (with Relapsing-Remitting and Progressive MS Sub-Sections) and Clinically Isolated Syndrome

In the recent study performed by Dorst et al. [42], a general well tolerance was observed with 5 mild infections in the PE group and 4 mild allergic reactions in the IA group. Furthermore, courses of anemia and thrombocytopenia were documented with anemia being more frequent in the PE group and thrombocytopenia being more frequent in the IA group.

8.3. Multiple Sclerosis (with Relapsing-Remitting and Progressive MS Sub-Sections) and Neuromyelitis Optica

In our studies the complication rate was about 3.7% in over 780 apheresis cycles. Furthermore, we could not detect any differences regarding the safety profile of IA versus PE [44,79].

All in all, both IA and PE have a high tolerability regarding the safety profile. It should be added that the majority of the documented side effects are to be considered as mild. However, the use of IA and PE should be reserved to specialized centers familiar with technical procedure and experienced with this specialized patient population to ensure a high quality of treatment with low complication rates.

9. Treatment Predictors

9.1. General

One major predicting factor is the time to initiate apheresis treatment. Early initiation of apheresis correlates with a higher response rate as was shown by several study groups [44,60,80,88]. In the onset of sudden hearing loss, the early initiation of apheresis treatment was also beneficial [89].

Comparing the cumulative corticosteroid doses in apheresis-responders versus non-responders, no significant difference was shown, which makes a synergistic effect of apheresis and corticosteroids unlikely [44].

9.2. Multiple Sclerosis (with Relapsing-Remitting and Progressive MS Sub-Sections)

Magana et al. postulated the duration of the disease and preserved deep tendon reflexes as important clinical predictors [41]. A different approach was followed by the study group of Stork et al., who conducted a single-center cohort study with 69 MS patients, evaluating treatment response in relation to histopathologically defined immunopathological patterns of MS [34]. As early active demyelinating MS lesions can be divided in 3 different immunopathological patterns of demyelination, Stork et al. demonstrated that patients with pattern 1 and 2 are most likely to benefit from apheresis treatment, especially in patients with pattern 2 who show signs of a humoral immune response in particular. Patients with pattern 3 most likely do not benefit from apheresis treatment. During our studies, we also became aware of the fact that patients having a good response to apheresis treatment were significantly younger than non-responders [44]. This observation may be due to a decrease in remyelination efficiency, as proposed by Sim et al. [90]. A gender-related treatment benefit towards the female gender was identified in sub-groups of MS patients [44,91].

9.3. Neuromyelitis Optica

In a large study performed by Kleiter et al., it was shown that PE or IA exerts a better recovery from acute relapses in patients suffering from neuromyelitis optica if they had isolated myelitis [92]. More recent studies focused on the plasma anti-aquaporin-4 immunoglobulin G antibody as a positive predictor for treatment success with PE or IA in patients suffering from neuromyelitis optica spectrum disorder [12]. In both studies, particularly, patients with a positive anti-aquaporin-4 immunoglobulin G antibody responded well to the treatment with PE and IA. In addition to that, no advantage was revealed for either PE or IA. The disease specificity of anti-aquaporin-4 immunoglobulin G antibody is almost at 100% and clinical studies with immunohistochemical evidence suggest that this antibody plays a central role in the pathogenesis of neuromyelitis optica spectrum disorder [93].

These predictors can thus be summarized according to various variables. Table 3 provides a compilation.

Table 3. Predictors of apheresis response. EDSS = Expanded Disability Status Scale; MRI = magnetic resonance imaging. * Pediatric patients only.

"Multiple Sclerosis" (with Relapsing-Remitting and Progressive MS Sub-Sections)			
Classification	Predictor	Citation	Meaning
Clinical signs and symptoms	EDSS ≤ 5	[43]	Indicates good apheresis response
	Preserved deep tendon reflexes	[41]	Indicates good apheresis response
Demographics	Younger age	[44]	Indicates good apheresis response
	Female	[37,91]	Indicates good apheresis response
Histological classification and localization	Gadolinium positive MRI lesions	[43]	Indicates good apheresis response
	Histological type 1 and 2 pattern	[34]	Indicates good apheresis response
	Histological type 3 pattern	[34]	Indicates poor apheresis response
Pre-treatment	No disease modifying drugs	[43]	Indicates good apheresis response
	Short duration of disease	[41]	Indicates good apheresis response
"Neuromyelitis Optica"			
Classification	Predictor	Citation	Meaning
Histological classification and localization	Isolated myelitis	[85]	Indicates good apheresis response
Laboratory values	Anti-aquaporin-4 IgG positive	[12]	Indicates good apheresis response
"Mixed"			
Classification	Predictor	Citation	Meaning
Apheresis	Early initiation	[44,60,80,88]	Indicates good apheresis response
Clinical signs and symptoms	Lower baseline scores on the EDSS, visual outcome, and gait scales	[94] *	Indicates good apheresis response
Pre-treatment	Cumulative corticosteroid doses	[44]	Irrelevant for apheresis response

10. Therapeutic Efficacy and Time Course

As for the time course of the therapeutic effect, the current literature agrees on regular neurological follow-ups after 6 months, manifesting a continuous and maximal clinical effect of the apheresis treatment [41,44,60,80]. Therapeutic effects over such a long period of time suggest immunomodulatory actions of apheresis rather than antibody removal on its own [95]. Those immunomodulatory actions happen most likely at the level of Th-cells and CNS-associated proteins, like the myelin basic protein. The prolonged therapeutic effect can be thought of as a clinical correlate of the immunomodulatory components of therapeutic apheresis. Furthermore, the duration of the apheresis induced therapeutic effect can be involved in the treatment process of initiating or changing disease-modifying drugs.

11. Conclusions

The focus of this current issue is the use and comparison of immunoadsorption and plasma exchange in the treatment of multiple sclerosis with the main concern of acute relapses.

Based on the studies of the current literature and performance of a meta-analysis, including 690 studies, 40 observational and 1 randomized with a total of 1383 patients, plasma exchange and immunoadsorption are treatment options of equal effectivity for acute glucocorticosteroid-unresponsive multiple sclerosis relapses.

For the meta-analysis randomized-controlled trials, prospective cohort studies, retrospective studies, and case series with sufficient information on therapy response of plasma exchange or immunoadsorption were included. Studies with heterogeneous mixing multiple sclerosis, clinically isolated syndrome, and/or neuromyelitis optica patients regarding therapy response were not included if the treatment response was not specified separately in the individual indications.

Plasma exchange has a therapy response of 76.6% in relapsing-remitting multiple sclerosis (RRMS) and clinically isolated syndrome (CIS), 53.9% in progressive multiple sclerosis (PMS), 71.5% in isolated optic neuritis, and 72.5% in neuromyelitis optica (NMO). Immunoadsorption (IA) has a therapy response of 80.6% in relapsing-remitting multiple sclerosis and clinically isolated syndrome and 100% in neuromyelitis optica.

Early treatment initiation with a median of 2–3 weeks and a patient age below 50 are considered to be beneficial regarding a treatment success. In addition to that, a treatment count of 5 to 7 with one plasma volume is also beneficial for treatment success, whereas patients suffering from progressive multiple sclerosis have a lower beneficial rate of apheresis therapy. Both immunoadsorption and plasma exchange have a high safety profile and a high tolerability regarding side effects.

Nevertheless, data situation is too heterogeneous regarding procedures and technical implementation to be finally assessed.

Author Contributions: Conceptualization, M.J.K.; Formal analysis, M.W.; Methodology, M.W.; Supervision, M.J.K.; Validation, M.L. and M.J.K.; Visualization, M.L.; Writing—original draft, M.L.; Writing—review & editing, M.W. and M.J.K. All authors have read and agreed to the published version of the manuscript.

Acknowledgments: This publication is dedicated to the work of G. A. Müller, who always promoted apheresis therapy during his time as a full professor at the chair of Nephrology Göttingen, Germany.

Abbreviations

ASFA	American society for apheresis
CIS	Clinical isolated syndrome
Ig	Immunoglobulin
IL	Interleukin
IFNγ	Interferon gamma
NMO	Neuromyelitis optica
MS	Multiple Sclerosis
PE	Plasma exchange
PPMS	Primary-Progressive MS
PRMS	Progressive-Relapsing MS
RRMS	Relapsing remitting MS
SPMS	Secondary-Progressive MS
Th	T helper
Treg	T regulatory
TNF-α	Tumor necrosis factor alpha
VA	Visual acuity
VEP	Visual evoked potential

References

1. Brucklacher-Waldert, V.; Stuerner, K.; Kolster, M.; Wolthausen, J.; Tolosa, E. Phenotypical and functional characterization of T helper 17 cells in multiple sclerosis. *Brain A J. Neurol.* **2009**, *132 Pt 12*, 3329–3341. [CrossRef]
2. Loma, I.; Heyman, R. Multiple sclerosis: Pathogenesis and treatment. *Curr. Neuropharmacol.* **2011**, *9*, 409–416. [CrossRef]
3. Leray, E.; Moreau, T.; Fromont, A.; Edan, G. Epidemiology of multiple sclerosis. *Rev. Neurol.* **2016**, *172*, 3–13. [CrossRef]
4. Compston, A.; Coles, A. Multiple sclerosis. *Lancet* **2008**, *372*, 1502–1517. [CrossRef]
5. Toosy, A.T.; Mason, D.F.; Miller, D.H. Optic neuritis. *Lancet Neurol.* **2014**, *13*, 83–99. [CrossRef]
6. Thompson, A.J.; Banwell, B.L.; Barkhof, F.; Carroll, W.M.; Coetzee, T.; Comi, G.; Correale, J.; Fazekas, F.; Filippi, M.; Freedman, M.S.; et al. Diagnosis of multiple sclerosis: 2017 revisions of the McDonald criteria. *Lancet Neurol.* **2018**, *17*, 162–173. [CrossRef]
7. Correale, J.; Villa, A. Role of CD8+ CD25+ Foxp3+ regulatory T cells in multiple sclerosis. *Ann. Neurol.* **2010**, *67*, 625–638. [CrossRef]

8.   Schoenborn, J.R.; Wilson, C.B. Regulation of interferon-gamma during innate and adaptive immune responses. *Adv. Immunol.* **2007**, *96*, 41–101.

9.   Minty, A.; Chalon, P.; Derocq, J.M.; Dumont, X.; Guillemot, J.C.; Kaghad, M.; Labit, C.; Leplatois, P.; Liauzun, P.; Miloux, B.; et al. Interleukin-13 is a new human lymphokine regulating inflammatory and immune responses. *Nature* **1993**, *362*, 248–250. [CrossRef]

10. Zhu, J.; Paul, W.E. CD4 T cells: Fates, functions, and faults. *Blood* **2008**, *112*, 1557–1569. [CrossRef]

11. Ghasemi, N.; Razavi, S.; Nikzad, E. Multiple Sclerosis: Pathogenesis, Symptoms, Diagnoses and Cell-Based Therapy. *Cell J.* **2017**, *19*, 1–10.

12. Nishimura, H.; Enokida, H.; Sakamoto, T.; Takahashi, T.; Hayami, H.; Nakagawa, M. Immunoadsorption plasmapheresis treatment for the recurrent exacerbation of neuromyelitis optica spectrum disorder with a fluctuating anti-aquaporin-4 antibody level. *J. Artif. Organs* **2018**, *21*, 378–382. [CrossRef]

13. Ouyang, W.; Kolls, J.K.; Zheng, Y. The biological functions of T helper 17 cell effector cytokines in inflammation. *Immunity* **2008**, *28*, 454–467. [CrossRef]

14. Lee, G.R. The Balance of Th17 versus Treg Cells in Autoimmunity. *Int. J. Mol. Sci.* **2018**, *19*, 730. [CrossRef]

15. Egg, R.; Reindl, M.; Deisenhammer, F.; Linington, C.; Berger, T. Anti-MOG and anti-MBP antibody subclasses in multiple sclerosis. *Mult. Scler. J.* **2001**, *7*, 285–289. [CrossRef]

16. Dendrou, C.A.; Fugger, L.; Friese, M.A. Immunopathology of multiple sclerosis. *Nat. Rev. Immunol.* **2015**, *15*, 545–558. [CrossRef]

17. Grigoriadis, N.; van Pesch, V. A basic overview of multiple sclerosis immunopathology. *Eur. J. Neurol.* **2015**, *22*, 3–13. [CrossRef]

18. Howell, O.W.; Reeves, C.A.; Nicholas, R.; Carassiti, D.; Radotra, B.; Gentleman, S.M.; Serafini, B.; Aloisi, F.; Roncaroli, F.; Magliozzi, R.; et al. Meningeal inflammation is widespread and linked to cortical pathology in multiple sclerosis. *Brain A J. Neurol.* **2011**, *134*, 2755–2771. [CrossRef]

19. Stern, J.N.H.; Yaari, G.; Vander Heiden, J.A.; Church, G.; Donahue, W.F.; Hintzen, R.Q.; Huttner, A.J.; Laman, J.D.; Nagra, R.M.; Nylander, A.; et al. B cells populating the multiple sclerosis brain mature in the draining cervical lymph nodes. *Sci. Transl. Med.* **2014**, *6*, 248ra107. [CrossRef]

20. Lucchinetti, C.; Bruck, W.; Parisi, J.; Scheithauer, B.; Rodriguez, M.; Lassmann, H. Heterogeneity of multiple sclerosis lesions: Implications for the pathogenesis of demyelination. *Ann. Neurol.* **2000**, *47*, 707–717. [CrossRef]

21. Wingerchuk, D.M.; Lennon, V.A.; Lucchinetti, C.F.; Pittock, S.J.; Weinshenker, B.G. The spectrum of neuromyelitis optica. *Lancet Neurol.* **2007**, *6*, 805–815. [CrossRef]

22. Bevan, C.; Gelfand, J.M. Therapeutic Management of Severe Relapses in Multiple Sclerosis. *Curr. Treat. Options Neurol.* **2015**, *17*, 17. [CrossRef] [PubMed]

23. Sellebjerg, F.; Barnes, D.; Filippini, G.; Midgard, R.; Montalban, X.; Rieckmann, P.; Selmaj, K.; Visser, L.H.; Sorensen, P.S. EFNS guideline on treatment of multiple sclerosis relapses: Report of an EFNS task force on treatment of multiple sclerosis relapses. *Eur. J. Neurol.* **2005**, *12*, 939–946. [CrossRef] [PubMed]

24. Wiendl, H.; Toyka, K.V.; Rieckmann, P.; Gold, R.; Hartung, H.P.; Hohlfeld, R. Basic and escalating immunomodulatory treatments in multiple sclerosis: Current therapeutic recommendations. *J. Neurol.* **2008**, *255*, 1449–1463. [PubMed]

25. Schroder, A.; Linker, R.A.; Gold, R. Plasmapheresis for neurological disorders. *Expert Rev. Neurother.* **2009**, *9*, 1331–1339. [CrossRef]

26. Padmanabhan, A.; Connelly-Smith, L.; Aqui, N.; Balogun, R.A.; Klingel, R.; Meyer, E.; Pham, H.P.; Schneiderman, J.; Witt, V.; Wu, Y.; et al. Guidelines on the Use of Therapeutic Apheresis in Clinical Practice—Evidence-Based Approach from the Writing Committee of the American Society for Apheresis: The Eighth Special Issue. *J. Clin. Apher.* **2019**, *34*, 171–354. [CrossRef]

27. Cortese, I.; Chaudhry, V.; So, Y.T.; Cantor, F.; Cornblath, D.R.; Rae-Grant, A. Evidence-based guideline update: Plasmapheresis in neurologic disorders: Report of the Therapeutics and Technology Assessment Subcommittee of the American Academy of Neurology. *Neurology* **2011**, *76*, 294–300. [CrossRef]

28. Paroder-Belenitsky, M.; Pham, H. *Immunoadsorption, Transfusion Medicine and Hemostasis*, 3rd ed.; Stacy Masucci: Cambridge, UK, 2019; pp. 497–500.

29. Available online: https://www.kompetenznetz-multiplesklerose.de/wp-content/uploads/2016/02/dgn-kknms_ms-ll_20140813.pdf (accessed on 20 May 2020).

30. Navarro-Martinez, R.; Cauli, O. Therapeutic Plasmapheresis with Albumin Replacement in Alzheimer's Disease and Chronic Progressive Multiple Sclerosis: A Review. *Pharmaceuticals* **2020**, *13*, 28. [CrossRef]

31. Koziolek, M.; Muhlhausen, J.; Friede, T.; Ellenberger, D.; Sigler, M.; Huppke, B.; Gartner, J.; Muller, G.A.; Huppke, P. Therapeutic apheresis in pediatric patients with acute CNS inflammatory demyelinating disease. *Blood Purif.* **2013**, *36*, 92–97. [CrossRef]

32. Koziolek, M.J.; Tampe, D.; Bahr, M.; Dihazi, H.; Jung, K.; Fitzner, D.; Klingel, R.; Muller, G.A.; Kitze, B. Immunoadsorption therapy in patients with multiple sclerosis with steroid-refractory optical neuritis. *J. Neuroinflamm.* **2012**, *9*, 80. [CrossRef]

33. Jamshidian, A.; Kazemi, M.; Shaygannejad, V.; Salehi, M. The Effect of Plasma Exchange on the Expression of FOXP3 and RORC2 in Relapsed Multiple Sclerosis Patients. *Iran. J. Immunol.* **2015**, *12*, 311–318. [PubMed]

34. Stork, L.; Ellenberger, D.; Beissbarth, T.; Friede, T.; Lucchinetti, C.F.; Bruck, W.; Metz, I. Differences in the Reponses to Apheresis Therapy of Patients With 3 Histopathologically Classified Immunopathological Patterns of Multiple Sclerosis. *JAMA Neurol.* **2018**, *75*, 428–435. [CrossRef] [PubMed]

35. Khatri, B.O.; McQuillen, M.P.; Harrington, G.J.; Schmoll, D.; Hoffmann, R.G. Chronic progressive multiple sclerosis: Double-blind controlled study of plasmapheresis in patients taking immunosuppressive drugs. *Neurology* **1985**, *35*, 312–319. [CrossRef]

36. Weiner, H.L.; Dau, P.C.; Khatri, B.O.; Petajan, J.H.; Birnbaum, G.; McQuillen, M.P.; Fosburg, M.T.; Feldstein, M.; Orav, E.J. Double-blind study of true vs. sham plasma exchange in patients treated with immunosuppression for acute attacks of multiple sclerosis. *Neurology* **1989**, *39*, 1143–1149. [CrossRef]

37. Weinshenker, B.G.; O'Brien, P.C.; Petterson, T.M.; Noseworthy, J.H.; Lucchinetti, C.F.; Dodick, D.W.; Pineda, A.A.; Stevens, L.N.; Rodriguez, M. A randomized trial of plasma exchange in acute central nervous system inflammatory demyelinating disease. *Ann. Neurol.* **1999**, *46*, 878–886. [CrossRef]

38. Habek, M.; Barun, B.; Puretic, Z.; Brinar, V.V. Treatment of steroid unresponsive relapse with plasma exchange in aggressive multiple sclerosis. *Ther. Apher. Dial.* **2010**, *14*, 298–302. [CrossRef]

39. Schilling, S.; Linker, R.A.; Konig, F.B.; Koziolek, M.; Bahr, M.; Muller, G.A.; Paulus, W.; Gartner, J.; Bruck, W.; Chan, A.; et al. Plasma exchange therapy for steroid-unresponsive multiple sclerosis relapses: Clinical experience with 16 patients. *Der Nervenarzt* **2006**, *77*, 430–438. [CrossRef]

40. Trebst, C.; Reising, A.; Kielstein, J.T.; Hafer, C.; Stangel, M. Plasma exchange therapy in steroid-unresponsive relapses in patients with multiple sclerosis. *Blood Purif.* **2009**, *28*, 108–115. [CrossRef]

41. Magana, S.M.; Keegan, B.M.; Weinshenker, B.G.; Erickson, B.J.; Pittock, S.J.; Lennon, V.A.; Rodriguez, M.; Thomsen, K.; Weigand, S.; Mandrekar, J.; et al. Beneficial plasma exchange response in central nervous system inflammatory demyelination. *Arch. Neurol.* **2011**, *68*, 870–878. [CrossRef]

42. Dorst, J.; Fangerau, T.; Taranu, D.; Eichele, P.; Dreyhaupt, J.; Michels, S.; Schuster, J.; Ludolph, A.C.; Senel, M.; Tumani, H. Safety and efficacy of immunoadsorption versus plasma exchange in steroid-refractory relapse of multiple sclerosis and clinically isolated syndrome: A randomised, parallel-group, controlled trial. *EClinicalMedicine* **2019**, *16*, 98–106. [CrossRef]

43. Ehler, J.; Koball, S.; Sauer, M.; Mitzner, S.; Hickstein, H.; Benecke, R.; Zettl, U.K. Response to Therapeutic Plasma Exchange as a Rescue Treatment in Clinically Isolated Syndromes and Acute Worsening of Multiple Sclerosis: A Retrospective Analysis of 90 Patients. *PLoS ONE* **2015**, *10*, e0134583. [CrossRef]

44. Lipphardt, M.; Muhlhausen, J.; Kitze, B.; Heigl, F.; Mauch, E.; Helms, H.J.; Muller, G.A.; Koziolek, M.J. Immunoadsorption or plasma exchange in steroid-refractory multiple sclerosis and neuromyelitis optica. *J. Clin. Apher.* **2019**, *34*, 381–391. [CrossRef]

45. Deschamps, R.; Gueguen, A.; Parquet, N.; Saheb, S.; Driss, F.; Mesnil, M.; Vignal, C.; Aboab, J.; Depaz, R.; Gout, O. Plasma exchange response in 34 patients with severe optic neuritis. *J. Neurol.* **2016**, *263*, 883–887. [CrossRef]

46. Ruprecht, K.; Klinker, E.; Dintelmann, T.; Rieckmann, P.; Gold, R. Plasma exchange for severe optic neuritis: Treatment of 10 patients. *Neurology* **2004**, *63*, 1081–1083. [CrossRef]

47. Yucesan, C.; Arslan, O.; Arat, M.; Yucemen, N.; Ayyildiz, E.; Ilhan, O.; Mutluer, N. Therapeutic plasma exchange in the treatment of neuroimmunologic disorders: Review of 50 cases. *Transfus. Apher. Sci.* **2007**, *36*, 103–107. [CrossRef]

48. Meca-Lallana, J.E.; Hernandez-Clares, R.; Leon-Hernandez, A.; Genoves Aleixandre, A.; Cacho Perez, M.; Martin-Fernandez, J.J. Plasma exchange for steroid-refractory relapses in multiple sclerosis: An observational, MRI pilot study. *Clin. Ther.* **2013**, *35*, 474–485. [CrossRef]

49. Ehler, J.; Koball, S.; Sauer, M.; Hickstein, H.; Mitzner, S.; Benecke, R.; Zettl, U.K. Therapeutic plasma exchange in glucocorticosteroid-unresponsive patients with Clinically Isolated Syndrome. *Ther. Apher. Dial.* **2014**, *18*, 489–496. [CrossRef]

50. Faissner, S.; Nikolayczik, J.; Chan, A.; Hellwig, K.; Gold, R.; Yoon, M.S.; Haghikia, A. Plasmapheresis and immunoadsorption in patients with steroid refractory multiple sclerosis relapses. *J. Neurol.* **2016**, *263*, 1092–1098. [CrossRef]

51. Correia, I.; Ribeiro, J.J.; Isidoro, L.; Batista, S.; Nunes, C.; Macario, C.; Borges, C.; Tomaz, J.; Sousa, L. Plasma exchange in severe acute relapses of multiple sclerosis—Results from a Portuguese cohort. *Mult. Scler. Relat. Disord.* **2018**, *19*, 148–152. [CrossRef]

52. Hauser, S.L.; Dawson, D.M.; Lehrich, J.R.; Beal, M.F.; Kevy, S.V.; Weiner, H.L. Immunosuppression and plasmapheresis in chronic progressive multiple sclerosis. Design of a clinical trial. *Arch. Neurol.* **1983**, *40*, 687–690. [CrossRef]

53. Medenica, R.D.; Mukerjee, S.; Huschart, T.; Corbitt, W. Interferon inhibitor factor predicting success of plasmapheresis in patients with multiple sclerosis. *J. Clin. Apher.* **1994**, *9*, 216–221. [CrossRef]

54. Giedraitiene, N.; Kaubrys, G.; Kizlaitiene, R.; Bagdonaite, L.; Griskevicius, L.; Valceckiene, V.; Stoskus, M. Therapeutic Plasma Exchange in Multiple Sclerosis Patients with Abolished Interferon-beta Bioavailability. *Med. Sci. Monit.* **2015**, *21*, 1512–1519.

55. Roesner, S.; Appel, R.; Gbadamosi, J.; Martin, R.; Heesen, C. Treatment of steroid-unresponsive optic neuritis with plasma exchange. *Acta Neurol. Scand.* **2012**, *126*, 103–108. [CrossRef]

56. Merle, H.; Olindo, S.; Jeannin, S.; Valentino, R.; Mehdaoui, H.; Cabot, F.; Donnio, A.; Hage, R.; Richer, R.; Smadja, D.; et al. Treatment of optic neuritis by plasma exchange (add-on) in neuromyelitis optica. *Arch. Ophthalmol.* **2012**, *130*, 858–862. [CrossRef]

57. Watanabe, S.; Nakashima, I.; Misu, T.; Miyazawa, I.; Shiga, Y.; Fujihara, K.; Itoyama, Y. Therapeutic efficacy of plasma exchange in NMO-IgG-positive patients with neuromyelitis optica. *Mult. Scler.* **2007**, *13*, 128–132. [CrossRef]

58. Wang, K.C.; Wang, S.J.; Lee, C.L.; Chen, S.Y.; Tsai, C.P. The rescue effect of plasma exchange for neuromyelitis optica. *J. Clin. Neurosci.* **2011**, *18*, 43–46. [CrossRef]

59. Lim, Y.M.; Pyun, S.Y.; Kang, B.H.; Kim, J.; Kim, K.K. Factors associated with the effectiveness of plasma exchange for the treatment of NMO-IgG-positive neuromyelitis optica spectrum disorders. *Mult. Scler.* **2013**, *19*, 1216–1218. [CrossRef]

60. Kim, S.H.; Kim, W.; Huh, S.Y.; Lee, K.Y.; Jung, I.J.; Kim, H.J. Clinical efficacy of plasmapheresis in patients with neuromyelitis optica spectrum disorder and effects on circulating anti-aquaporin-4 antibody levels. *J. Clin. Neurol.* **2013**, *9*, 36–42. [CrossRef]

61. Abboud, H.; Petrak, A.; Mealy, M.; Sasidharan, S.; Siddique, L.; Levy, M. Treatment of acute relapses in neuromyelitis optica: Steroids alone versus steroids plus plasma exchange. *Mult. Scler.* **2016**, *22*, 185–192. [CrossRef]

62. Aungsumart, S.; Apiwattanakul, M. Clinical outcomes and predictive factors related to good outcomes in plasma exchange in severe attack of NMOSD and long extensive transverse myelitis: Case series and review of the literature. *Mult. Scler. Relat. Disord.* **2017**, *13*, 93–97. [CrossRef]

63. Srisupa-Olan, T.; Siritho, S.; Kittisares, K.; Jitprapaikulsan, J.; Sathukitchai, C.; Prayoonwiwat, N. Beneficial effect of plasma exchange in acute attack of neuromyelitis optica spectrum disorders. *Mult. Scler. Relat. Disord.* **2018**, *20*, 115–121. [CrossRef]

64. Jiao, Y.; Cui, L.; Zhang, W.; Zhang, Y.; Wang, W.; Zhang, L.; Tang, W.; Jiao, J. Plasma Exchange for Neuromyelitis Optica Spectrum Disorders in Chinese Patients and Factors Predictive of Short-term Outcome. *Clin. Ther.* **2018**, *40*, 603–612. [CrossRef]

65. Mori, S.; Kurimoto, T.; Ueda, K.; Nakamura, M. Short-term effect of additional apheresis on visual acuity changes in patients with steroid-resistant optic neuritis in neuromyelitis optica spectrum disorders. *Jpn. J. Ophthalmol.* **2018**, *62*, 525–530. [CrossRef]

66. Kumar, R.; Paul, B.S.; Singh, G.; Kaur, A. Therapeutic Efficacy of Plasma Exchange in Neuromyelitis Optica. *Ann. Indian Acad. Neurol.* **2018**, *21*, 140–143.

67. Kleiter, I.; Gahlen, A.; Borisow, N.; Fischer, K.; Wernecke, K.D.; Hellwig, K.; Pache, F.; Ruprecht, K.; Havla, J.; Kumpfel, T.; et al. Apheresis therapies for NMOSD attacks: A retrospective study of 207 therapeutic interventions. *Neurol. Neuroimmunol. Neuroinflamm.* **2018**, *5*, e504. [CrossRef]

68. Song, W.; Qu, Y.; Huang, X. Plasma exchange: An effective add-on treatment of optic neuritis in neuromyelitis optica spectrum disorders. *Int. Ophthalmol.* **2019**, *39*, 2477–2483. [CrossRef]

69. De Andres, C.; Anaya, F.; Gimenez-Roldan, S. Plasma immunoadsorption treatment of malignant multiple sclerosis with severe and prolonged relapses. *Rev. Neurol.* **2000**, *30*, 601–605.

70. Heigl, F.; Hettich, R.; Arendt, R.; Durner, J.; Koehler, J.; Mauch, E. Immunoadsorption in steroid-refractory multiple sclerosis: Clinical experience in 60 patients. *Atheroscler. Suppl.* **2013**, *14*, 167–173. [CrossRef]

71. Mauch, E.; Zwanzger, J.; Hettich, R.; Fassbender, C.; Klingel, R.; Heigl, F. Immunoadsorption for steroid-unresponsive multiple sclerosis-relapses: Clinical data of 14 patients. *Der Nervenarzt* **2011**, *82*, 1590–1595. [CrossRef]

72. Trebst, C.; Bronzlik, P.; Kielstein, J.T.; Schmidt, B.M.; Stangel, M. Immunoadsorption therapy for steroid-unresponsive relapses in patients with multiple sclerosis. *Blood Purif.* **2012**, *33*, 1–6. [CrossRef]

73. Hoffmann, F.; Kraft, A.; Heigl, F.; Mauch, E.; Koehler, J.; Harms, L.; Kumpfel, T.; Kohler, W.; Ehrlich, S.; Bayas, A.; et al. Tryptophan immunoadsorption during pregnancy and breastfeeding in patients with acute relapse of multiple sclerosis and neuromyelitis optica. *Ther. Adv. Neurol. Disord.* **2018**, *11*. [CrossRef] [PubMed]

74. Moldenhauer, A.; Haas, J.; Wascher, C.; Derfuss, T.; Hoffmann, K.T.; Kiesewetter, H.; Salama, A. Immunoadsorption patients with multiple sclerosis: An open-label pilot study. *Eur. J. Clin. Investig.* **2005**, *35*, 523–530. [CrossRef] [PubMed]

75. Schimrigk, S.; Adibi, I.; Eberl, A.; Selka, I.; Galle, J.; Schmidt, S.; Fritz, H.G.; Fassbender, C.; Klingel, R.; Fuchtemann, D.; et al. Immunoadsorption as Relapse Escalation Therapy for Multiple Sclerosis. *Aktuel. Neurol.* **2012**, *39*, 174–179.

76. Schimrigk, S.; Faiss, J.; Kohler, W.; Gunther, A.; Harms, L.; Kraft, A.; Ehrlich, S.; Eberl, A.; Fassbender, C.; Klingel, R.; et al. Escalation Therapy of Steroid Refractory Multiple Sclerosis Relapse with Tryptophan Immunoadsorption—Observational Multicenter Study with 147 Patients. *Eur. Neurol.* **2016**, *75*, 300–306. [CrossRef] [PubMed]

77. Faissner, S.; Nikolayczik, J.; Chan, A.; Gold, R.; Yoon, M.S.; Haghikia, A. Immunoadsorption in patients with neuromyelitis optica spectrum disorder. *Ther. Adv. Neurol. Disord.* **2016**, *9*, 281–286. [CrossRef]

78. Hohenstein, B.; Passauer, J.; Ziemssen, T.; Julius, U. Immunoadsorption with regenerating systems in neurological disorders –A single center experience. *Atheroscler. Suppl.* **2015**, *18*, 119–123. [CrossRef]

79. Muhlhausen, J.; Kitze, B.; Huppke, P.; Muller, G.A.; Koziolek, M.J. Apheresis in treatment of acute inflammatory demyelinating disorders. *Atheroscler. Suppl.* **2015**, *18*, 251–256. [CrossRef]

80. Llufriu, S.; Castillo, J.; Blanco, Y.; Ramio-Torrenta, L.; Rio, J.; Valles, M.; Lozano, M.; Castella, M.D.; Calabia, J.; Horga, A.; et al. Plasma exchange for acute attacks of CNS demyelination: Predictors of improvement at 6 months. *Neurology* **2009**, *73*, 949–953. [CrossRef]

81. Bramlage, C.P.; Schroder, K.; Bramlage, P.; Ahrens, K.; Zapf, A.; Muller, G.A.; Koziolek, M.J. Predictors of complications in therapeutic plasma exchange. *J. Clin. Apher.* **2009**, *24*, 225–231. [CrossRef]

82. Mokrzycki, M.H.; Kaplan, A.A. Therapeutic plasma exchange: Complications and management. *Am. J. Kidney Dis.* **1994**, *23*, 817–827. [CrossRef]

83. Samtleben, W.; Blumenstein, M.; Liebl, L.; Gurland, H.J. Membrane plasma separation for treatment of immunologically mediated diseases. *Trans. Am. Soc. Artif. Intern. Organs* **1980**, *26*, 12–16. [PubMed]

84. Sprenger, K.B.; Rasche, H.; Franz, H.E. Membrane plasma separation: Complications and monitoring. *Artif. Organs* **1984**, *8*, 360–363. [PubMed]

85. Kohler, W.; Bucka, C.; Klingel, R. A randomized and controlled study comparing immunoadsorption and plasma exchange in myasthenic crisis. *J. Clin. Apher.* **2011**, *26*, 347–355. [CrossRef] [PubMed]

86. Zollner, S.; Pablik, E.; Druml, W.; Derfler, K.; Rees, A.; Biesenbach, P. Fibrinogen reduction and bleeding complications in plasma exchange, immunoadsorption and a combination of the two. *Blood Purif.* **2014**, *38*, 160–166. [CrossRef]

87. Schneider-Gold, C.; Krenzer, M.; Klinker, E.; Mansouri-Thalegani, B.; Mullges, W.; Toyka, K.V.; Gold, R. Immunoadsorption versus plasma exchange versus combination for treatment of myasthenic deterioration. *Ther. Adv. Neurol. Disord.* **2016**, *9*, 297–303. [CrossRef]

88. Keegan, M.; Pineda, A.A.; McClelland, R.L.; Darby, C.H.; Rodriguez, M.; Weinshenker, B.G. Plasma exchange for severe attacks of CNS demyelination: Predictors of response. *Neurology* **2002**, *58*, 143–146. [CrossRef]

89. Heigl, F.; Hettich, R.; Suckfuell, M.; Luebbers, C.W.; Osterkorn, D.; Osterkorn, K.; Canis, M. Fibrinogen/LDL apheresis as successful second-line treatment of sudden hearing loss: A retrospective study on 217 patients. *Atheroscler. Suppl.* **2009**, *10*, 95–101. [CrossRef]

90. Sim, F.J.; Zhao, C.; Penderis, J.; Franklin, R.J. The age-related decrease in CNS remyelination efficiency is attributable to an impairment of both oligodendrocyte progenitor recruitment and differentiation. *J. Neurosci.* **2002**, *22*, 2451–2459. [CrossRef]

91. Freedman, M.S.; De Stefano, N.; Barkhof, F.; Polman, C.H.; Comi, G.; Uitdehaag, B.M.; Casset-Semanaz, F.; Hennessy, B.; Lehr, L.; Stubinski, B.; et al. Patient subgroup analyses of the treatment effect of subcutaneous interferon beta-1a on development of multiple sclerosis in the randomized controlled REFLEX study. *J. Neurol.* **2014**, *261*, 490–499. [CrossRef]

92. Kleiter, I.; Gahlen, A.; Borisow, N.; Fischer, K.; Wernecke, K.D.; Wegner, B.; Hellwig, K.; Pache, F.; Ruprecht, K.; Havla, J.; et al. Neuromyelitis optica: Evaluation of 871 attacks and 1153 treatment courses. *Ann. Neurol.* **2016**, *79*, 206–216. [CrossRef]

93. Zekeridou, A.; Lennon, V.A. Aquaporin-4 autoimmunity. *Neurol. Neuroimmunol. Neuroinflamm.* **2015**, *2*, e110. [CrossRef] [PubMed]

94. Savransky, A.; Rubstein, A.; Rios, M.H.; Vergel, S.L.; Velasquez, M.C.; Sierra, S.P.; Marcarian, G.; Alba, R.; Pugliese, A.M.; Tenembaum, S. Prognostic indicators of improvement with therapeutic plasma exchange in pediatric demyelination. *Neurology* **2019**, *93*, 2065–2073. [CrossRef] [PubMed]

95. Goto, H.; Matsuo, H.; Nakane, S.; Izumoto, H.; Fukudome, T.; Kambara, C.; Shibuya, N. Plasmapheresis affects T helper type-1/T helper type-2 balance of circulating peripheral lymphocytes. *Ther. Apher.* **2001**, *5*, 494–496. [CrossRef] [PubMed]

Permissions

The contributors of this book come from diverse backgrounds, making this book a truly international effort. This book will bring forth new frontiers with its revolutionizing research information and detailed analysis of the nascent developments around the world.

We would like to thank all the contributing authors for lending their expertise to make the book truly unique. They have played a crucial role in the development of this book. Without their invaluable contributions this book wouldn't have been possible. They have made vital efforts to compile up to date information on the varied aspects of this subject to make this book a valuable addition to the collection of many professionals and students.

This book was conceptualized with the vision of imparting up-to-date information and advanced data in this field. To ensure the same, a matchless editorial board was set up. Every individual on the board went through rigorous rounds of assessment to prove their worth. After which they invested a large part of their time researching and compiling the most relevant data for our readers.

The editorial board has been involved in producing this book since its inception. They have spent rigorous hours researching and exploring the diverse topics which have resulted in the successful publishing of this book. They have passed on their knowledge of decades through this book. To expedite this challenging task, the publisher supported the team at every step. A small team of assistant editors was also appointed to further simplify the editing procedure and attain best results for the readers.

Apart from the editorial board, the designing team has also invested a significant amount of their time in understanding the subject and creating the most relevant covers. They scrutinized every image to scout for the most suitable representation of the subject and create an appropriate cover for the book.

The publishing team has been an ardent support to the editorial, designing and production team. Their endless efforts to recruit the best for this project, has resulted in the accomplishment of this book. They are a veteran in the field of academics and their pool of knowledge is as vast as their experience in printing. Their expertise and guidance has proved useful at every step. Their uncompromising quality standards have made this book an exceptional effort. Their encouragement from time to time has been an inspiration for everyone.

The publisher and the editorial board hope that this book will prove to be a valuable piece of knowledge for researchers, students, practitioners and scholars across the globe.

List of Contributors

Alexander J. Davies, Janev Fehmi and Simon Rinaldi
Nuffield Department of Clinical Neurosciences, University of Oxford, Oxford OX3 9DU, UK

Makbule Senel, Hayrettin Tumani, Frank Fillies, Katharina Althaus and Johannes Dorst
Department of Neurology, University of Ulm, 89081 Ulm, Germany

Claudia Celletti, Roberta Mollica and Filippo Camerota
Physical Medicine and Rehabilitation, Umberto I University Hospital, 00161 Rome, Italy

Cristina Ferrario
Department of Mechanic, Politecnico di Milano, 20124 Milan, Italy
Department of Electronics, Information and Bioengineering (DEIB) Politecnico di Milano, 20133 Milan, Italy

Manuela Galli
Department of Electronics, Information and Bioengineering (DEIB) Politecnico di Milano, 20133 Milan, Italy

Stefan Kayser
Pentracor GmbH, 16761 Hennigsdorf, Germany

Patrizia Brunner
iAdsorb GmbH, 10787 Berlin, Germany

Ahmed Sheriff
Pentracor GmbH, 16761 Hennigsdorf, Germany
Medizinische Klinik m.S. Gastroenterologie/Infektiologie/Rheumatologie, Charité Universitätsmedizin, 12203 Berlin, Germany

Tanya J. W. McDonald and Mackenzie C. Cervenka
Department of Neurology, Johns Hopkins University School of Medicine, 600 North Wolfe Street, Meyer 2-147, Baltimore, MD 21287, USA

Nooshin Haji Ghassemi, Julius Hannink, Nils Roth and Björn M. Eskofier
Machine Learning and Data Analytics Lab, Department of Computer Science, Friedrich-Alexander-University Erlangen-Nürnberg (FAU), Carl-Thiersch-Strasse 2b, D-91052 Erlangen, Germany

Heiko Gaßner, Franz Marxreiter and Jochen Klucken
Department of Molecular Neurology, University Hospital Erlangen, Schwabachanlage 6, D-91054 Erlangen, Germany

Pietro Caliandro
Unità Operativa Complessa Neurologia, Fondazione Policlinico Universitario A. Gemelli IRCCS, Largo A. Gemelli, 8, 00168 Rome, Italy

Carmela Conte and Chiara Iacovelli
IRCCS Fondazione Don Carlo Gnocchi, Piazzale Morandi, 6, 20121 Milan, Italy

Antonella Tatarelli
Department of Occupational and Environmental Medicine, Epidemiology and Hygiene, INAIL, via Fontana Candida, 1, 00078 Monte Porzio Catone, Italy

Stefano Filippo Castiglia
Department of Medical and Surgical Sciences and Biotechnologies, Sapienza University of Rome, Piazzale Aldo Moro, 5, 00185 Rome, Italy

Giuseppe Reale
Department of Neurosciences, Università Cattolica del Sacro Cuore, Largo F. Vito, 1, 00168 Rome, Italy

Mariano Serrao
Department of Medical and Surgical Sciences and Biotechnologies, Sapienza University of Rome, Piazzale Aldo Moro, 5, 00185 Rome, Italy
Policlinico Italia, Movement Analysis Laboratory, Piazza del Campidano, 6, 00162 Rome, Italy

Kazutaka Ueda and Masayuki Nakao
Department of Mechanical Engineering, Graduate School of Engineering, The University of Tokyo, 7-3-1 Hongo, Bunkyo-ku, Tokyo 113-8656, Japan

Sylvia Stracke
Department for Internal Medicine A, Nephrology, University Medicine Greifswald, Ferdinand-Sauerbruch-Straße, 17475 Greifswald, Germany

Sandra Lange
Institute of Diagnostic Radiology and Neuroradiology, University Medicine Greifswald, 17475 Greifswald, Germany

Sarah Bornmann, Antje Vogelgesang and Felix von Podewils
Department of Neurology, University Medicine Greifswald, 17475 Greifswald, Germany

Holger Kock
Strategic Research Management, University Medicine Greifswald, 17475 Greifswald, Germany

Lara Schulze and Johanna Klinger-König
Department of Psychiatry and Psychotherapy, University Medicine Greifswald, 17475 Greifswald, Germany

Susanne Böhm
Coordinating Centre for Clinical Trials, University Medicine Greifswald, 17475 Greifswald, Germany

Agnes Föel
Department of Neurology, University Medicine Greifswald, 17475 Greifswald, Germany
German Center for Neurodegenerative Diseases (DZNE), 17475 Rostock/Greifswald, partner site Greifswald, Germany

Hans J. Grabe
Department of Psychiatry and Psychotherapy, University Medicine Greifswald, 17475 Greifswald, Germany
German Center for Neurodegenerative Diseases (DZNE), 17475 Rostock/Greifswald, partner site Greifswald, Germany

Stefan Gross and Marcus Dörr
Department of Internal Medicine B, University Medicine Greifswald, Ferdinand-Sauerbruch-Straße, 17475 Greifswald, Germany
German Centre for Cardiovascular Research (DZHK), 17475 Greifswald, Germany

Katrin Wenzel and Gerd Wallukat
Berlin Cures GmbH, 13125 Berlin, Germany

Alexander Dressel
Department of Neurology, Carl-Thiem-Klinikum, 03048 Cottbus, Germany

Rudolf Kunze
Science Office, Hessenhagen 2, 17268 Flieth-Stegelitz, Germany

Sönke Langner
Institute of Diagnostic Radiology and Neuroradiology, University Medicine Greifswald, 17475 Greifswald, Germany
Institute of Diagnostic and Interventional Radiology, University Medicine Rostock, 18057 Rostock Germany

Steffen Pfeuffer, Leoni Rolfes, Tobias Ruck, Matthias Schilling, Nico Melzer, Heinz Wiendl and Sven G. Meuth
Neurology Clinic and Institute for Translational Neurology, University of Muenster, 48149 Münster, Germany

Eike Bormann and Cristina Sauerland
Institute of Biostatistics and Clinical Research, University of Muenster, 48149 Münster, Germany

Marcus Brand
Department of Internal Medicine D, University of Muenster 48149 Münster, Germany

Refik Pul and Christoph Kleinschnitz
Department of Neurology, University Duisburg-Essen, 45147 Essen, Germany

Milagros Fuentes-Albero
Children's Mental Health Center, Hospital Arnau de Villanova, 46015 Valencia, Spain

María Isabel Martínez-Martínez and Omar Cauli
Department of Medicine and Nursing, University of Valencia, 46010 Valencia, Spain

Christopher Buckley, M. Encarna Micó-Amigo and Silvia Del Din
Institute of Neuroscience/Institute for Ageing, Newcastle University, Newcastle Upon Tyne NE4 5PL, UK

Michael Dunne-Willows
EPSRC Centre for Doctoral Training in Cloud Computing for Big Data, Newcastle University, Newcastle Upon Tyne NE4 5PL, UK

Alan Godfrey
Department of Computer and Information Science, Northumbria University, Newcastle upon Tyne NE1 8ST, UK

Aodhán Hickey
Department of Health Intelligence, HSC Public Health Agency, Belfast BT2 7ES, Northern Ireland

Sue Lord
Institute of Neuroscience/Institute for Ageing, Newcastle University, Newcastle Upon Tyne NE4 5PL, UK
Auckland University of Technology, 55 Wellesley St E, Auckland 1010, New Zealand

Lynn Rochester
Institute of Neuroscience/Institute for Ageing, Newcastle University, Newcastle Upon Tyne NE4 5PL, UK
The Newcastle upon Tyne Hospitals NHS Foundation Trust, Newcastle Upon Tyne NE7 7DN, UK

Sarah A. Moore
Institute of Neuroscience/Institute for Ageing, Newcastle University, Newcastle Upon Tyne NE4 5PL, UK
Institute of Neuroscience (Stroke Research Group), Newcastle University, 3-4 Claremont Terrace, Newcastle upon Tyne NE2 4AE, UK
Stroke Northumbria, Northumbria Healthcare NHS Foundation Trust, Rake Lane, North Shields, Tyne and Wear NE29 8NH, UK

Jens Dreyhaupt
Institute for Epidemiology and Medical Biometry, University of Ulm, 89081 Ulm, Germany

Mariachiara Ricci, Franco Giannini and Giovanni Saggio
Department of Electronic Engineering, University of Rome "Tor Vergata", 00133 Rome, Italy

Giulia Di Lazzaro, Antonio Pisani, Simona Scalise, Mohammad Alwardat and Chiara Salimei
Department of Systems Medicine, University of Rome "Tor Vergata", 00133 Rome, Italy

Rosa Rössling and Harald Prüss
Department of Neurology and Experimental Neurology, Charité–Universitätsmedizin Berlin, Charitéplatz 1, 10117 Berlin, Germany
German Center for Neurodegenerative Diseases (DZNE) Berlin, 10117 Berlin, Germany

Lorenza Angelini and Claudia Mazzà
Department of Mechanical Engineering, University of Sheffield, Sheffield S1 3JD, UK
Insigneo Institute for in silico Medicine, University of Sheffield, Sheffield S1 3JD, UK

Krishnan Padmakumari Sivaraman Nair
Insigneo Institute for in silico Medicine, University of Sheffield, Sheffield S1 3JD, UK
Academic Department of Neuroscience, Sheffield NIHR Neuroscience BRC, Sheffield Teaching Hospital NHS Foundation Trust, Sheffield S10 2JF, UK

Ilaria Carpinella, Davide Cattaneo, Maurizio Ferrarin and Elisa Gervasoni
IRCCS Fondazione Don Carlo Gnocchi, 20121 Milan, Italy

Basil Sharrack
Academic Department of Neuroscience, Sheffield NIHR Neuroscience BRC, Sheffield Teaching Hospital NHS Foundation Trust, Sheffield S10 2JF, UK

David Paling
Sheffield Institute of Translational Neuroscience, Sheffield Teaching Hospitals NHS Foundation Trust, Sheffield S10 2JF, UK

Mark Lipphardt, Manuel Wallbach and Michael J. Koziolek
Department of Nephrology and Rheumatology, University Medical Center Göttingen, Robert-Koch-Str. 40, D-37075 Goettingen, Germany

Index

Printed in the USA
CPSIA information can be obtained
at www.ICGtesting.com
JSHW051359091023
49903JS00006B/206

9 781646 466139